LIPPINCOTT

NCLEX-PN®
Alternate-Format
Questions

Third Edition

Wolters Kluwer

Health

Philadelphia · Baltimore · New York · London
Buenos Aires · Hong Kong · Sydney · Tokyo

Product Director: Peter Darcy
Product Manager: Renee Gagliardi
Product Development Editor: Bernadette Enneg
Design Coordinator: Joan Wendt
Production Project Manager: Cynthia Rudy
Illustration Coordinator: Jennifer Clements
Manufacturing Coordinator: Kathleen Brown
Production Service: SPi Global

3rd edition

Library of Congress Cataloging-in-Publication Data
Rupert, Diana L., author.
  Lippincott NCLEX-PN alternate format questions / Diana L. Rupert. — Third edition.
      p. ; cm.
  NCLEX-PN alternate format questions
  Preceded by: NCLEX-PN 250 new-format questions. 2nd ed. 2006.
  Includes bibliographical references and index.
  ISBN 978-1-4698-4535-7 (paperback : alk. paper)
  I. NCLEX-PN 250 new-format questions. Preceded by (work): II. Title. III. Title: NCLEX-PN alternate format questions.
  [DNLM: 1. Nursing, Practical—United States—Examination Questions. WY 18.2]
  RT55
  610.7306'93076—dc23
                                                                    2013051126

Care has been taken to confirm the accuracy of the information presented and to describe generally accepted practices. However, the authors, editors, and publisher are not responsible for errors or omissions or for any consequences from application of the information in this book and make no warranty, expressed or implied, with respect to the currency, completeness, or accuracy of the contents of the publication. Application of the information in a particular situation remains the professional responsibility of the practitioner; the clinical treatments described and recommended may not be considered absolute and universal recommendations.

The authors, editors, and publisher have exerted every effort to ensure that drug selection and dosage set forth in this text are in accordance with current recommendations and practice at the time of publication. However, in view of ongoing research, changes in government regulations, and the constant flow of information relating to drug therapy and drug reactions, the reader is urged to check the package insert for each drug for any change in indications and dosage and for added warnings and precautions. This is particularly important when the recommended agent is a new or infrequently employed drug.

Some drugs and medical devices presented in this publication have Food and Drug Administration (FDA) clearance for limited use in restricted research settings. It is the responsibility of the health care provider to ascertain the FDA status of each drug or device planned for use in their clinical practice.

RRS1510

ACKNOWLEDGMENTS

Many thanks to Renee Gagliardi and Bernadette Enneg and the staff at Lippincott who have helped in the development of this book.

Also, thanks to my family: My husband Cliff whose love and support is greatly appreciated. My children: Jeff and Amy (and baby Rupert on the way), Mike and Amy, Patrick and Taylor who provide me with so much joy. Thanks Dad and Mom for always being there to support me. I love you all.

ABOUT THE AUTHOR

Dr. Diana Rupert is an alumnus of Indiana University of Pennsylvania. She began her nursing career 23 years ago as a pediatric nurse before moving to home health and then education. She has 15 years of teaching experience, including practical nursing programs, a diploma nursing program, baccalaureate, and masters nursing programs.

Dr. Rupert is the administrator at the Indiana County Technology Center, School of Practical Nursing, Indiana, PA, and an assistant professor at Indiana University of Pennsylvania. She has presented on NCLEX topics via webinar, workshops, and small group sessions and is the author of three books for NCLEX preparation.

CONTENTS

CONTENTS

PART ONE

Preparing for the NCLEX®

Passing the National Council Licensure Examination (NCLEX®) is an important landmark in your career as a nurse. The first step on your way to passing the NCLEX is to understand what it is and how it is administered.

NCLEX Structure

The NCLEX is a test written by nurses who, like most of your nursing instructors, have an advanced degree and clinical expertise in a particular area. Only one small difference distinguishes nurses who write NCLEX questions: they are trained to write questions in a style particular to the NCLEX.

If you have completed an accredited nursing program, you have already taken numerous tests written by nurses with backgrounds and experiences similar to those of the nurses who write for the NCLEX. The test-taking experience you have already gained will help you pass the NCLEX. So your NCLEX review should be just that—a review.

The NCLEX is designed for one purpose: to determine whether it is appropriate for you to receive a license to practice as a nurse. By passing the NCLEX, you demonstrate that you possess the minimum level of knowledge necessary for a competent entry level practitioner to practice nursing safely.

If you completed your nursing education in a foreign country, you must follow certain guidelines to be eligible to work as a registered nurse (RN) in the United States. (See *Guidelines for international nurses*, page 3.)

In nursing school, you probably took separate courses, such as pharmacology, nursing leadership, and health assessment, as well as courses that addressed adult health, pediatric, maternal–neonatal, and psychiatric nursing. In contrast, the NCLEX is integrated, meaning that different subjects are mixed together.

As you answer NCLEX questions, you may encounter patients in any stage of life, from neonatal to geriatric. These patients—clients, in NCLEX terminology—may be of any background, may be completely well or extremely ill, and may have any of a variety of disorders.

Client Needs

The NCLEX draws questions from four categories of *client needs* that were developed by the National Council of State Boards of Nursing (NCSBN), the organization that sponsors and manages the NCLEX. Client needs categories ensure that a wide variety of topics appears on every NCLEX.

The NCSBN develops client needs categories after conducting a practice analysis. The practice analysis assists the NCSBN in evaluating the validity of the test plan. The NCSBN conducts a practice analysis every 3 years from a random sample of LPN/VNs who passed the NCLEX-PN. All aspects of nursing care observed in the study were broken down into four main categories, some of which were broken down further into subcategories. (See *Client needs categories*, page 4.)

Integrated Processes

Integrated throughout the client needs categories and subcategories are four key processes that are fundamental to the practice of nursing:

- **Nursing process**—a scientific, clinical reasoning approach to client care that includes assessment, analysis, planning, implementation, and evaluation
- **Caring**—an atmosphere of mutual respect and trust that exists between the nurse and the client in which the nurse provides encouragement, support, hope, and compassion to help the client achieve desired outcomes
- **Communication and documentation**—nonverbal and verbal exchanges or interactions among the nurse and the client, the client's significant other, and the health care team, and the validation of client care in written and electronic records that reflect standards of practice and accountability in the provision of care
- **Teaching and learning**—making possible the gaining of knowledge, attitudes, and skills to promote a change in behavior.

NCLEX Test Plan

The four client needs categories and their corresponding subcategories provide the basic framework for the NCLEX test plan. Question writers and the other people who compile the examination use the NCLEX test plan to ensure that the content and distribution of test questions cover the full spectrum of nursing activities and competencies across all client care settings.

Critical Thinking

Although NCLEX questions cover all levels of cognitive abilities—from basic nursing knowledge to comprehension, application, analysis, synthesis, and evaluation—most are written at the application or higher cognitive levels, which require critical thinking. Critical thinking relies on the nurse's knowledge, skills, and ability to solve the problem. Test-taking strategies are provided for all rationales in this book to help you focus on where or how to find the correct answer to each question as you study for the NCLEX.

In order to become eligible to work as an PN In the United States, you will need to complete several steps. In addition to passing the NCLEX-PN, you may need to obtain a certificate and credentials evaluation from the Commission on Graduates of Foreign Nursing Schools (CGFNS®) and acquire a visa. Since requirements differ from state to state, it is important that you first contact the board of nursing in the state where you want to practice nursing.

CGFNS Certification Program

Most states require that you obtain CGFNS certification. This certification requires the following:

- A review and authentication of your credentials, including your nursing education, registration, and licensure
- A passing score on the CGFNS Qualifying Examination of nursing knowledge
- A passing score on an English language proficiency test

In order to be eligible to take the CGFNS Qualifying Examination, you must complete a minimum number of classroom and clinical practice hours in medical–surgical nursing, maternal–neonatal nursing, pediatric nursing, and psychiatric and mental health nursing from a government-approved nursing school. You must also be registered as a first-level nurse in your country of education, and currently hold a license as an RN in some jurisdiction.

The CGFNS Qualifying Examination is a paper-and-pencil test that includes 260 multiple-choice questions. It is administered under controlled testing conditions. Because the test is designed to predict your likelihood of successfully passing the NCLEX-PN examination, it is based on the NCLEX-PN test plan.

You may select from three English proficiency examinations: Test of English as a Foreign Language (TOEFL®), Test of English for International Communication (TOEIC®), or International English Language Testing System (IELTS). Each test has different passing scores and the scores are valid for up to 2 years.

CGFNS Credentials Evaluation Service

This evaluation is a comprehensive report that analyzes and compares your education and licensure with U.S. standards. It is prepared by the CGFNS for a state board of nursing, an immigration office, an employer, or a university. It requires that you complete an application, submit appropriate documentation, and pay a fee.

More information about the CGFNS certification program and credentials evaluation service is available at *www.cgfns.org*.

Visa

You cannot legally immigrate to work in the United States without an occupational visa (temporary or permanent) from the United States Citizenship and Immigration Services (USCIS). The visa process is separate from the CGFNS certification process, although some of the same steps are involved. Some visas require prior CGFNS certification and a *VisaScreen®* Certificate from the International Commission on Healthcare Professions. The *VisaScreen* program involves the following:

- A credentials review of your nursing education and current registration or licensure
- Successful completion of either the CGFNS certification program or the NCLEX-PN
- A passing score on an approved English language proficiency examination

Once you successfully complete all parts of the *VisaScreen* program, you will receive a certificate to present to the USCIS. The visa-granting process can take up to a year.

You can obtain more detailed information about visa application at *www.uscis.gov*.

Testing by Computer

Like many standardized tests today, the NCLEX is administered by computer. That means you will not be filling in empty circles, sharpening pencils, or erasing frantically. It also means that you must become familiar with computer tests, if you are not already. Fortunately, the skills required to take the NCLEX on a computer are simple enough to allow you to focus on the questions, not the keyboard.

When you take the test, depending on the question format, you will be presented with a question and four or more possible answers, a blank space in which you have to enter your answer, a figure on which you will click the mouse to select the correct area of the figure, a series of charts or exhibits to view in order to select the correct response, items you must prioritize by dragging and dropping them in place, an audio recording to listen to in order to select the correct response, or a question and four graphic options.

The NCLEX is a *computer-adaptive test*, meaning that the computer reacts to the answers you give, supplying more difficult questions if you answer correctly and slightly easier questions if you answer incorrectly.

Each question on the NCLEX is assigned a category based on client needs. This chart lists client needs categories and subcategories and the percentages of each type of question that appears on an NCLEX:

Category	Subcategories	Percentage of NCLEX Questions
Safe and effective care environment	• Coordinated care • Safety and infection control	16%–22% 10%–16%
Health promotion and maintenance		7%–13%
Psychosocial integrity		8%–14%
Physiological integrity	• Basic care and comfort • Pharmacological therapies • Reduction of risk potential • Physiological adaptation	7%–13% 11%–17% 10%–16% 7%–13%

Each test is thus uniquely adapted to the individual test-taker.

You have a great deal of flexibility with the amount of time you spend on individual questions. The examination lasts a maximum of 5 hours so do not waste time. If you fail to answer a set number of questions within the 5 hours, the computer will determine that you lack minimum competency.

Most students have plenty of time to complete the test, so take as much time as you need to get the question right without wasting time. Keep moving at a decent pace to help maintain concentration.

If you find as you progress through the test that the questions seem to be increasingly difficult, it is a good sign. The more questions you answer correctly, the more difficult the questions become.

Some students, though, knowing that questions get progressively harder, focus on the degree of difficulty of subsequent questions to try to figure out if they are answering questions correctly. Avoid the temptation to do this, as this may get you off track. Stay focused on selecting the best answer for each question put before you.

The computer test finishes when one of these events occurs:

• You demonstrate minimum competency, according to the computer program.
• You demonstrate a lack of minimum competency, according to the computer program.
• You have answered the maximum number of questions (205 total questions).
• You have used the maximum time allowed (5 hours).

Alternate-Format Questions

In April 2004, the NCSBN added alternate-format items to the examination. These currently include seven types:

• Multiple response–multiple choice
• Fill in the blank
• Hotspot
• Chart or exhibit
• Drag and drop
• Audio
• Graphic options

However, most of the questions on the NCLEX are four-option, multiple-choice items with only one correct answer. Certain strategies can help you understand and answer any type of NCLEX question.

The NCSBN has not established a percentage of alternate-format items to be administered to each candidate. In fact, your examination may contain only one alternate-format item. So relax; the standard, four-option, multiple-choice format questions compose the bulk of the test.

Multiple-Response, Multiple-Choice Question

The first type of alternate-format item is the *multiple-response, multiple-choice question*. Unlike a traditional multiple-choice question, each multiple-response, multiple-choice question has one or more correct answers for every question, and it will contain four to six answer options. You will recognize this type of question because it will ask you to select *all* that apply—not just the best answer (as may be requested in the more traditional multiple-choice questions).

Keep in mind that for each multiple-response, multiple-choice question, you must select at least one answer and you must select all correct answers for the item to be counted as correct. On the NCLEX, there is no partial credit in the scoring of these items.

Fill-in-the-blank Question

The second type of alternate-format item is the *fill in the blank*. These questions require you to provide the answer yourself, rather than select it from a list of options. You will perform a calculation, then type your answer (a number without any words, units of measurement, commas, or spaces) in the blank space provided after the question. Rules for rounding are included in the question stem if appropriate. A calculator button is provided so you can easily do your calculations electronically.

Hotspot Question

The third type of alternate-format item is a question that asks you to identify an area on an illustration or graphic. For these so-called *"hotspot" questions*, the computerized examination will ask you to place your cursor and click over the correct area on an illustration. Try to be as precise as possible when marking the location. As with the fill in the blanks, the identification questions on the computerized examination may require extremely precise answers to be considered correct.

Chart/Exhibit Question

The fourth type of alternate-format item is the *chart/exhibit* format. Here you will be given a problem and an exhibit that contains additional information you will need in order to answer the question. By clicking on the EXHIBIT button, you can access a series of three screens to review. Your answer can then be chosen from four multiple-choice answer options.

Drag-and-drop Question

The fifth type of alternate-format item involves prioritizing, or placing in correct order, a series of statements using a *drag-and-drop* technique. You will decide which of the given options is first, click and hold it with the mouse, then drag it into the first box given beneath and drop it into place. You will repeat this process until you have placed all the available options in the lower boxes.

Audio Question

The sixth type of alternate-format item involves listening with a set of headphones to an *audio* clip in order to answer the question. Your answer is chosen from four multiple-choice answer options.

Graphic Option Question

The final type of alternate-format item is the *graphic option* question. You will be presented with a question and options that are graphics instead of text.

Understanding the Question

NCLEX questions are usually long. As a result, it is easy to feel overwhelmed with information. To focus on the question, apply proven strategies for answering NCLEX questions, including the following:

- Determining what the question is asking
- Determining relevant facts about the client
- Rephrasing the question in your mind
- Choosing the best option(s) before entering your answer

Determine What the Question is Asking

Read the question twice. If the answer is not apparent, rephrase the question in simpler, more personal terms. Breaking down the question into easier, less intimidating terms may help you to focus more accurately on the correct answer.

(*Text continues on page 8*)

Sometimes, getting used to the test format is as important as knowing the material covered. Try your hand at these sample questions and you will have a leg up when you take the real test!

Sample Four-Option, Multiple-Choice Question

The oncoming nurse is receiving shift report from the departing nurse. When discussing the care of a client, the following arterial blood gas (ABG) results are noted: pH 7.16; $PaCO_2$, 80 mm Hg; PaO_2, 46 mm Hg; HCO_3^-, 24 mEq/L; SaO_2, 81%. For which condition would the nurses' plan care?

☐ **1.** Metabolic acidosis

☐ **2.** Metabolic alkalosis

☐ **3.** Respiratory acidosis

☐ **4.** Respiratory alkalosis

Answer: 3

Sample Multiple-Response, Multiple-Choice Question

The nurse is caring for a 45-year-old married client who has undergone hemicolectomy for colon cancer. The client has two children. Which concepts about families should the nurse keep in mind when providing care for this client? Select all that apply:

☐ **1.** Illness in one family member can affect all members.

☐ **2.** Family roles do not change because of illness.

☐ **3.** A family member may have more than one role in the family.

☐ **4.** Children typically are not affected by adult illness.

☐ **5.** The effects of an illness on a family depend on the stage of the family's life cycle.

☐ **6.** Changes in sleeping and eating patterns may be signs of stress in a family.

Answer: 1, 3, 5, 6

Sample Fill-in-the-Blank Calculation Question

An infant who weighs 8 kg is to receive ampicillin 25 mg/kg I.V. every 6 hours. How many milligrams should the nurse administer per dose? Record your answer using a whole number.

_____ mg

Answer: 200

Sample Hotspot Question

An elderly client has a history of aortic stenosis. Identify the area where the nurse should place the stethoscope to best hear the murmur.

Answer:

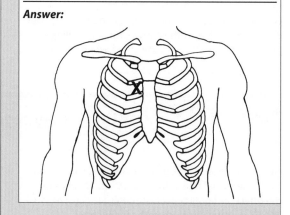

Sample Chart/Exhibit Question

A 3-year-old client is being treated for severe status asthmaticus. After reviewing the progress notes (shown below), the nurse should determine that this client is being treated for which condition?

Progress Notes

4/5/10	Pt. was acutely restless, diaphoretic, and
0600	with SOB at 0530. Dr. T. Smith notified
	and ordered ABG analysis. ABG drawn from
	R radial artery. Stat results as follows: pH
	7.28, PaCO₂ 55 mm Hg, HCO₃⁻ 26 mEg/L. Dr.
	Smith with pt. now. ———— J. Collins, LPN.

☐ **1.** Metabolic acidosis.

☐ **2.** Respiratory alkalosis.

☐ **3.** Respiratory acidosis.

☐ **4.** Metabolic alkalosis.

Answer: 3

Sample Drag-and-Drop Question

When teaching an antepartal client about the passage of the fetus through the birth canal during labor, the nurse describes the cardinal mechanisms of labor. Place these events in the sequence in which they occur. Use all the options.

1. Flexion

2. External rotation

3. Descent

4. Expulsion

5. Internal rotation

6. Extension

Answer: 3, 1, 5, 6, 2, 4

Sample Audio Question

Listen to the audio clip. What sound do you hear in the lung bases of this client with heart failure?

☐ **1.** Crackles

☐ **2.** Rhonchi

☐ **3.** Wheezes

☐ **4.** Pleural friction rub

Answer: 1

Sample Graphic Option Question

Which electrocardiogram strip should the nurse document as atrial flutter?

☐ **1.**

☐ **2.**

☐ **3.**

☐ **4.**

Answer: 4

For example, a question might read:"A client with a history of heart failure is admitted to the coronary care unit with pulmonary edema. The client is intubated and placed on a mechanical ventilator. Which assessment finding is essential for the LPN to report to the RN following the administration of a bolus dose of furosemide (Lasix) I.V.?"

The options for this question—numbered from 1 to 4—may be:

☐ **1.** Daily weight.

☐ **2.** 24-Hour intake and output.

☐ **3.** Serum sodium levels.

☐ **4.** Hourly urine output.

Read the question again, ignoring all details except what is being asked. Focus on the last line of the question. It asks you to select the appropriate assessment for monitoring a client who received a bolus of furosemide I.V.

Determine Which Facts About the Client are Relevant

Next, sort out the relevant client information. Start by asking whether any of the information provided about the client is not relevant to the facts needed to answer the question. For instance, do you need to know that the client has been admitted to the coronary care unit? Probably not; the reaction to I.V. furosemide will not be affected by the location in the hospital.

Determine what you do know about the client. In the example, you know that

- the client has just received an I.V. bolus of furosemide, a crucial fact;
- the client has pulmonary edema, the most fundamental aspect of the client's underlying condition;

- the client is intubated and placed on a mechanical ventilator, suggesting that the pulmonary edema is serious;
- the client has a history of heart failure, a fact that may or may not be relevant.

Rephrase the Question

After you have determined relevant information about the client and the question being asked, consider rephrasing the question to make it clearer. Eliminate jargon and put the question in simpler, more personal terms. Here is how you might rephrase the question in the example:"My client has pulmonary edema. The client requires intubation and mechanical ventilation. The client has a history of heart failure. The client received an I.V. bolus of furosemide. What assessment parameter should I monitor and report to the RN?"

Choose the Best Option

Armed with all the information you now have, it is time to select an option. You know that the client received an I.V. bolus of furosemide, a diuretic. You know that monitoring fluid intake and output is a key nursing intervention for a client taking a diuretic, a fact that eliminates options 1 and 3 (daily weight and serum sodium levels), narrowing the answer down to option 2 or 4 (24-hour intake and output or hourly urine output).

You also know that the drug was administered by I.V. bolus, suggesting a rapid effect. (In fact, furosemide administered by I.V. bolus takes effect almost immediately.) Monitoring the client's 24-hour intake and output would be appropriate for assessing the effects of repeated doses of furosemide. Hourly urine output, however, is most appropriate in this situation because it monitors the immediate effect of this rapid-acting drug.

Key Strategies

Regardless of the type of question, four key strategies will help you determine the correct answer for each question. (See *Strategies for success*.) These strategies are as follows:

- Considering the nursing process
- Referring to Maslow's hierarchy of needs

- Reviewing patient safety
- Reflecting on principles of therapeutic communication
- Considering the standards of care

Keeping a few main strategies in mind as you answer each NCLEX question can help ensure greater success. These five strategies are critical for answering NCLEX questions correctly:

- If the question asks what you should do in a situation, use the nursing process to determine which step in the process would be next.
- If the question asks what the client needs, use Maslow's hierarchy to determine which need to address first.
- If the question indicates that the client does not have an urgent physiologic need, focus on the patient's safety.
- If the question involves communicating with a patient, use the principles of therapeutic communication.
- If the question involves a nursing procedure, consider the standards of care.

Nursing Process

One of the ways to answer a question is to apply the nursing process. Steps in the nursing process include

- assessment;
- analysis;
- planning;
- implementation;
- evaluation.

The nursing process may provide insights that help you analyze a question. According to the nursing process, assessment comes before analysis, which comes before planning, which comes before implementation, which comes before evaluation.

You are halfway to the correct answer when you encounter a four-option, multiple-choice question that asks you to assess the situation and then provides two assessment options and two implementation options. You can immediately eliminate the implementation options, which then gives you, at worst, a 50-50 chance of selecting the correct answer. Use the following sample question to apply the nursing process:

A client returns from an endoscopic procedure during which the client was sedated. Before offering the client food, which action should the nurse take?

☐ **1.** Assess the client's respiratory status.

☐ **2.** Check the client's gag reflex.

☐ **3.** Place the client in a side-lying position.

☐ **4.** Have the client drink a few sips of water.

According to the nursing process, the nurse must assess a client before performing an intervention. Does the question indicate that the client has been properly assessed? No, it does not. Therefore, you can eliminate options 3 and 4 because they are both interventions.

That leaves options 1 and 2, both of which are assessments. Your nursing knowledge should tell you the correct answer—in this case, option 2. The sedation required for an endoscopic procedure may impair the client's gag reflex, so you would assess the gag reflex before giving food to the client to reduce the risk of aspiration and airway obstruction.

Why not select option 1, assessing the client's respiratory status? You might select this option but the question is specifically asking about offering the client food, an action that would not be taken if the client's respiratory status were at all compromised. In this case, you are making a judgment based on the phrase "Before offering the client food." If the question were trying to test your knowledge of respiratory depression following an endoscopic procedure, it probably would not mention a function—such as giving food to a client—that clearly occurs only after the client's respiratory status has been stabilized.

Maslow's Hierarchy

Knowledge of Maslow's hierarchy of needs can be a vital tool for establishing priorities on the NCLEX. Maslow's theory states that physiologic needs are the most basic human needs of all. Only after physiologic needs have been met can safety concerns be addressed. Only after safety concerns are met can concerns involving love and belonging be addressed, and so forth. Apply the principles of Maslow's hierarchy of needs to the following sample question:

A client complains of severe pain 2 days after surgery. Which action should the nurse perform first?

☐ **1.** Offer reassurance of less pain to the client.

☐ **2.** Allow the client time to verbalize feelings.

☐ **3.** Check the client's vital signs.

☐ **4.** Administer an analgesic.

In this example, two of the options—3 and 4—address physiologic needs. Options 1 and 2 address psychosocial concerns. According to Maslow, physiologic needs must be met before psychosocial needs, so you can eliminate options 1 and 2.

Now, use your nursing knowledge to choose the best answer from the two remaining options. In this case, option 3 is correct because the client's vital signs should be checked before administering an analgesic (assessment before intervention). When prioritizing according to Maslow's hierarchy, remember your ABCs—airway, breathing, and circulation—to help you further prioritize. Check for a patent airway before addressing breathing. Check breathing before checking the health of the cardiovascular system.

Just because an option appears on the NCLEX does not mean it is a viable choice for the client referred to in the question. Always examine your choice in light of your knowledge and experience. Ask yourself, "Does this choice make sense for this client?" Allow yourself to eliminate choices—even those that might normally take priority—if they do not make sense for a particular client's situation.

Patient Safety

As you might expect, patient safety takes high priority on the NCLEX. You will encounter many questions that can be answered by asking yourself, "Which answer will best ensure the safety of this client?" Use patient safety criteria for situations involving laboratory values, drug administration, or nursing care procedures.

You may encounter a question in which some options address the client and others address the equipment. When in doubt, select an option relating to the client; never place equipment before a client.

For instance, suppose a question asks what the nurse should do first when entering a client's room where an infusion pump alarm is sounding. If two options deal with the infusion pump, one with the infusion tubing, and another with the client's catheter insertion site, select the one relating to the client's catheter insertion site. Always check the client first; the equipment can wait.

Therapeutic Communication

Some NCLEX questions focus on the nurse's ability to communicate effectively with the client. Therapeutic communication incorporates verbal or nonverbal responses and involves

- listening to the client;
- understanding the client's needs;
- promoting clarification and insight about the client's condition.

Like other NCLEX questions, those dealing with therapeutic communication require choosing the best response. First, eliminate options that indicate the use of poor therapeutic communication techniques, such as those in which the nurse

- tells the client what to do without regard to the client's feelings or desires (the "do this" response);
- asks a question that can be answered "yes" or "no," or with another one-syllable response;
- seeks reasons for the client's behavior;
- implies disapproval of the client's behavior;
- offers false reassurances;
- attempts to interpret the client's behavior rather than allowing the client to verbalize his own feelings;
- offers a response that focuses on the nurse, not the client.

When answering NCLEX questions, look for responses that

- allow the client time to think and reflect;
- encourage the client to talk;
- encourage the client to describe a particular experience;
- reflect that the nurse has listened to the client, such as through paraphrasing the client's response.

Avoiding Pitfalls

Even the most knowledgeable students can get tripped up on certain NCLEX questions. (See *A tricky question*.) Students commonly cite three areas that can be difficult for unwary test-takers:

- Knowing the difference between the NCLEX and the "real world"
- Delegating care
- Knowing laboratory values

The NCLEX occasionally asks a particular kind of question called the "further teaching" question, which involves patient-teaching situations. These questions can be tricky. You will have to choose the response that suggests that the patient has *not* learned the correct information. Here is an example:

A client undergoes a total hip replacement. Which statement by the client indicates that he requires further teaching?

☐ **1.** "I'll need to keep several pillows between my legs at night."

☐ **2.** "I'll need to remember not to cross my legs. It's such a bad habit."

☐ **3.** "The occupational therapist is showing me how to use a 'sock puller' to help me get dressed."

☐ **4.** "I don't know if I'll be able to get off that low toilet seat at home by myself."

The answer you should choose here is option 4 because it indicates that the client has a poor understanding of the precautions required after a total hip replacement and that he needs further teaching. *Remember:* If you see the phrase *further teaching* or *further instruction*, you are looking for a wrong answer by the patient.

NCLEX Versus the Real World

Some students who take the NCLEX have extensive practical experience in health care. For example, many test-takers have worked as nursing assistants. In one of those capacities, test-takers might have been exposed to less than optimum clinical practice and may carry those experiences over to the NCLEX.

Take the NCLEX with the understanding that what happens in the real world may differ from what the NCLEX and your nursing instructors say should happen.

If you have had practical experience in health care, you may know a quicker way to perform a procedure or tricks to get by when you do not have the right equipment. Situations such as staff shortages may force you to improvise. On the NCLEX, such scenarios can lead to trouble. Always check your practical experiences against textbook evidence-based nursing care, taking care to select the response that follows the textbook.

Delegating Care

On the NCLEX, you may encounter questions that assess your ability to delegate care. Delegating care involves coordinating the efforts of other health care workers to provide effective care for your client. On the NCLEX, you may be asked to assign duties to

- direct care workers, such as nursing assistants and personal care aides;
- other support staff, such as nutrition assistants and housekeepers.

In addition, you will be asked to decide when to notify a physician, a social worker, or another hospital staff member. In each case, you will have to decide when, where, and how to delegate.

As a general rule, it is acceptable to delegate actions that involve stable clients or standard, unchanging procedures. Bathing, feeding, dressing, and transferring clients are examples of procedures that can be delegated.

Be careful not to delegate complicated or complex activities. In addition, do not delegate activities that involve assessment, evaluation, or your own nursing judgment. On the NCLEX and in the real world, these duties fall squarely on your shoulders. Make sure that you take primary responsibility for assessing and evaluating the client and for making decisions about the client's care. Never hand off those responsibilities to someone with less training.

Deciding when to notify a physician, a social worker, or another hospital staff member is an important element of nursing care. On the NCLEX, however, choices that involve notifying the physician are

- Blood urea nitrogen: 8 to 25 mg/dL
- Creatinine: 0.6 to 1.5 mg/dL
- Sodium: 135 to 145 mmol/L
- Potassium: 3.5 to 5.5 mEq/L
- Chloride: 97 to 110 mmol/L
- Glucose (fasting plasma): 65 to 115 mg/dL
- Hemoglobin
  Male: 13.8 to 17.2 g/dL
  Female: 12.1 to 15.1 g/dL
- Hematocrit
  Male: 40.7% to 50.3%
  Female: 36.1% to 44.3%

usually incorrect. Remember that the NCLEX wants to see you, the nurse, at work.

If you are sure the correct answer is to notify the physician, it is essential to make sure that the client's safety has been addressed before notifying a physician or another staff member. On the NCLEX, the client's safety has a higher priority than notifying other health care providers.

Knowing Laboratory Values

Some NCLEX questions supply laboratory results without indicating normal levels. As a result, answering questions involving laboratory values requires you to have the normal range of the most common laboratory values memorized to make an informed decision. (See *Normal laboratory values on page 11.*)

Study Preparations

If you are like most people preparing to take the test, you are probably feeling nervous, anxious, or concerned. Keep in mind that most test-takers pass the NCLEX the first time around.

Passing the test will not happen by accident, though; you will need to prepare carefully and efficiently. To help jump-start your preparations:

- determine your strengths and weaknesses;
- create a study schedule;
- set realistic goals;
- find an effective study space;
- think positively;
- start studying sooner rather than later.

Strengths and Weaknesses

Most students recognize that, even at the end of their nursing studies, they know more about some topics than others. Because the NCLEX covers a broad range of material, you should make some decisions about how intensively you will review each topic.

Base those decisions on a list. Divide a sheet of paper in half vertically. On one side, list topics you think you know well. On the other side, list topics you need to review. Pay no attention if one side is longer than the other. When you are done studying, you will feel strong in every area.

To make sure your list reflects a comprehensive view of all the areas you studied in school, look at the contents page in the front of this book. For each topic listed, place it in the "know well" column or "needs review" column. Separating content areas this way shows immediately which topics need less study time and which topics need more time.

Scheduling Study Time

Study when you are most alert. Most people can identify a period of the day when they feel most alert. If you feel most alert and energized in the morning, for example, set aside sections of time in the morning for topics that need a lot of review. Then you can use the evening,

a time of lesser alertness, for topics that need some refreshing. The opposite is true as well; if you are more alert in the evening, study difficult topics at that time.

Set up a basic schedule for studying. Using a calendar or organizer, determine how much time remains before you will take the NCLEX. (See *2 to 3 months before the NCLEX.*) Fill in the remaining days

2 TO 3 MONTHS BEFORE THE NCLEX

With 2 to 3 months remaining before you plan to take the examination, take these steps:

- Establish a study schedule. Set aside ample time to study and also leave time for social activities, exercise, family or personal responsibilities, and other matters.
- Become knowledgeable about the NCLEX-PN examination, its content, the types of questions it asks, and the testing format.
- Begin studying your notes, texts, and other study materials.
- Take some NCLEX practice questions to help you diagnose strengths and weaknesses as well as to become familiar with NCLEX-style questions.

with specific times and topics to be studied. For example, you might schedule the respiratory system on a Tuesday morning and the gastrointestinal system that afternoon. Remember to schedule difficult topics during your most alert times.

Keep in mind that you should not fill each day with studying. Be realistic and set aside time for normal activities. Try to create ample study time before the NCLEX and then stick to the schedule.

Part of creating a schedule means setting goals you can accomplish. You no doubt studied a great deal in nursing school, and by now you have a sense of your own capabilities. Ask yourself, "How much can I cover in a day?" Set that amount of time aside and then stay on task. You will feel better about yourself—and your chances of passing the NCLEX—when you meet your goals regularly.

Study Space

Find a space conducive to effective learning and then study there. Whatever you do, do not study with a television on in the room. Instead, find a quiet, inviting study space that

- is located in a quiet, convenient place, away from normal traffic patterns;
- contains a solid chair that encourages good posture (avoid studying in bed; you will be more likely to fall asleep and not accomplish your goals);
- uses comfortable, soft lighting with which you can see clearly without eye strain;
- has a temperature between 65°F and 70°F;
- contains flowers or green plants, familiar photos or paintings, and easy access to soft, instrumental background music.

Consider taping positive messages around your study space. Make signs with words of encouragement, such as "You can do it!" "Keep studying!" and "Remember the goal!" These upbeat messages can help keep you going when your attention begins to waver.

When you are faced with reviewing the amount of information covered by the NCLEX, it is easy to become distracted and lose your concentration. When you lose concentration, you make less effective use of valuable study time. To help stay focused, keep these tips in mind:

- Alternate the order of the subjects you study during the day to add variety to your study. Try alternating between topics you find most interesting and those you find least interesting.
- Approach your studying with enthusiasm, sincerity, and determination.
- Once you have decided to study, begin immediately. Do not let anything interfere with your thought processes once you have begun.
- Concentrate on accomplishing one task at a time, to the exclusion of everything else.
- Do not try to do two things at once, such as studying and watching television or conversing with friends.
- Work continuously without interruption for a while, but do not study for such a long period that the whole experience becomes grueling or boring.
- Allow time for periodic breaks to give yourself a change of pace. Use these breaks to ease your transition into studying a new topic.

- When studying in the evening, wind down from your studies slowly. Do not progress directly from studying to sleeping.

Taking Care of Yourself

Never neglect your physical and mental well-being in favor of longer study hours. Maintaining physical and mental health is critical for success in taking the NCLEX. (See *4 to 6 weeks before the NCLEX*, page 14.)

You can increase your likelihood of passing the test by following these simple health rules:

- Get plenty of rest. You cannot think deeply or concentrate for long periods when you are tired.
- Drink enough noncaffeinated beverages. Mild dehydration increases the effort required to concentrate and reason while distracting attention through feelings of fatigue and thirst.
- Eat nutritious meals. Maintaining your energy level is impossible when you are undernourished.
- Exercise regularly. Regular exercise helps you work harder and think more clearly. As a result, you will study more efficiently and increase the likelihood of success.

With 4 to 6 weeks remaining before you plan to take the examination, take these steps:

- Focus on your areas of weakness. That way, you will have time to review these areas again before the test date.
- Find a study partner or form a study group.
- Take a practice test to gauge your skill level early.
- Take time to eat, sleep, exercise, and socialize to avoid burnout.

If you are having trouble concentrating but would rather push through than take a break, try making your studying more active by reading out loud. Active studying can renew your powers of concentration. By reading review material out loud to yourself, you are engaging your ears as well as your eyes—and making your studying a more active process. Hearing the material out loud also fosters memory and subsequent recall.

You can also rewrite in your own words a few of the more difficult concepts you are reviewing. Explaining these concepts in writing forces you to think through the material and can jump-start your memory.

Study Schedule

When you were creating your schedule, you might have asked yourself, "How long should I study? One hour at a stretch? Two hours? Three?" To make the best use of your study time, you will need to answer those questions.

Optimum Study Time

Experts are divided about the optimum length of study time. Some say you should study no more than 1 hour at a time several times a day. Their reasoning: you remember the material you study at the beginning and end of a session best and tend to remember less material studied in the middle of the session.

Other experts say you should hold longer study sessions because you lose time in the beginning, when you are just getting warmed up, and again at the end, when you are cooling down. Therefore, say those experts, a long, concentrated study period will allow you to cover more material.

So what is the answer? It does not matter as long as you determine what is best for *you*. At the beginning of your NCLEX study schedule, try study periods of varying lengths. Pay close attention to those that seem more successful.

Remember that you are a trained nurse who is competent at assessment. Think of yourself as a patient, and assess your own progress. Then implement the strategy that works best for you.

Finding Time to Study

So does that mean that short sections of time are useless? Not at all. We all have spaces in our day that might otherwise be dead time. (See *1 week before the NCLEX*.) These are perfect times to review for the NCLEX but not to cover new material because by the time you get deep into new material, your time will be over. Always keep some flashcards or a small notebook handy for situations when you have a few extra minutes.

With 1 week remaining before the NCLEX, take these steps:

- Take a review test to measure your progress.
- Record key ideas and principles on note cards or audiotapes.
- Rest, eat well, and avoid thinking about the examination during nonstudy times.
- Treat yourself to one special event. You have been working hard, and you deserve it!

You will be amazed how many short sessions you can find in a day and how much reviewing you can do in 5 minutes. The following places offer short stretches of time you can use:

- Eating breakfast
- Waiting for, or riding on, a train or bus
- Waiting in line at the bank, post office, bookstore, or other places

Creative Studying

Even when you study in a perfect study space and concentrate better than ever, studying for the NCLEX can get a little, well, dull. Even people with terrific study habits occasionally feel bored or sluggish. That is why it is important to have some creative tricks in your study bag to liven up your studying during those downtimes.

Creative studying does not have to be hard work. It involves making efforts to alter your study habits a bit. Some techniques that might help include studying with a partner or group and creating flash cards or other audiovisual study tools.

Study Partners

Studying with a partner or group of students can be an excellent way to energize your studying. Working with a partner allows you to test each other on the material you have reviewed. Your partner can give you encouragement and motivation. Perhaps most important, working with a partner can provide a welcome break from solitary studying.

Exercise some care when choosing a study partner or assembling a study group. A partner who does not fit your needs will not help you make the most of your study time. Look for a partner who

- possesses similar goals to yours. For example, someone taking the NCLEX at approximately the same date who feels the same sense of urgency as you do might make an excellent partner.
- possesses about the same level of knowledge as you. Tutoring someone can sometimes help you learn, but partnering should be give-and-take so both partners can gain knowledge.
- can study without excess chatting or interruptions. Socializing is an important part of creative study, but remember, you have still got to pass the NCLEX—so stay serious!

Audiovisual Tools

Flash cards and other audiovisual tools foster retention and make learning and reviewing fun.

Flash cards can provide you with an excellent study tool. The process of writing material on a flash card will help you remember it. In addition, flash cards are small and easily portable, perfect for those 5-minute slivers of time that show up during the day.

Creating a flash card should be fun. Use magic markers, highlighters, and other colorful tools to make them visually stimulating. The more effort you put into creating your flash cards, the better you will remember the material contained on the cards.

Flowcharts, drawings, diagrams, and other image-oriented study aids can also help you learn material more effectively. Substituting images for text can be a great way to give your eyes a break and recharge your brain. Remember to use vivid colors to make your creations visually engaging.

If you learn more effectively when you hear information rather than see it, consider recording key ideas using a handheld tape recorder. Recording information helps promote memory because you say the information aloud when taping and then listen to it when playing it back. Like flash cards, tapes are portable and perfect for those short study periods during the day. (See *The day before the NCLEX.*)

THE DAY BEFORE THE NCLEX

With 1 day before the NCLEX, take these steps:

- Drive to the test site, review traffic patterns, and find out where to park. If your route to the test site occurs during heavy traffic or if you are expecting bad weather, set aside extra time to ensure prompt arrival.
- Do something relaxing during the day.
- Avoid concentrating on the test.
- Rest, eat, and drink well, and avoid dwelling on the NCLEX during nonstudy periods.
- Call a supportive friend or relative for some last-minute words of encouragement.

Practice Tests

Practice questions should constitute an important part of your NCLEX study strategy. Practice questions can improve your studying by helping you review material and familiarizing yourself with the exact style of questions you will encounter on the NCLEX.

Consider working through some practice questions as soon as you begin studying for the NCLEX. For example, you might try a half-dozen questions from each chapter in this book.

If you score well, you probably know the material contained in that chapter fairly well and can spend less time reviewing that particular topic. If you have trouble with the questions, spend extra study time on that topic.

Practice questions can also provide an excellent means of marking your progress. Do not worry if you have trouble answering the first few practice questions you take; you will need time to adjust to the way the questions are asked. Eventually you will become accustomed to the question format and begin to focus more on the questions themselves.

If you make practice questions a regular part of your study regimen, you will be able to notice areas in which you are improving. You can then adjust your study time accordingly.

As you near the examination date, continue to answer practice questions, and also set aside time to take an entire NCLEX practice test. That way, you will know exactly what to expect. (See *The day of the NCLEX*.) The more you know ahead of time, the better you are likely to do on the NCLEX.

Taking an entire practice test is also a way to gauge your progress. When you find yourself answering questions correctly, it will give you the confidence you need to conquer the real NCLEX.

THE DAY OF THE NCLEX

On the day of the NCLEX, take these steps:
- Get up early.
- Wear comfortable clothes, preferably with layers you can adjust to fit the room temperature.
- Drink a glass of water and eat a small nutritious breakfast.
- Make sure you have proper identification and your authorization to test.
- Leave your house early.
- Arrive at the test site at least 30 minutes prior to the scheduled time.
- Listen carefully to the instructions given before entering the test room.
- Succeed, succeed, *succeed!*

PART TWO

Fundamentals of Nursing

1. A nurse is developing a care plan for a client with an injury to the frontal lobe of the brain. Which nursing interventions should be included as part of the care plan? Select all that apply.

- ☐ **1.** Keep instructions simple and brief because the client will have difficulty concentrating.
- ☐ **2.** Speak clearly and slowly because the client will have difficulty hearing.
- ☐ **3.** Assist with bathing because the client will have vision disturbances.
- ☐ **4.** Orient the client to person, place, and time as needed because of memory problems.
- ☐ **5.** Assess vital signs frequently because vital bodily functions are affected.

Answer: 1, 4

Rationale: Damage to the frontal lobe affects personality, memory, reasoning, concentration, and motor control of speech. Damage to the temporal lobe, not the frontal lobe, causes hearing and speech problems. Damage to the occipital lobe causes vision disturbances. Damage to the brain stem affects vital functions.

Test-taking strategy: Analyze to determine what the question asks for, which is the nursing interventions needed when caring for a client with an injury to the frontal lobe of the brain. Recall the physiologic functions of the different areas of the brain to understand what type of damage has occurred. "Select all that apply" questions require considering each option to decide its merit. Compare each option in relation to the functions of the frontal lobe and deficits that arise following injury. Review the functions of specific sections of the brain if you had difficulty answering this question.

Client needs category: Physiological integrity
Client needs subcategory: Basic care and comfort
Cognitive level: Applying

2. A nurse, assigned to a client with emphysema, is providing shift report. Which nursing interventions would be appropriate to include? Select all that apply.

- ☐ **1.** The nurse should reduce fluid intake to less than 850 mL per shift.
- ☐ **2.** The nurse should teach diaphragmatic, pursed-lip breathing.
- ☐ **3.** The nurse should administer low-flow oxygen.
- ☐ **4.** The nurse should keep the client in a supine position as much as possible.
- ☐ **5.** The nurse should encourage alternating activity with rest periods.
- ☐ **6.** The nurse should teach the use of postural drainage and chest physiotherapy.

Answer: 2, 3, 5, 6

Rationale: The nurse provides report on nursing interventions required for a client with emphysema. Diaphragmatic, pursed-lip breathing strengthens respiratory muscles and enhances oxygenation in clients with emphysema. Low-flow oxygen should be administered because a client with emphysema has chronic hypercapnia and a hypoxic respiratory drive. Alternating activity with rest allows to perform activities without excessive distress. If the client has difficulty mobilizing copious secretions, the nurse should teach the client and family members how to perform postural drainage and chest physiotherapy. Fluid intake should be increased to 3,000 mL/day, if not contraindicated, to liquefy secretions and facilitate their removal. The client should be placed in high Fowler's position to improve ventilation.

Test-taking strategy: Analyze to determine what the question asks for, which is the essential nursing interventions to include when nurses discuss care in the shift report. Recall the pathophysiology of emphysema and the client's physical needs created by the disease process. "Select all that apply" questions require considering each option to decide its merit. Consider each nursing intervention against the ability to improve the respiratory status of a client with emphysema. Review the care of a client with emphysema if you had difficulty answering this question.

Client needs category: Safe and effective care environment

Client needs subcategory: Coordinated care

Cognitive level: Applying

---

3. A nurse is caring for a client who underwent surgical repair of a detached retina in the right eye. Which nursing interventions should the nurse perform? Select all that apply.

☐ **1.** Place the client in a prone position.
☐ **2.** Approach the client from the left side.
☐ **3.** Encourage deep breathing and coughing.
☐ **4.** Discourage bending down.
☐ **5.** Orient the client to the environment.
☐ **6.** Administer a stool softener.

Answer: 2, 4, 5, 6

Rationale: The nurse should approach the client from the left side—the unaffected side—to avoid startling. The nurse should also discourage the client from bending down, deep breathing, hard coughing and sneezing, and other activities that can increase intraocular pressure during the postoperative period. The client should be oriented to the environment to reduce the risk of injury. Stool softeners should be administered to discourage straining during defecation. The client should lie on the back or on the unaffected side to reduce intraocular pressure in the affected eye.

Test-taking strategy: Analyze to determine what information the question asks for, which is the postoperative care following repair of a detached retina. "Select all that apply" questions require considering each option to decide its merit. Recall the pathophysiology of a detached retina and the surgical intervention needed. Consider potential complications and nursing interventions essential in preventing those complications. Review postoperative care of a client with a detached retina if you had difficulty answering this question.

Client needs category: Physiological integrity

Client needs subcategory: Reduction of risk potential

Cognitive level: Applying

4. A nurse is planning care for a client with hyper-thyroidism. Which nursing interventions are appropriate? Select all that apply.

☐ **1.** Instill isotonic eyedrops as necessary.
☐ **2.** Provide several small, well-balanced meals.
☐ **3.** Provide rest periods.
☐ **4.** Keep the environment warm.
☐ **5.** Encourage frequent visitors and conversation.
☐ **6.** Weigh the client daily.

Answer: 1, 2, 3, 6

Rationale: Hyperthyroidism is a condition where the thyroid gland makes too much thyroid hormone causing physical and metabolic changes. If the client has exophthalmos (a sign of hyperthyroidism), the conjunctivae should be moistened often with isotonic eyedrops. Hyperthyroidism results in increased appetite, which can be satisfied by frequent, small, well-balanced meals. The nurse should provide the client with rest periods to reduce metabolic demands. The client should be weighed daily to check for weight loss, a possible consequence of hyperthyroidism. Because metabolism is increased in hyperthyroidism, heat intolerance and excitability result. Therefore, the nurse should provide a cool and quiet environment, not a warm and busy one, to promote client comfort.

Test-taking strategy: Analyze to determine what the question asks for, which is the nursing interventions necessary in the care of a client with hyperthyroidism. Recall the signs and symptoms and pathophysiology of hyperthyroidism. "Select all that apply" questions require considering each option to decide its merit. Consider each nursing intervention against its ability to reduce the potential side effects. Review nursing care of a client with hyperthyroidism if you had difficulty answering this question.

Client needs category: Physiological integrity
Client needs subcategory: Basic care and comfort
Cognitive level: Applying

---

5. A client has a tumor of the posterior pituitary gland. A nurse planning care should include which nursing interventions? Select all that apply.

☐ **1.** Weigh the client daily.
☐ **2.** Restrict fluids.
☐ **3.** Measure urine specific gravity.
☐ **4.** Encourage intake of coffee or tea.
☐ **5.** Monitor intake and output.

Answer: 1, 3, 5

Rationale: The pituitary gland is divided into the anterior and posterior sections with each section secreting specific hormones. Tumors of the posterior pituitary gland can lead to diabetes insipidus due to deficiency of vasopressin, also called antidiuretic hormone (ADH). Decreased ADH reduces the kidneys' ability to concentrate urine, resulting in excessive urination, thirst, and fluid intake. To monitor fluid balance, the nurse should weigh the client daily, measure urine specific gravity, and monitor intake and output. The nurse should also encourage fluids to keep intake equal to output and prevent dehydration. Coffee, tea, and other fluids that have a diuretic effect should be avoided.

Test-taking strategy: Analyze to determine what the question asks for, which is nursing interventions in the care of a client with a posterior pituitary tumor. Focus on the pathophysiology and implications of a tumor of the posterior pituitary gland. Recall that the posterior pituitary secretes oxytocin and vasopressin (ADH). Vasopressin stimulates water retention and raises blood pressure. Review the role of the posterior pituitary and manifestations caused by a tumor if you had difficulty answering this question.

Client needs category: Physiological integrity

Client needs subcategory: Basic care and comfort

Cognitive level: Applying

---

6. A nurse is preparing to administer an intramuscular (I.M.) injection in the deltoid muscle. In which anatomical location would the nurse administer this injection?

Answer:

Rationale: To locate the deltoid muscle, find the lower edge of the acromial process and the point on the lateral arm in line with the axilla. The needle should be inserted 1″ to 2″ (usually two or three fingerbreadths) below the acromial process, and at a 90° angle, or slightly angled, toward the process.

Test-taking strategy: Analyze to determine what information the question asks for, which is the location for an I.M. injection in the deltoid muscle. Focus on the anatomy of the upper arm and the location of the deltoid muscle and recall the process for administering an I.M. injection. Recall that the deltoid I.M. injection site is triangular in shape, with the base of the triangle on the lower edge of the acromial process. Visualize the process for completing the I.M. injection. Review the skill of completing an I.M. injection in the deltoid site if you had difficulty answering this question.

Client needs category: Physiological integrity

Client needs subcategory: Pharmacological therapies

Cognitive level: Applying

7. A nurse is performing a fecal occult blood test using a Hemoccult slide for a client with a possible lower gastrointestinal bleed. Place the steps for performing the fecal occult blood test in the correct order.

1.	Allow the specimens to dry for 3 minutes.
2.	Put on gloves.
3.	Apply a drop of Hemoccult developing solution to boxes A and B on the slide's reverse side.
4.	Place a stool smear on box A of the slide.
5.	Apply a stool smear from another part of the specimen to box B on the slide.
6.	Put a drop of Hemoccult developing solution on each control dot on the slide's reverse side.

Answer: 2, 4, 5, 1, 6, 3

Rationale: After receiving the stool specimen from the client, the nurse should put on gloves and then follow the other steps in the order listed above. Before using the developer, the nurse should check the expiration date; the nurse should discard the developer if the date has expired. A blue reaction after 30 to 60 seconds indicates a positive result.

Test-taking strategy: Analyze to determine what information the question asks for, which is the correct sequence for performing a fecal occult blood test using a Hemoccult slide. Recall the process of standard precautions and visualize the sequence of steps to be performed. Review the skill of performing a fecal occult blood test using a Hemoccult slide if you had difficulty answering this question.

Client needs category: Health promotion and maintenance

Client needs subcategory: None

Cognitive level: Applying

---

8. A nurse is caring for a client with a hiatal hernia. The client complains of abdominal and sternal pain after eating. The pain makes it difficult for the client to sleep. Which instructions should the nurse recommend when teaching this client? Select all that apply.

- ☐ **1.** Avoid constrictive clothing.
- ☐ **2.** Lie down for 30 minutes after eating.
- ☐ **3.** Decrease the intake of caffeine and spicy foods.
- ☐ **4.** Eat three meals per day.
- ☐ **5.** Sleep with the upper body elevated.
- ☐ **6.** Maintain a normal body weight.

Answer: 1, 3, 5, 6

Rationale: A hiatal hernia occurs when a portion of the stomach pushes through the diaphragm. A hiatal hernia may cause abdominal and sternal pain after eating. The discomfort is associated with reflux of gastric contents. To reduce gastric reflux, the nurse should instruct the client to avoid constrictive clothing, caffeine, and spicy foods; sleep with the upper body elevated; lose weight, if obese; remain upright for 2 hours after eating; and eat small, frequent meals.

Test-taking strategy: Analyze to determine what information the question asks for, which is selecting instructions to provide a client experiencing pain after eating. Focus on the pathophysiology of hiatal hernia and recall the clinical manifestations of this disorder. Relate the cause of the disorder to instructions that would reduce the symptoms by preventing the reflux of gastric contents. Review methods to decrease the symptoms of hiatal hernia if you had difficulty answering this question.

Client needs category: Physiological integrity

Client needs subcategory: Basic care and comfort

Cognitive level: Analyzing

9. A nurse is caring for a client diagnosed with heart failure. When assessing for lower extremity perfusion and edema, indicate with an X where the nurse would assess the left dorsalis pedis pulse.

Answer:

Rationale: Many peripheral pulse sites may be used to assess pulse and circulatory status by palpation. The dorsalis pedis pulse can be palpated on the medial dorsal surface of the foot when the client's toes are pointed down. This pulse can be difficult to palpate and may seem to be absent in healthy clients.

Test-taking strategy: Use knowledge of medical terminology to determine the site for palpation. If unsure of the location of dorsalis pedis, break the word apart. Dorsalis means dorsal aspect. Focus on the location of the dorsalis pedis pulse and recall the correct finger placement when performing the assessment. Review peripheral pulse sites if you had difficulty answering this question.

Client needs category: Physiological integrity
Client needs subcategory: Physiological adaptation
Cognitive level: Understanding

---

10. A client with renal failure is placed on a potassium-restricted diet. For lunch, the client consumed 6 oz of hamburger on a bun, one cup of cooked broccoli, a raw pear, and iced tea. Using the chart provided, calculate how many milliequivalents of potassium were in this meal.

☐ **1.** 24.4
☐ **2.** 30
☐ **3.** 31.4
☐ **4.** 37

Answer: 4

Rationale: According to the chart, 4 oz of beef contains 11.2 mEq of potassium. Add 5.6 mEq for the additional 2 oz for a total of 16.8 mEq of potassium in the beef. The amount of potassium in one cup of broccoli is 14 mEq. A pear has 6.2 mEq. Thus, the total amount of potassium in this meal is 37 mEq. The iced tea and bun do not contain significant amounts of potassium and, therefore, are not listed on the chart.

Test-taking strategy: Analyze to determine what information the question asks for, which is the amount of potassium in the following meal. Use basic math skills to calculate the totals requested. Pay particular attention to using prudent strategies for addition such as making sure to maintain number alignment, maintain placement of decimals, and proofread work. Double-check to make sure that you included all of the mEq of potassium noted in the chart with no error in transcription.

Client needs category: Physiological integrity
Client needs subcategory: Physiological adaptation
Cognitive level: Analyzing

Intake and Output

DIETARY SOURCES OF POTASSIUM

Foods and Beverages	Serving Size	Amount of Potassium (mEq)
Meats		
Beef	4 oz (112 g)	11.2
Chicken	4 oz	12.0
Scallops	5 large	30.0
Vegetables		
Broccoli (cooked)	1/2 cup	7.0
Carrots (raw)	1 large	8.8
Potatoes (baked)	1 small	15.4
Tomatoes (raw)	1 medium	10.4
Fruits		
Bananas	1 medium	12.8
Cantaloupe	6 oz	13.0
Pears (raw)	1 medium	6.2
Beverages		
Orange juice	1 cup	11.4
Prune juice	1 cup	14.4
Tomato juice	1 cup	11.6
Milk (whole or skim)	1 cup	8.8

11. A nurse is teaching a client with left leg weakness to walk with a cane. The nurse should include which nursing points about safe cane use in the client teaching? Select all that apply.

☐ **1.** Place the cane 8″ to 10″ from the base of the little toe.

☐ **2.** Hold the cane on the uninvolved side of the body.

☐ **3.** Adjust the cane so that the handle is level with the hip bone.

☐ **4.** Walk by moving the involved leg, then the cane, and then the uninvolved leg.

☐ **5.** Shorten the stride length on the involved side.

☐ **6.** Avoid leaning on the cane to get in and out of a chair.

Answer: 2, 3, 6

Rationale: To ambulate safely, a client with leg weakness should hold the cane in the hand opposite the involved leg with the handle level adjacent to the hip bone. The client should not lean on the cane to get in or out of a chair because of the risk of falls. The cane base should be placed 4″ to 6″ from the base of the little toe. When walking, the client should move the cane and involved leg simultaneously, alternating with the uninvolved leg in equal length strides and timing.

Test-taking strategy: Analyze to determine what information the question asks for, which is nursing points necessary for the safe use of a cane. Recall the placement of the cane in relation to the involved side and the importance of ensuring patient safety. Consider the potential for losing balance, which is important in the geriatric population. Review ambulation with an assistive device if you had difficulty answering this question.

Client needs category: Physiological integrity

Client needs subcategory: Reduction of risk potential

Cognitive level: Analyzing

---

12. A nurse is caring for a client who is recovering from an illness requiring prolonged bed rest. Based on the nursing documentation below, which procedure would the nurse implement next?

Progress Notes
2/10/10 1015 — Pt. instructed in contraction of back extensors, hip extensors, knee extensors, and ankle flexors and extensors. Pt. able to demonstrate correct technique without joint motion or muscle lengthening. c/o being "a little tired" after holding each contraction 5 seconds and repeating three times. Instructed to repeat exercises three times daily; pt. verbalized understanding of all information given. ————————F. Brown, LPN

☐ **1.** Performing active range-of-motion exercises of the legs

☐ **2.** Performing isometric exercises of the legs

☐ **3.** Providing assistance walking the client to the bathroom

☐ **4.** Performing passive range-of-motion exercises of the legs

Answer: 1

Rationale: Active range-of-motion exercises involve moving the client's joints through their full range of motion; they require some muscle strength and endurance. The client should have received passive range-of-motion exercises since admission to maintain joint flexibility and should have been taught isometric exercises to build strength and endurance for transfers and ambulation. Walking to the bathroom would be unsafe without the ability to first dangle the legs over the bedside and transfer from bed to chair.

Test-taking strategy: Look at the key word "next" indicating that the client has reached a point when there is a clear next step in progress. Focus on the types of exercise being discussed with the client and review the correct sequence of activities when advancing the client's mobility status. Recall the dangers of progressing too quickly or regressing in ability. Review the range-of-motion exercises and isometric exercises if you had difficulty answering this question.

Client needs category: Physiological integrity

Client needs subcategory: Reduction of risk potential

Cognitive level: Analyzing

13. The nurse is providing care for a client who has had a stroke. Since the onset of symptoms, the client has been experiencing left-sided hemianopsia. Which nursing interventions would be appropriate? Select all that apply.

- ☐ **1.** Place the client's belongings on the right side of the bed.
- ☐ **2.** Approach the client from the left side.
- ☐ **3.** Refuse to acknowledge the condition to promote the client's independence.
- ☐ **4.** Stand on the right side of the bed when providing care.
- ☐ **5.** Provide the client with an eye patch for the right eye.
- ☐ **6.** Dim the lights in the room to prevent eye strain.

Answer: 1, 4

Rationale: Hemianopsia is a condition in which the client has lost half of the visual field. It is most often associated with a stroke. In this case, the stroke has affected the client's left side; therefore, placing belongings on the right side of the bed will enable the client to best see them. Standing on the right side of the bed when providing care will ensure the client is able to see the nurse. Approaching the client from the left side is counterproductive because the client would not be able to adequately see the nurse. Using an eye patch or dimming the lights will not help with treating or managing the condition.

Test-taking strategy: Analyze to determine what information the question asks for, which is nursing interventions for a client with left-sided hemianopsia. Begin by thinking of the visual deficits and how these impact the client's ability to complete activities. Recall the clinical effects of hemianopsia and consider the client's basic need to have meaningful interactions with the nursing staff and environment. Also differentiate between a deficit on the right side and one on the left side. Review the care of a client with hemianopsia if you had difficulty answering this question.

Client needs category: Physiological integrity

Client needs subcategory: Basic needs and comfort

Cognitive level: Analyzing

14. The physician writes an order that a client may have 12 oz of clear liquids at each meal and may supplement this with an additional 10 oz at each shift (7-3, 3-11, and 11-7). How many milliliters should the nurse document for the day shift (7-3) if the client took in all of the ordered volumes? Record your answer using a whole number.

_____ milliliters

Answer: 1020

Rationale: The nurse must add all the volumes together, knowing that 1 oz equals 30 mL. There are two meals in the day shift (7-3).

$$12 \text{ oz} \times 30 \text{ mL} = 360 \text{ mL}$$
$$360 \text{ mL} \times 2 \text{ meals} = 720 \text{ mL}$$
$$10 \text{ oz (supplement)} \times 30 \text{ mL} = 300 \text{ mL}$$
$$720 \text{ mL} + 300 \text{ mL} = 1{,}020 \text{ mL}.$$

Test-taking strategy: Analyze to determine what information the question asks for, which is the total volume of intake for the day shift. Begin by considering the times of each meal and adding the supplemental amount. Also, review ounce to milliliter equivalents. Last, double-check your math calculation.

Client needs category: Physiological integrity

Client needs subcategory: Basic care and comfort

Cognitive level: Applying

15. The nurse is recording the intake and output for a client with the following: D_5NSS 1,000 mL; urine 450 mL; emesis 125 mL; Jackson Pratt drain #1 35 mL; Jackson Pratt drain #2 32 mL; and Jackson Pratt drain #3 12 mL. How many milliliters should the nurse document as the client's output? Record your answer using a whole number.

_____ milliliters

Answer: 654

Rationale: The nurse must add all the output volumes together:

$$450 \text{ mL} + 125 \text{ mL} + 35 \text{ mL} + 32 \text{ mL} + 12 \text{ mL} = 654 \text{ mL}.$$

D_5NSS 1,000 mL is considered input, not output.

Test-taking strategy: Analyze to determine what information the question asks for, which is the client's total output. Begin by determining output versus input. Next, add the amounts keeping the columns in proper alignment. Last, double-check your math calculation.

Client needs category: Physiological integrity

Client needs subcategory: Basic care and comfort

Cognitive level: Applying

Basic Psychosocial Needs

1. A client has just been diagnosed with terminal cancer and is being transferred to home hospice care. The client's daughter tells the nurse, "I don't know what to say to my mother if she asks me if she's going to die." Which responses by the nurse would be appropriate? Select all that apply.

☐ **1.** "Tell your mother not to worry. She still has some time left."

☐ **2.** "Let's talk about your mother's illness and how it will progress."

☐ **3.** "You sound like you have some questions about your mother dying. Let's talk about that."

☐ **4.** "Don't worry, hospice will take care of your mother."

☐ **5.** "Tell me how you're feeling about your mother dying."

Answer: 2, 3, 5

Rationale: Talking about death is an uncomfortable situation. Conveying information clearly and openly can alleviate fears and strengthen the individual's sense of control. Encouraging verbalization of feelings helps build a therapeutic relationship based on trust and reduces anxiety. Advising the daughter not to worry, or having her tell her mother that, ignores her feelings and discourages further communication.

Test-taking strategy: Begin by determining which responses promote open, therapeutic communication. Also, consider the psychosocial needs of the family of a dying client. Eliminate responses that do not answer the client's question or are condescending. Review therapeutic communication skills if you had difficulty answering this question.

Client needs category: Psychosocial integrity

Client needs subcategory: None

Cognitive level: Analyzing

2. While providing care to a married client, the nurse notes multiple blue, purple, and yellow ecchymotic areas on the arms and trunk. When the nurse asks about these bruises, the client responds, "I tripped." What actions should the nurse take? Select all that apply.

- ☐ **1.** Document the client's statement and complete a body map indicating the size, color, shape, location, and type of injuries.
- ☐ **2.** Contact the local authorities to report suspicions of abuse.
- ☐ **3.** Assist the client in developing a safety plan for times of increased violence.
- ☐ **4.** Call the client's spouse to arrange a meeting to discuss the situation.
- ☐ **5.** Instruct the client to leave the abusive situation as soon as possible.
- ☐ **6.** Provide the client with telephone numbers of local shelters and safe houses.

Answer: 1, 3, 6

Rationale: The nurse should objectively document the assessment findings. A detailed description of physical findings of abuse in the medical record is essential if legal action is pursued. All individuals, men or women, suspected of being abuse victims should be counseled on a safety plan, which consists of recognizing escalating violence within the family, formulating a plan to exit quickly, and knowing the telephone numbers of local shelters and safe houses. The nurse should not report this suspicion of abuse because the client is a competent adult who has the right to self-determination. Contacting the client's spouse without consent violates confidentiality. The nurse should respond to the client in a nonthreatening manner that promotes trust, rather than ordering the client to break off the relationship.

Test-taking strategy: Analyze to determine what information the question asks for, which is nursing actions to take when a client is suspected of being an abuse victim. Consider actions reflecting objectivity and remain nonjudgmental while developing trust with the client. Review the nurse's responsibilities when caring for a potential abuse victim and consider the client's age to determine appropriate actions. Review the Nurse's Code of Ethics and Standards of Care if you had difficulty answering this question.

Client needs category: Psychosocial integrity

Client needs subcategory: None

Cognitive level: Analyzing

---

3. A nurse is caring for a terminally ill client. The nurse assesses the client for identification of the psychosocial stage of acceptance. Place the following five stages of death and dying described by Elisabeth Kübler-Ross in the order in which they most often occur.

1. Bargaining
2. Denial and isolation
3. Acceptance
4. Anger
5. Depression

Answer: 2, 4, 1, 5, 3

Rationale: Elisabeth Kübler-Ross outlined similarities to psychosocial responses to impending death or loss. Duration during each stage may vary or even overlap from individual to individual. According to Kübler-Ross, the five stages of death and dying are denial and isolation, anger, bargaining, depression, and acceptance.

Test-taking strategy: The key words are "in order" assuming that there is a progression or sequence. Critically think through the options to place each in a particular order. Begin with denial being the first and ending with acceptance if you are arranging by simply the definition of the words. Review the stages of death and dying and work of Elisabeth Kübler-Ross if you had difficulty answering this question.

Client needs category: Psychosocial integrity

Client needs subcategory: None

Cognitive level: Applying

4. A client with chronic renal failure was recently told by the physician of being a poor candidate for a transplant because of chronic uncontrolled hypertension and diabetes mellitus. Now the client tells the nurse, "I want to go off dialysis. I'd rather not live than be on this treatment for the rest of my life." Which responses are appropriate? Select all that apply.

☐ **1.** Take a seat next to the client and sit quietly to reflect on what was said.

☐ **2.** Say to the client, "We all have days when we don't feel like going on."

☐ **3.** Leave the room to allow the client privacy to collect thoughts.

☐ **4.** Say to the client, "You're feeling upset about the news you got about the transplant."

☐ **5.** Say to the client, "The treatments are only 3 days a week. You can live with that."

Answer: 1, 4

Rationale: Silence is a therapeutic communication technique that allows the nurse and client to reflect on what has taken place or been said. By waiting quietly and attentively, the nurse encourages the client to initiate and maintain a conversation. By reflecting on the client's implied feelings, the nurse promotes communication. Using such platitudes as "We all have days when we don't feel like going on" fails to address the client's needs. The nurse should not leave the client alone abruptly stopping therapeutic communication. Reminding the client of the treatment frequency does not address the feelings.

Test-taking strategy: Analyze to determine what information the question asks for, which is responses to a statement to end life-sustaining treatment. Recall the principles of patient advocacy and therapeutic communication. Review the care of the client under emotional stress and principles of therapeutic communication if you had difficulty answering this question.

Client needs category: Psychosocial integrity

Client needs subcategory: None

Cognitive level: Analyzing

---

5. A nurse is caring for a client with advanced cancer. After reading the nursing note below, determine the nurse's next intervention.

Progress Notes	
1/7/10 1545	Pt. states, "The doctor says my chemotherapy isn't working anymore. They can only treat my symptoms now. I don't want to die in the hospital, I want to be in my own bed."
	————————————R. Daly, LPN

☐ **1.** Reread the Patient's Bill of Rights to the client.

☐ **2.** Call the client's spouse to discuss the client's statements.

☐ **3.** Tell the client that only in the hospital can there be adequate pain relief.

☐ **4.** Explain the use of an advance directive to express the client's wishes.

Answer: 4

Rationale: An advance directive is a legal document used as a guideline for life-sustaining medical care of a client with an advanced disease or disability who can no longer indicate his own wishes. This document can include a living will, which instructs the health care provider to administer no life-sustaining treatment, and a durable power of attorney for health care, which names another person to act on the client's behalf for medical decisions if the client cannot act for himself. The Patient's Bill of Rights does not specifically address the client's wishes regarding future care. Calling the spouse is a breach of the client's right to confidentiality. Stating that only a hospital can provide adequate pain relief in a terminal situation demonstrates inadequate knowledge of the resources available in the community through hospice and home care agencies in collaboration with the client's health care provider.

Test-taking strategy: Use the process of elimination to select the option that is the most important "next" step to be taken by the nurse. Focus on the needs of a client who is making difficult medical decisions, consider referrals available to the nurse, and review the use of advance directives. Eliminate options focused on the nurse and spouse or those that tell the client what should be done. Review the principles of advanced directives and Patient's Bill of Rights if you had difficulty answering this question.

Client needs category: Psychosocial integrity

Client needs subcategory: None

Cognitive level: Applying

---

6. The nurse is caring for a client whose cultural background is different. Which nursing actions are appropriate? Select all that apply.

- ☐ **1.** Consider that nonverbal cues, such as eye contact, may have a different meaning in different cultures.
- ☐ **2.** Respect the client's cultural beliefs.
- ☐ **3.** Ask the client if there are cultural or religious requirements that should be considered in the plan of care.
- ☐ **4.** Explain the nurse's beliefs so that the client will understand the differences.
- ☐ **5.** Understand that all cultures experience pain in the same way.

Answer: 1, 2, 3

Rationale: Nonverbal cues may have different meanings in different cultures. In one culture, eye contact may be a sign of disrespect; in another, eye contact may show respect and attentiveness. The nurse should always respect the client's cultural beliefs and ask if there are cultural or religious requirements. This may include food choices or restrictions, body coverings, or time for prayer. The nurse should attempt to understand the client's culture; it is not the client's responsibility to understand the nurse's culture. The nurse should never impose his or her own beliefs on clients. Culture influences a client's expression of pain. For example, pain may be openly expressed in one culture and quietly endured in another.

Test-taking strategy: Analyze to determine what information the question asks for, which is nursing actions for a client from a different culture. Recall the implications of culturally sensitive care and the nurse's responsibilities when delivering such care to clients. Select the responses that encourage discussion of cultural practices that influence client family behaviors and care. Review culturally sensitive nursing actions if you had difficulty answering this question.

Client needs category: Psychosocial integrity

Client needs subcategory: None

Cognitive level: Analyzing

7. A nurse is caring for a middle-aged client who has undergone a hemicolectomy for colon cancer. The client has two children. Which concepts about families should the nurse consider when providing care for this client? Select all that apply.

- ☐ **1.** Illness in one family member can affect all members.
- ☐ **2.** Family roles do not change because of illness.
- ☐ **3.** A family member may perform more than one role at a time.
- ☐ **4.** Children typically are not affected by adult illness.
- ☐ **5.** The effects of an illness on a family depend on the stage of the family's life cycle.
- ☐ **6.** Changes in sleeping and eating patterns may be signs of stress in a family.

Answer: 1, 3, 5, 6

Rationale: Illness in one family member can affect all family members, even children. Each member of a family may have several roles to perform. A middle-aged client, for example, may have the roles of father/mother, husband/wife, wage earner, child care provider, and housekeeper. When one family member cannot fulfill a role because of illness, the roles of the other family members are affected. Families move through certain predictable life cycles (such as birth of a baby, a growing family, adult children leaving home, and grandparenting). The impact of illness on the family depends on the stage of the life cycle as family members take on different roles and the family structure changes. Illness produces stress in families; changes in eating and sleeping patterns are signs of stress.

Test-taking strategy: Analyze to determine what information the question asks for, which is considerations regarding family that may influence the client's care. Select options that impact family dynamics and roles of the family members. Review the impact of stress and illness on the family and recall the manifestations that may result from stress if you had difficulty answering this question.

Client needs category: Health promotion and maintenance

Client needs subcategory: None

Cognitive level: Analyzing

---

8. A nurse is assessing a newly admitted client. In the family assessment, who should be considered as part of the client's family? Select all that apply.

- ☐ **1.** People related by blood or marriage
- ☐ **2.** People whom the client views as family
- ☐ **3.** People who live in the same house
- ☐ **4.** People whom the nurse thinks are important to the client
- ☐ **5.** People of the same racial background who live in the same house as the client
- ☐ **6.** People who provide for the physical and emotional needs of the client

Answer: 2, 6

Rationale: When providing care to a client, the nurse should consider family members to be all the people whom the client views as family. Family members may also include those people who provide for the physical and emotional needs of the client. The traditional definition of a family has changed and may include people not related by blood or marriage, those of a different racial background, and those who may not live in the same house as the client. Family members are defined by the client, not by the nurse.

Test-taking strategy: Analyze to determine what information the question asks for, which is who is considered to be family. "Select all that apply" questions require considering each option to decide its merit. Recall the components of a family group and consider the changes that have taken place in society relating to family members. Review the definition of family if you had difficulty answering this question.

Client needs category: Health promotion and maintenance

Client needs subcategory: None

Cognitive level: Analyzing

9. A nurse is working with the family of a client who has Alzheimer's disease. The nurse notes that the client's spouse is too exhausted to provide care all alone. The adult children live too far away to provide relief on a weekly basis. Which nursing interventions would be helpful? Select all that apply.

☐ **1.** Calling a family meeting to tell the absent children that they must participate in caregiving

☐ **2.** Suggesting that the spouse seek psychological counseling to help cope with exhaustion

☐ **3.** Recommending community resources for adult day care and respite care

☐ **4.** Encouraging the spouse to talk about the difficulties involved in caring for a loved one

☐ **5.** Asking whether friends or church members can help with errands or provide short periods of relief

☐ **6.** Recommending that the client be placed in a long-term care facility

Answer: 3, 4, 5

Rationale: Many community services exist for Alzheimer's clients and their families. Encouraging use of these resources may make it possible to keep the client at home and to alleviate the spouse's exhaustion. The nurse can also support the caregiver by urging him or her to talk about the difficulties faced in caring for a spouse. Friends and church members may be able to help provide care to the client, allowing the caregiver time for rest, exercise, or an enjoyable activity. Arranging a family meeting to tell the children to participate more would probably be ineffective and might evoke anger or guilt. Counseling might be helpful, but it would not alleviate the caregiver's physical exhaustion or address the client's immediate needs. A long-term care facility is not an option until the family is ready to make that decision.

Test-taking strategy: Analyze to determine what information the question asks for, which is determining nursing interventions helpful for a caregiving spouse. Think of the nurse's role when offering emotional support to individuals struggling with the stressors associated with caring for the chronically ill. Select the options that meet the needs identified as "relief" for exhaustion and help in providing "sole" care. Review roles of the nurse for patient advocacy, and ethical standards if you had difficulty answering this question.

Client needs category: Psychosocial integrity

Client needs subcategory: None

Cognitive level: Analyzing

---

10. The home health nurse is completing the admission paperwork for a new client diagnosed with osteomyelitis who will be receiving home service I.V. therapy for the next month. The client is 32 years old and happily married. Which of the following findings will warrant further investigation? Select all that apply.

☐ **1.** The client reports having many hobbies and interests outside of the home.

☐ **2.** The client voices concerns about recovering quickly to return to work in the next month.

☐ **3.** The client talks repeatedly about death.

☐ **4.** The client spends a great deal of time reflecting back on teen years.

☐ **5.** The client is talkative about the spouse and children.

Answer: 3, 4

Rationale: At age 32, the client is in the middle adult stage of life. The repeated discussions about death and reflections back on life are not appropriate or expected for this stage of development and should be investigated further. An interest in civic responsibilities and the establishment of hobbies is expected. During this developmental period, the greatest concern typically relates to establishing gainful employment and significant relationships. This is being demonstrated by the client's willingness to discuss family, which includes spouse and children.

Test-taking strategy: The key phrase in this question is "warrant further investigation," indicating that there is a nursing concern. Consider each option for a statement that is inconsistent with the client's developmental stage. Review Erikson's developmental stages if you had difficulty answering this question.

Client needs category: Psychosocial integrity

Client needs subcategory: None

Cognitive level: Analyzing

1. A physician prescribes I.V. normal saline solution to be infused at a rate of 150 mL/hour for a client. How many liter(s) of solution will the client receive during an 8-hour shift? Record your answer using one decimal place.

_____ liters

Answer: 1.2

Rationale: The ordered infusion rate is 150 mL/hour. The nurse should multiply 150 mL by 8 hours to determine the total volume in milliliters the client will receive during an 8-hour shift (1,200 mL). Then the nurse should convert milliliters to liters by dividing by 1,000. The total volume in liters that the client will receive in 8 hours is 1.2 L.

Test-taking strategy: Analyze to determine what information the question asks for, which is the volume of I.V. solution to be received in an 8-hour period. Consider the information presented in the question to determine how to set up the math calculation. Proofread your math calculation for accuracy. Review basic drug calculations and basic conversions if you had difficulty answering this question.

Client needs category: Physiological integrity

Client needs subcategory: Pharmacological therapies

Cognitive level: Applying

---

2. A client is prescribed heparin 6,000 units subcutaneously every 12 hours for deep vein thrombosis prophylaxis. The pharmacy dispenses a vial containing 10,000 units/1 mL. How many milliliter(s) of heparin should the nurse administer? Record your answer using one decimal place.

_____ milliliter(s)

Answer: 0.6

Rationale: The dose dispensed by the pharmacy is 10,000 units/1 mL, and the desired dose is 6,000 units. The nurse should use the following equations to determine the amount of heparin to administer:

Dose on hand/quantity on hand = dose desired/X

$$10,000 \text{ units}/1 \text{ mL} = 6,000 \text{ units}/X$$
$$10,000 \text{ units} \times X = 6,000 \text{ units} \times 1 \text{ mL}$$
$$X = 6,000 \text{ units} \times 1 \text{ mL}/10,000 \text{ units}$$
$$X = 0.6 \text{ mL}.$$

Test-taking strategy: Analyze to determine what information the question asks for, which is the amount of milliliters for a dose of medication. One method of calculation is the ratio and proportion method to set up this problem. When using this method, ensure that units divided by milliliters of medication is maintained on both sides of the equation. Review basic drug calculations if you had difficulty answering this question.

Client needs category: Physiological integrity

Client needs subcategory: Pharmacological therapies

Cognitive level: Applying

3. A nurse is ordered to administer ampicillin 125 mg I.M. every 6 hours to a 10-kg child with a respiratory tract infection. The drug label reads, "The recommended dose for a client weighing less than 40 kg is 25 to 50 mg/kg/day I.M. or I.V. in equally divided doses at 6- to 8-hour intervals." The drug concentration is 125 mg/5 mL. Which nursing interventions are appropriate at this time? Select all that apply.

- ☐ **1.** Draw up 10 mL of ampicillin to administer.
- ☐ **2.** Administer the medication at 10 a.m., 2 p.m., 6 p.m., and 10 p.m.
- ☐ **3.** Assess the client for allergies to penicillin.
- ☐ **4.** Administer the medication because the dosage is within the recommended range.
- ☐ **5.** Question the prescriber about the order exceeding the recommended dosage.
- ☐ **6.** Obtain a sputum culture, if ordered, before administering the medication.

Answer: 3, 4, 6

Rationale: Because ampicillin is a penicillin antibiotic, the nurse should assess the client for penicillin allergies before administering this drug. The ampicillin dose is within the recommended range for a 10-kg client: 50 mg/kg × 10 kg = 500 mg. A dose of 500 mg divided by four (given every 6 hours) = 125 mg. Cultures should be obtained before antibiotics are given. The nurse should draw up 5 mL—not 10 mL—to administer the correct dose, according to the concentration on the label. The correct dosing schedule is every 6 to 8 hours, not every 4 hours.

Test-taking strategy: Analyze to determine what information the question asks for, which is appropriate interventions for a pediatric client to receive an antibiotic. To begin, a nurse must determine the safe dosage for the 10-kg pediatric client and review medication administration (antibiotic) safety practices as well. Review pediatric drug calculations and dosage guidelines for pediatric antibiotics if you had difficulty answering this question.

Client needs category: Physiological integrity

Client needs subcategory: Pharmacological therapies

Cognitive level: Analyzing

---

4. A cardiologist prescribes digoxin (Lanoxin) 125 µg by mouth every morning for a client diagnosed with heart failure. The pharmacy dispenses tablets that contain 0.25 mg each. How many tablet(s) should the nurse administer in each dose? Record your answer using one decimal place.

_____ tablet(s)

Answer: 0.5

Rationale: The nurse should begin by converting 125 µg to milligrams:

$$125 \ µg/1,000 = 0.125 \ mg.$$

Then the nurse should use the following formula to calculate the drug dosage:

Dose on hand/quantity on hand = dose desired/X

$$0.25 \ mg/1 \ tablet = 0.125 \ mg/X$$
$$0.25 \times X = 0.125 \times 1 \ tablet$$
$$X = 0.5 \ tablet$$

Test-taking strategy: Analyze to determine what information the question asks for, which is the number of tablets in each dose. Use knowledge of drug calculations and the calculation method of ratio and proportion to set up this problem. Ensure that conversions to milligrams are completed first before inserting into the milligram per tablet proportion. Proofread your math calculation for accuracy. Review basic drug calculations and basic conversions if you had difficulty answering this question.

Client needs category: Physiological integrity

Client needs subcategory: Pharmacological therapies

Cognitive level: Applying

5. A 75-year-old client is admitted to the hospital with lower gastrointestinal bleeding. His hemoglobin on admission to the emergency department is 7.3 g/dL. The physician prescribes 2 units of packed red blood cells to infuse over 2 hours each. Each unit of packed red blood cells contains 250 mL. The blood administration set has a drip factor of 10 gtt/mL. What flow rate will the registered nurse set and the licensed practical nurse maintain? Round your answer to the nearest whole number.

_____ gtt/minute

Answer: 21

Rationale: Each unit of packed red blood cells contains 250 mL, which should infuse over 2 hours (120 minutes). Therefore, the rate per minute is:

$$250 \text{ mL}/120 \text{ minutes} = 2.08 \text{ mL/minute}.$$

Multiply by the drip factor to determine the flow rate:

$$2.08 \text{ mL} \times 10 \text{ gtt} = 20.8 \text{ gtt/minute}$$
$$(\text{round up to } 21 \text{ gtt/minute}).$$

Critical thinking strategy: Analyze to determine what information the question asks for, which is the drop rate per minute of blood. Recall that this is a two-step calculation as the nurse must calculate the milliliter per minute before placing into the drip rate formula. Proofread your math calculation for accuracy. Review I.V. drug calculations and basic conversions if you had difficulty answering this question.

Client needs category: Physiological integrity

Client needs subcategory: Pharmacological therapies

Cognitive level: Applying

---

6. A nurse is preparing a teaching plan for a client who was prescribed enalapril maleate (Vasotec) for the treatment of hypertension. Which instructions should the nurse include in the teaching plan? Select all that apply.

☐ **1.** Instruct the client to avoid salt substitutes.
☐ **2.** Tell the client that light-headedness is a common adverse effect that does not need to be reported.
☐ **3.** Inform the client of a potential sore throat for the first few days of therapy.
☐ **4.** Advise the client to report facial swelling or difficulty breathing immediately.
☐ **5.** Tell the client that blood tests will be necessary every 3 weeks for 2 months and periodically after that.
☐ **6.** Advise the client not to change the position suddenly to minimize orthostatic hypotension.

Answer: 1, 4, 6

Rationale: The nurse should tell the client to avoid salt substitutes because they may contain potassium, which can cause light-headedness and syncope. Facial swelling or difficulty breathing should be reported immediately because they may be signs of angioedema, which would require discontinuation of the drug. The client should also be advised to change the position slowly to minimize orthostatic hypotension. The nurse should tell the client to report light-headedness, especially during the first few days of therapy, so dosage adjustments can be made. The client should also report signs of infection, such as sore throat and fever, because the drug may decrease the white blood cell (WBC) count. Because this effect is generally seen within 3 months, the WBC count and differential should be monitored periodically.

Test-taking strategy: Analyze to determine what information the question asks for, which is instructions for the teaching plan of a client beginning enalapril maleate. Recall the classes of antihypertensives and, specifically, angiotensin-converting enzyme (ACE) inhibitors and relate the type of adverse reactions to expect. This information, along with the dosage, would formulate the basis for a teaching plan. Review the drug classification of ACE inhibitors if you had difficulty answering this question.

Client needs category: Physiological integrity

Client needs subcategory: Pharmacological therapies

Cognitive level: Analyzing

7. A client returns to the room from the postanesthesia care unit after undergoing a appendectomy. The physician orders 1 L of dextrose 5% in half-normal saline solution to infuse at 125 mL/hour. The drop factor of the available I.V. tubing is 15 gtt/mL. What is the drip rate in drops per minute? Round your answer to the nearest whole number.

_____ gtt/minute

Answer: 31

Rationale: The flow rate is 125 mL/hour, or 125 mL/60 minutes. Use the following equation to determine the drip rate:

125 mL/60 minutes × 15 gtt/1 mL = 31.25 gtt/minute (round down to 31 gtt/minute).

Test-taking strategy: Analyze to determine what information the question asks for, which is the drip rate per minute of I.V. fluid. Recall how to calculate I.V. drip rates and proofread the math calculation. Rounding is completed to the nearest complete drop. Review I.V. drip rate calculations if you had difficulty answering this question.

Client needs category: Physiological integrity

Client needs subcategory: Pharmacological therapies

Cognitive level: Applying

---

8. After undergoing small-bowel resection, a client is prescribed metronidazole (Flagyl) 500 mg I.V. The mixed I.V. solution contains 100 mL. The nurse is to administer the drug over 30 minutes. The drop factor of the available I.V. tubing is 15 gtt/mL. What is the drip rate in drops per minute? Record your answer using a whole number.

_____ drops/minute

Answer: 50

Rationale: The nurse should use the following equation to calculate the drip rate:

Total quantity/administration time × gtt/min = X

100 mL/30 min × 15 gtt/min = X

$$X = \frac{1,500 \text{ gtt}}{30 \text{ min}}$$

$X = 50$ gtt/minute

Test-taking strategy: Analyze to determine what information the question asks for, which is the drip rate per minute of a secondary infusion. Recall the standard formula. Proofread the math calculation. Review the calculation of I.V. drip rates if you had difficulty answering this question.

Client needs category: Physiological integrity

Client needs subcategory: Pharmacological therapies

Cognitive level: Applying

9. A client with an I.V. complains of pain at the insertion site. Assessment of the site reveals a vein that is red, warm, and hard. Which actions should the nurse take? Select all that apply.

☐ **1.** Slow the infusion rate while notifying the physician.

☐ **2.** Discontinue the infusion at the affected site.

☐ **3.** Restart the infusion distal to the discontinued I.V. site.

☐ **4.** Assess the client for skin sloughing.

☐ **5.** Apply warm soaks to the I.V. site.

☐ **6.** Document the assessment, nursing actions taken, and the client's response.

Answer: 2, 5, 6

Rationale: Redness, warmth, pain, and a hard, cordlike vein at the I.V. insertion site suggest that the client has phlebitis. The nurse should discontinue the I.V. infusion and insert a new I.V. catheter proximal to or above the discontinued site or in the other arm. Applying warm soaks to the site reduces inflammation. The nurse should document the assessment of the I.V. site, the actions taken, and client's response to the situation. Slowing the infusion rate would not reduce the phlebitis. Restarting the infusion at a site distal to the phlebitis may contribute to the inflammation. Skin sloughing is not a symptom of phlebitis; it is associated with extravasation of certain toxic medications.

Test-taking strategy: Analyze to determine what information the question asks for, which is the nursing actions needed when a client complains of symptoms at the I.V. site. "Select all that apply" questions require considering each option to decide its merit. Recall the assessment findings associated with I.V. sites and the interventions for an abnormal assessment. Note that the symptoms stated are also symptoms of irritation and phlebitis, requiring nursing intervention. Review I.V. site management if you had difficulty answering this question.

Client needs category: Physiological integrity

Client needs subcategory: Pharmacological therapies

Cognitive level: Applying

---

10. When administering medication, the nurse ensures client safety by following the rights of medication administration. Identify the "rights of medication administration." Select all that apply.

☐ **1.** Right room

☐ **2.** Right client

☐ **3.** Right dose

☐ **4.** Right medication

☐ **5.** Right time

☐ **6.** Right route

Answer: 2, 3, 4, 5, 6

Rationale: A nurse must always implement safe nursing practices when administering medications. Following the rights of medication administration helps protect the client from medication errors. Safe procedure includes confirming the right client, dose, medication, time, and route. Confirming the room number does not guarantee that the right client will receive the correct medication.

Test-taking strategy: Analyze to determine what information the question asks for, which is safety guidelines for medication administration. Recall the standards of practice guidelines for medication administration. Logically consider what would ensure safe medication administration. Review the rights of medication administration if you had difficulty answering this question.

Client needs category: Physiological integrity

Client needs subcategory: Pharmacological therapies

Cognitive level: Remembering

11. A client is to be started on a Lasix (furosemide). Which interventions should be included in the teaching plan? Select all that apply.

- ☐ **1.** Advise the client to reduce dietary sodium intake.
- ☐ **2.** Encourage the use of salt substitutes.
- ☐ **3.** Tell the client to alert the physician about any visible edema.
- ☐ **4.** Instruct the client to take the medication as directed.
- ☐ **5.** Suggest taking the medication just before bedtime to establish a routine.

Answer: 1, 3, 4

Rationale: Lasix (furosemide) is a loop diuretic. Patient teaching focuses on actions related to the fluid gradient and electrolyte balance. Reducing dietary sodium intake will help increase the effectiveness of diuretic medication and may allow smaller doses to be ordered. Diuretics are commonly prescribed to control fluid accumulation in the body; therefore, the presence of edema may indicate the need for the physician to adjust the therapy. Compliance is very important with diuretics. In order to effectively monitor therapy, the nurse should encourage the client to take the medication exactly as prescribed. Salt substitutes are not recommended because they contain potassium instead of sodium and may cause serious cardiovascular effects. Diuretics cause an increased urine output, which may interfere with the client's sleep if taken at bedtime.

Test-taking strategy: Analyze to determine what information the question asks for, which is pharmacologic actions and use of diuretics and the educational needs of clients taking these drugs. Recall the nature of diuretics and consider potential side effects to guide the teaching content. Review diuretic therapy and patient teaching if you had difficulty answering this question.

Client needs category: Health promotion and maintenance

Client needs subcategory: None

Cognitive level: Analyzing

12. A client receives a short-acting insulin and an intermediate-acting insulin before breakfast at 0800. Using the chart below, when should the nurse expect the onset of the intermediate-acting insulin to take effect?

Medication Administration Record

Insulin type	Onset	Peak	Duration
Lispro (Humalog)	15–30 minutes	1–2 hours	4–5 hours
Humulin Regular	20–60 minutes	2–4 hours	8–10 hours
Humulin NPH	1–2 hours	4–8 hours	10–20 hours
Glargine (Lantus)	1–2 hours	Relatively flat	20–24 hours

☐ **1.** 1500
☐ **2.** 1300
☐ **3.** 1000
☐ **4.** 0830

Answer: 3

Rationale: The timing of insulin's effects varies according to the type. Referring to the chart, the nurse would note that the onset of action for the intermediate-acting insulin (Humulin NPH) is 1 to 2 hours. Because the administration time was 0800, the effects should begin 1 to 2 hours after administration, at approximately 1000.

Test-taking strategy: Analyze to determine what information the question asks for, which is identifying the onset of intermediate-acting insulin. Begin by identifying which insulin in the table is classified as an intermediate-acting insulin. Note that rapid-acting, short-acting, intermediate-acting, and long-acting insulins are documented, respectively. It is important for the nurse to recognize the onset of action to determine when blood sugar levels decline. Once the intermediate-acting insulin is selected, read the chart to confirm the onset of action and calculate the time using military time. Review administration of various types of insulin if you had difficulty answering this question.

Client needs category: Physiological integrity

Client needs subcategory: Pharmacological therapies

Cognitive level: Analyzing

---

13. A client has an I.V. line in place for 3 days and begins to complain of discomfort at the insertion site. Based on the client's progress notes below, what condition has most likely occurred?

Progress Notes

02/15/10 0730	I.V. site assessed and found to have blanching around the site, swelling, and coolness to the touch. Laboratory results include a white blood cell count within normal limits.————————————— —————————Sue Thompson, LPN

☐ **1.** Infiltration
☐ **2.** Phlebitis
☐ **3.** Infection
☐ **4.** Infection and infiltration

Answer: 1

Rationale: The assessment findings of pallor, swelling, skin that is cool to the touch at the I.V. insertion site, and a normal WBC count all indicate infiltration. The infusion should be discontinued and restarted in a different site. Phlebitis would be evidenced by redness at the cannula tip and along the vein. Infection would be evidenced by an elevated WBC count.

Test-taking strategy: Analyze to determine what information the question asks for, which is potential diagnosis of I.V. site complications. Focus on the symptoms noted in the question and nurses' documentation for clues that either validate or eliminate options. Use the process of elimination to make the correct selection. Review the signs and symptoms of I.V. complications if you had difficulty answering this question.

Client needs category: Physiological integrity

Client needs subcategory: Pharmacological therapies

Cognitive level: Applying

14. A client is prescribed an I.V. solution of 1,000 mL to be infused from 0800 to 2000. The nurse will use an infusion pump that delivers in milliliters per hour. At what rate should the nurse set the pump to deliver the solution? Record your answer using a whole number.

_____ milliliters/hour

Answer: 83

Rationale: First, determine how many hours the infusion needs to run. 0800 to 2000 is 12 hours. Use the following equation to determine the milliliters per hour:

$$\frac{\text{Volume to infuse}}{\text{Infusion time}} = \text{Flow rate per hour}$$

$$\frac{1,000 \text{ mL}}{12 \text{ hours}} = 83.3 \text{ mL/hour (rounded to 83 mL/hour)}$$

The pump should be set to deliver 83 mL/hour.

Test-taking strategy: Analyze to determine what information the question asks for, which is the milliliters per hour that the infusion device is to be set. Use the standard formula calculating the milliliters per hour. Review calculations of I.V. drip rates if you had difficulty answering this question.

Client needs category: Physiological integrity

Client needs subcategory: Pharmacological therapies

Cognitive level: Applying

---

15. A nurse enters a client's semiprivate room and prepares to administer the 0900 medications. Place the following steps in chronological sequence to indicate the safe measures to take when administering these medications. Use all the options.

1. Administer the medications.
2. Obtain the correct unit-dose medications.
3. Confirm the client's identity.
4. Check the client's medication administration record (MAR) for the 0900 medications.
5. Open the unit-dose packages.

Answer: 4, 2, 3, 5, 1

Rationale: Following sequential steps helps ensure safe medication administration. The nurse should first check to see which medications the client is due to receive at 0900 and then obtain them. Next, the nurse should confirm the client's identity according to facility protocol. Once the client is properly identified, the nurse should open the drug packages at the bedside, administer the medications to the client, and document administration.

Test-taking strategy: Analyze to determine what information the question asks for, which is medication administration safety practices. Consider the step-by-step process to obtain the medication through documenting the medication for a logical flow of events. Recall the most logical process to note any errors in administration. Review medication administration techniques if you had difficulty answering this question.

Client needs category: Physiological integrity

Client needs subcategory: Pharmacological therapies

Cognitive level: Analyzing

16. The nurse prepares to administer medications into a client's jejunostomy tube. Identify the area where the nurse would assess the tube to be located.

Answer:

Rationale: A jejunostomy tube is often placed for long-term nutritional support. The tubes are inserted surgically in the jejunum and are not easily dislodged. The jejunum is the immediate portion of the small intestine that connects proximally with the duodenum and distally with the ileum.

Test-taking strategy: Analyze to determine what information the question asks for, which is the location of the jejunostomy tube. Use knowledge of medical terminology to identify that jejunostomy relates to jejunum, which is the small intestine. Review the anatomy of the gastrointestinal system and the correct placement for a jejunostomy tube if you had difficulty answering this question.

Client needs category: Health promotion and maintenance

Client needs subcategory: None

Cognitive level: Applying

Basic Physical Assessment

1. A client who was involved in a motor vehicle accident is admitted to the intensive care unit. The emergency department admission record indicates that the client was hit in the right temporal lobe. A nurse would expect the client to demonstrate the following abnormalities? Select all that apply.

- ☐ **1.** Difficulty comprehending language
- ☐ **2.** Decreased hearing
- ☐ **3.** Aphasia
- ☐ **4.** Amnesia for recent events
- ☐ **5.** Ataxic gait
- ☐ **6.** Personality changes

Answer: 1, 2, 4

Rationale: The temporal lobe controls hearing, language comprehension, and the storage and recall of memories; therefore, the client would likely have difficulty comprehending language, diminished hearing, and amnesia for recent events. Aphasia and personality changes might be expected from injury to the frontal lobe. An ataxic gait would indicate injury primarily to the cerebellum.

Test-taking strategy: Analyze to determine what information the question asks for, which is deficits that may occur when there is damage to the temporal lobe of the brain. Recall the anatomy and physiology of the brain and the specific function of each section, focusing particularly on the temporal lobe. Review the temporal lobe functions if you had difficulty answering this question.

Client needs category: Physiological integrity

Client needs subcategory: Physiological adaptation

Cognitive level: Analyzing

2. A nurse is assessing a client who reports burning on urination and a low-grade fever. On physical examination, the nurse notes right-sided costovertebral tenderness. On the anatomical position drawing, identify the area of client tenderness.

Answer:

Rationale: To determine whether costovertebral tenderness (a sign of glomerulonephritis) is present, the nurse should percuss the costovertebral angle (the angle over each kidney that is formed by the lateral and downward curve of the lowest rib and the vertebral column). Since the kidney lies directly below this area, tapping disturbs the inflamed tissue causing pain. The costovertebral angle can be percussed by placing the palm of one hand over the costovertebral angle and striking it with the fist of the other hand.

Test-taking strategy: Analyze to determine what information the question asks for, which is to document right-sided costovertebral tenderness on the anatomical drawing. Note that the question infers burning on urination, suggesting a urinary/kidney problem narrowing the area for percussion. Review the assessment techniques for the renal system and the clinical manifestations of the findings if you had difficulty answering this question.

Client needs category: Physiological integrity

Client needs subcategory: Physiological adaptation

Cognitive level: Applying

3. A client presents to the emergency department with liver failure and obvious jaundice. When palpating a client's abdomen, identify the area that would provide the most essential information?

Answer:

Rationale: Palpation of the liver in the right upper quadrant would provide essential information on the organ's status. Palpation in a systematic manner identifies masses, enlargement, and degree of tenderness. The nurse can best palpate the liver by standing on the client's right side and placing the nurse's right hand on the client's abdomen, along the right midclavicular line. The nurse should point the fingers of the right hand toward the client's head, just under the right rib margin.

Test-taking strategy: Analyze to determine what information the question asks for, which is identifying an abdominal area that would provide "essential" assessment information. With the stem of the question noting liver failure, assessing the status of the liver would provide the "essential" information. Recall the anatomy in the abdominal cavity and, specifically, techniques for assessing the liver. Review the anatomy of the abdominal cavity if you had difficulty answering this question.

Client needs category: Physiological integrity
Client needs subcategory: Physiological adaptation
Cognitive level: Analyzing

4. While examining the hands of a client with osteoarthritis, a nurse notes Heberden's nodes on the second (index) finger. Identify the area on the finger where the nurse observes the node.

Answer:

Rationale: Heberden's nodes appear on the distal interphalangeal joints. Bouchard's nodes appear on the proximal interphalangeal joints. These bony and cartilaginous enlargements are usually hard and painless and typically occur in middle-aged and elderly clients with osteoarthritis.

Test-taking strategy: Analyze to determine what information the question asks for, which is the location of Heberden's nodes on the finger. Recall that osteoarthritis affects the joints of the body narrowing the selected areas. Review the anatomy of the hand and the pathophysiology of osteoarthritis if you had difficulty answering this question.

Client needs category: Physiological integrity
Client needs subcategory: Physiological adaptation
Cognitive level: Applying

5. A nurse is caring for a client diagnosed with herpes zoster. Place in chronological order the pathophysiological changes that the nurse would anticipate in assessing the progression of the disease.

1.	Fever, malaise, and red nodules appear in a dermatome distribution.
2.	The virus multiplies in the ganglia, causing deep pain, itching, and paresthesia or hyperesthesia.
3.	Vesicles crust and scab but no longer shed the virus.
4.	Residual antibodies from the initial infection mobilize but are ineffective.
5.	Vesicles appear, filled with either clear fluid or pus.
6.	Varicella-zoster virus is reactivated.

Answer: 6, 4, 1, 2, 5, 3

Rationale: Herpes zoster (shingles) is an acute inflammation caused by infection with the herpes virus varicella-zoster (chickenpox virus). After acquiring chickenpox, the virus remains inactive (dormant) in certain nerves of the body. The reason the virus becomes active is not clear. The pathophysiologic changes associated with this disorder follow a typical viral path and occur in the order described above.

Test-taking strategy: Analyze to determine what information the question asks for, which is the progression of the herpes zoster disease process. Recall the steps from the reactivation of the virus to the crusting which identifies the concluding stage of the disease. Review the pathophysiology of herpes zoster if you had difficulty answering this question.

Client needs category: Physiological integrity
Client needs subcategory: Physiological adaptation
Cognitive level: Analyzing

6. An elderly client has a history of aortic valve stenosis. Identify the area where the nurse should place the stethoscope to best hear the murmur.

Answer:

Rationale: Aortic stenosis occurs from a constriction that restricts blood flow through the heart and causes the left ventricle to enlarge. This enlargement can lead to heart failure and development of life-threatening irregular heartbeats. The murmur of aortic stenosis is low-pitched, rough, and rasping. It is heard best in the second intercostal space, to the right of the sternum.

Test-taking strategy: Analyze to determine what information the question asks for, which is identifying the site to assess a murmur in a client with aortic valve stenosis. Review the anatomy of the cardiovascular system and consider the pressure changes within the heart when stenosis occurs. Critically think about the nature of a murmur being a backflow of blood and the location in the noted area. Review anatomical structures of the heart and techniques for assessment if you had difficulty answering this question.

Client needs category: Physiological integrity
Client needs subcategory: Physiological adaptation
Cognitive level: Applying

7. A nurse is assessing a client who has a rash on the chest and upper arms. Which questions should the nurse ask in order to gain further information about the client's rash? Select all that apply.

☐ **1.** "When did the rash start?"
☐ **2.** "Are you allergic to any medications, foods, or pollen?"
☐ **3.** "How old are you?"
☐ **4.** "What have you been using to treat the rash?"
☐ **5.** "Have you recently traveled outside the country?"
☐ **6.** "Do you smoke cigarettes or drink alcohol?"

Answer: 1, 2, 4, 5

Rationale: The nurse should first find out when the rash began; this can assist with the correct diagnosis. The nurse should also ask about allergies; rashes can occur when a person changes medications, eats new foods, or contacts pollen. It is also important to find out how the client has been treating the rash; some topical ointments or oral medications may worsen it. The nurse should ask about recent travel; exposure to foreign foods and environments can cause a rash. The client's age and smoking and drinking habits would not provide further insight into the rash or its cause.

Test-taking strategy: Analyze to determine what information the question asks for, which is specific assessment questions when a client presents with a rash. "Select all that apply" questions require considering each option to decide its merit. Begin selection by asking the benefit of the information received from the question and how it may relate to a rash. Review the anatomy and pathophysiology of the integumentary system and history-taking techniques if you had difficulty answering this question.

Client needs category: Physiological integrity
Client needs subcategory: Physiological adaptation
Cognitive level: Analyzing

---

8. While assessing a client's spine for abnormal curvatures, a nurse notes kyphosis. Using a picture diagram to instruct the client about kyphosis, in which location would the nurse note the structural abnormality?

Answer:

Rationale: Kyphosis is characterized by an accentuated forward curve of the thoracic area of the spine, which leads to a hunchback or slouching position. In adults, kyphosis can be caused by degenerative joint disease, fractures, trauma, and spondylolisthesis. Symptoms stem from the location of the deformity and include mild back pain, rounded back appearance, tenderness and stiffness in the spine, and, in extreme cases, difficulty breathing,

Test-taking strategy: Analyze to determine what information the question asks for, which is location of kyphosis. Recall that the location of the deformity is located in the thoracic region, thus identifying the following regions on the illustration: cervical (neck), thoracic (upper back), lumbar (lower back), and sacral (tailbone). Review the anatomy of the musculoskeletal system and techniques for assessing the spinal column if you had difficulty answering this question.

Client needs category: Health promotion and maintenance

Client needs subcategory: None

Cognitive level: Applying

---

9. A nurse is auscultating a client's lungs. Identify the area on the client's vertebrae, representing the base of the lungs, where the nurse expects the breath sounds to stop at the end of expiration.

Answer:

Rationale: Based on posterior landmarks, the lungs extend from the cervical area to the level of the 10th thoracic vertebrae (T10) at the end of expiration.

Test-taking strategy: Analyze to determine what information the question asks for, which is the area of the lungs where the nurse anticipates to hear no further breath sounds. Recall that the lungs fill the thoracic cavity. Review the anatomy of the respiratory system and techniques for assessing the lungs if you had difficulty answering this question.

Client needs category: Health promotion and maintenance

Client needs subcategory: None

Cognitive level: Applying

10. A nurse is performing an otoscopic examination on a client with ear pain. If the nurse suspects a potential diagnosis of otitis media, in what location would evidence confirm the diagnosis?

Answer:

Rationale: Otitis media is a middle ear infection located between the tympanic membrane and the inner ear. When an infection occurs, pressure increases, causing a bulging and red appearance of the tympanic membrane. Rupture of the tympanic membrane can occur.

Test-taking strategy: Analyze to determine what information the question asks for, which is the location of confirming evidence of otitis media. Consider the structure of the ear including the outer, middle, and inner ear. Upon otoscopic examination, a nurse can confirm symptoms associated with a middle ear infection at the location of the tympanic membrane. Review the anatomy and pathophysiology of the ear and assessment techniques if you had difficulty answering this question.

Client needs category: Physiological integrity

Client needs subcategory: Physiological adaptation

Cognitive level: Analyzing

---

11. A nurse is performing a cardiac assessment on a client with a suspected murmur. In which location should the nurse place the stethoscope to auscultate Erb's point?

Answer:

Rationale: Erb's point is located at the third intercostal space, to the left of the sternum where S2 is best auscultated. Murmurs of both aortic and pulmonic origin may be heard at Erb's point.

Test-taking strategy: Analyze to determine what information the question asks for, which is the location of Erb's point. Recall that the places where valvular movement can be heard are not the actual anatomical location of the valves. Rather, the sounds represent the direction of blood flow. Review the anatomy of the cardiovascular system and techniques for assessing the heart if you had difficulty answering this question.

Client needs category: Health promotion and maintenance

Client needs subcategory: None

Cognitive level: Applying

12. A nurse is performing a head and neck assessment on a client who reports fatigue. When palpating lymph nodes, in which location would the nurse palpate the occipital lymph nodes?

Answer:

Rationale: Lymph nodes are part of the lymphatic system. Lymph nodes vary in size depending upon the body status. There are clusters of head and neck lymph nodes. Using the pads of the fingers, the nurse should palpate the area behind the ears bilaterally to assess the occipital lymph nodes.

Test-taking strategy: Analyze to determine what information the question asks for, which is the location where the nurse would palpate the occipital lymph nodes. Use medical terminology (occiput means back of head) to identify the location of the lymph nodes. Review the anatomy of the lymphatic system and techniques for assessing lymph nodes if you had difficulty answering this question.

Client needs category: Physiological integrity

Client needs subcategory: Physiological adaptation

Cognitive level: Applying

---

13. A client has been admitted with severe abdominal pain that has lasted for the past 4 hours. Place in chronological order the correct sequence for conducting an abdominal assessment. Use all of the options.

1. Auscultate the client's abdomen.
2. Perform light palpation.
3. Ask the client to urinate.
4. Percuss the client's abdomen.
5. Inspect the client's abdomen.

Answer: 3, 5, 1, 4, 2

Rationale: The nurse should begin the assessment by having the client empty the bladder first. This allows the nurse to hear abdominal sounds better during auscultation. Next, inspect the abdomen for unusual skin discoloration or movement. Because the client is in pain, the nurse should auscultate the abdomen before percussing it. Also, auscultation is usually performed before palpation and percussion since bowel sounds induced by percussion or palpation may mask abdominal bruits or pleural rubs. The nurse should then perform light palpation over the abdomen, leaving the painful area for last.

Test-taking strategy: Analyze to determine what information the question asks for, which is the sequence for conducting an abdominal assessment. Consider least disturbing to the abdomen first and leave painful procedures for last. Review techniques to use when assessing the abdomen if you had difficulty answering this question.

Client needs category: Physiological integrity

Client needs subcategory: Basic care and comfort

Cognitive level: Applying

14. The nurse is assessing a client's deep tendon reflexes. Which graphic shows assessing the biceps reflex?

☐ **1.**

☐ **2.**

☐ **3.**

☐ **4.**

Answer: 3

Rationale: To test the biceps reflex, the client's elbow is flexed at a 45° angle. The nurse places her thumb or index finger over the biceps tendon and strikes the digit with the pointed end of the reflex hammer, watching and feeling for the contraction of the biceps muscle and flexion of the forearm. Option 1 shows assessment of the patellar reflex. Option 2 shows assessment of the brachioradialis reflex. Option 4 shows assessment of the triceps reflex.

Test-taking strategy: Analyze to determine what information the question asks for, which is assessing the biceps reflex. Use the knowledge of anatomy to narrow the site of the reflex. Consider which illustration would elicit the bicep tendon. Review the location of bicep tendon and the proper technique for eliciting deep tendon reflexes if you had difficulty answering this question.

Client needs category: Physiological integrity

Client needs subcategory: Reduction of risk potential

Cognitive level: Analyzing

15. The nurse is assessing a client's respiratory pattern. Which graphic illustrates Kussmaul's respirations?

☐ 1.

☐ 2.

☐ 3.

☐ 4.

Answer: 2

Rationale: Kussmaul's breathing is characterized by rapid, deep breathing without pauses. Option 1 shows tachypnea (shallow breathing with an increased respiratory rate). Option 3 shows Cheyne-Stokes respirations (breaths gradually become faster and deeper than normal and then slower with intermittent periods of apnea). Option 4 shows hyperpnea (deep breathing at a normal rate).

Test-taking strategy: Analyze to determine what information the question asks for, which is characteristics of Kussmaul's breathing and eliminate the other patterns. Recall that Kussmaul's respirations are deep and labored breathing patterns often associated with severe metabolic acidosis. Relate to the disease process and need to reduce carbon dioxide in the blood. Review Kussmaul's breathing pattern if you had difficulty answering this question.

Client needs category: Physiological integrity

Client needs subcategory: Reduction of risk potential

Cognitive level: Analyzing

16. A nurse is instructing a female client on the proper hygiene of wiping after toileting from front to back in order to prevent contamination of the urethra. At which location of the genitourinary tract is it most likely to establish an infection from improper hygiene?

Answer

Rationale: Because of the structure of the female genitourinary tract, bacteria causing infection can be introduced into the urethra and travel to the bladder to cause a bladder infection. One cause of a bladder infection is improper hygiene during toileting. Keeping the perineum as clean as possible diminishes the possibility of bladder infections due to contamination.

Test-taking strategy: Analyze to determine what information the question asks for, which is area of the genitourinary tract prone to infection due to improper hygiene. Consider the structure of the genitourinary tract and what structure is closest to the urethra opening. Recall that the bladder is prior to the kidney. Review the structure of the genitourinary tract if you had difficulty answering this question.

Client needs category: Physiological integrity

Client needs subcategory: Reduction of risk potential

Cognitive level: Applying

Medical–Surgical Nursing

1. The nurse is evaluating an electrocardiogram (ECG) tracing. Which graphic shows the QT interval?

☐ 1.

☐ 2.

☐ 3.

☐ 4.

Answer: 1

Rationale: The QT interval extends from the beginning of the QRS complex to the end of the T wave. It measures the time needed for ventricular depolarization and repolarization. Option 2 shows the PR interval, which is measured from the beginning of the P wave to the beginning of the QRS complex. It tracks the atrial impulse from the sinus node through the atrioventricular (AV) node. Option 3 shows the ST segment, which represents the end of ventricular depolarization. Option 4 shows the QRS duration and represents impulse conduction through the ventricles.

Test-taking strategy: Analyze to determine what information the question asks for, which is identifying the QT interval. Recall the components of the ECG waveform and what each represents in the function of the heart's conduction system. Consider which waveform is first initiated and then follow the alphabetical sequence (P wave then QRS complex and lastly the T wave). Review the ECG waveform if you had difficulty answering this question.

Client needs category: Physiological integrity

Client needs subcategory: Reduction of risk potential

Cognitive level: Analyzing

---

2. A nurse is interpreting a client's ECG strip. If the PR interval measures four small blocks, how many seconds is the PR interval?

_____ seconds

Answer: 0.16

Rationale: Each small block on a telemetry strip graph represents 0.04 second. So multiply as follows:

4 blocks × 0.04 second = 0.16 second.

Test-taking strategy: Analyze to determine what information the question asks for, which is the PR interval documented in seconds. An interval is a portion of the baseline and at least one wave. Intervals are measured on the horizontal axis in seconds. Recall the standard rate of each small block and multiply. Review ECG measurements and focus on second per block calculations if you had difficulty answering this question.

Client needs category: Physiological integrity

Client needs subcategory: Reduction of risk potential

Cognitive level: Applying

3. A nurse is caring for a client with Raynaud's phenomenon secondary to systemic lupus erythematosus (SLE). Which of the client statements shows an understanding of the nurse's teaching about this disorder? Select all that apply.

☐ **1.** "My hands get pale, bluish, and feel numb and painful when I'm really stressed."

☐ **2.** "I can't continue to wash dishes and do my cleaning because of this problem."

☐ **3.** "I don't need to report any other skin problems with my fingers or hands to my practitioner."

☐ **4.** "I probably got this disorder because I have lupus."

☐ **5.** "This problem is caused by a temporary lack of circulation in my hands."

☐ **6.** "Medication might help treat this problem."

Answer: 1, 4, 5, 6

Rationale: Raynaud's phenomenon causes blanching, cyanosis, coldness, numbness, and throbbing pain in the hands when the client is exposed to cold or stress. It is caused by episodic vasospasm in the small peripheral arteries and arterioles and can affect the feet as well as the hands. The phenomenon is commonly associated with connective tissue diseases such as lupus and may be alleviated by calcium channel blockers or adrenergic blockers. It does not limit the client's ability to function, although the symptoms are bothersome. Keeping the hands warm and learning to manage stressful situations effectively reduces the frequency of episodes. The disorder can progress to skin ulcerations and even gangrene in some clients, so all skin changes should be reported to the practitioner promptly.

Test-taking strategy: Analyze to determine what information the question asks for, which is correct client statements related to the Raynaud's phenomenon. "Select all that apply" questions require considering each option to decide its merit. When assessing for correct statements, the true focus is correct information regarding Raynaud's phenomenon. Review the pathophysiology of Raynaud's phenomenon if you had difficulty answering this question.

Client needs category: Physiological integrity

Client needs subcategory: Physiological adaptation

Cognitive level: Analyzing

4. A nurse is evaluating the 12-lead ECG of a client experiencing an inferior wall myocardial infarction (MI). While conferring with the heath care team, which ECG changes associated with an evolving MI does the nurse correctly identify? Select all that apply.

☐ **1.** Notched T wave

☐ **2.** Presence of a U wave

☐ **3.** T-wave inversion

☐ **4.** Prolonged PR interval

☐ **5.** ST-segment elevation

☐ **6.** Pathologic Q wave

Answer: 3, 5, 6

Rationale: T-wave inversion, ST-segment elevation, and a pathologic Q wave are all signs of tissue hypoxia that occur during an MI. Ischemia results from inadequate blood supply to the myocardial tissue and is reflected by T-wave inversion. Injury results from prolonged ischemia and is reflected by ST-segment elevation. Q waves may become evident when the injury progresses to infarction. A notched T wave may indicate pericarditis in an adult client. A U wave may be apparent on a normal ECG; it represents repolarization of the Purkinje fibers. A prolonged PR interval is associated with first-degree AV block.

Test-taking strategy: Analyze to determine what information the question asks for, which is assessment of an MI and rhythm strip analysis. First, determine changes from a sinus rhythm and relate the changes to tissue ischemia. "Select all that apply" questions require considering each option to decide its merit. Review the clinical documentation of tissue hypoxia occurring during an MI if you had difficulty answering this question.

Client needs category: Physiological integrity

Client needs subcategory: Physiological adaptation

Cognitive level: Analyzing

5. A client with a bicuspid aortic valve has severe stenosis and is scheduled for valve replacement. While teaching the client about the condition and upcoming surgery, the nurse shows a heart illustration. Which valve should the nurse indicate as needing replacement?

Answer

Rationale: The aortic valve is located between the left ventricle and the aorta. It is one of the semilunar valves, which only has two leaflets instead of three. A person with a bicuspid aortic valve is at risk for aortic stenosis and aortic regurgitation. This impaired blood flow through the valve leads to increased pumping pressure of the left ventricle.

Test-taking strategy: Analyze to determine what information the question asks for, which is the location of the aortic valve. Consider the anatomy of the heart and knowledge of medical terminology to narrow the choices, if unsure. It may be helpful to visualize the path of blood flow to remind yourself of blood passing through valves. Review the placement of the aortic valve if you had difficulty answering this question.

Client needs category: Physiological integrity

Client needs subcategory: Physiological adaptation

Cognitive level: Applying

6. A nurse is awaiting the arrival of a client from the emergency department with a diagnosis of left ventricular myocardial infarction (MI). In caring for this client, the nurse should be alert for which signs and symptoms of left-sided heart failure? Select all that apply.

- ☐ **1.** Jugular vein distention
- ☐ **2.** Hepatomegaly
- ☐ **3.** Dyspnea
- ☐ **4.** Crackles
- ☐ **5.** Tachycardia
- ☐ **6.** Right upper quadrant pain

Answer: 3, 4, 5

Rationale: The right side of the heart is where the body deposits deoxygenated blood from the systematic circulation. Blood is then pumped from the right side of the heart to the lungs, where it exchanges CO_2 and picks up oxygen. Once the blood is oxygenated, it flows to the left side of the heart which pumps to the rest of the body. Signs and symptoms of left-sided heart failure include dyspnea, orthopnea, and paroxysmal nocturnal dyspnea; fatigue; nonproductive cough and crackles; hemoptysis; point of maximal impulse displaced toward the left anterior axillary line; tachycardia; S_3 and S_4 heart sounds; and cool, pale skin. Jugular vein distention, hepatomegaly, and right upper quadrant pain are all signs of right-sided heart failure.

Test-taking strategy: Analyze to determine what information the question asks for, which is signs and symptoms of left-sided heart failure. "Select all that apply" questions require considering each option to decide its merit. Consider where the blood flows and what would happen if the left heart muscle was inefficient with pumping blood. Review the pathophysiology of heart failure and review the differences between right- and left-sided heart failure if you had difficulty answering this question.

Client needs category: Physiological integrity

Client needs subcategory: Physiological adaptation

Cognitive level: Applying

---

7. A client is admitted to the emergency department after complaining of acute chest pain radiating down the left arm. The client appears anxious, dyspneic, and diaphoretic. Which laboratory studies would the nurse anticipate? Select all that apply.

- ☐ **1.** Hemoglobin and hematocrit (HCT)
- ☐ **2.** Serum glucose
- ☐ **3.** Creatine kinase (CK)
- ☐ **4.** Troponin T and troponin I
- ☐ **5.** Myoglobin
- ☐ **6.** Blood urea nitrogen (BUN)

Answer: 3, 4, 5

Rationale: With myocardial ischemia or infarction, levels of CK, troponin T, and troponin I typically rise because of cellular damage. Myoglobin elevation is an early indicator of myocardial damage. Hemoglobin, HCT, serum glucose, and BUN levels do not provide information related to myocardial ischemia.

Test-taking strategy: Analyze to determine what information the question asks for, which is anticipating laboratory testing for a client with certain symptoms. First note that the client is experiencing symptoms of myocardial ischemia or infarction. Next, determine which laboratory test would provide helpful data in confirming or disproving a diagnosis. Review laboratory studies that diagnose cardiac problems or diagnostic findings for an MI if you had difficulty answering this question.

Client needs category: Physiological integrity

Client needs subcategory: Reduction of risk potential

Cognitive level: Analyzing

8. A client is prescribed lisinopril (Zestril) for the treatment of hypertension. The client asks a nurse about possible adverse effects. Which common adverse effects of angiotensin-converting enzyme (ACE) inhibitors should the nurse include in the teaching? Select all that apply.

☐ **1.** Constipation
☐ **2.** Dry cough
☐ **3.** Headache
☐ **4.** Hyperglycemia
☐ **5.** Hypotension
☐ **6.** Indigestion

Answer: 2, 3, 5

Rationale: ACE is a potent vasoconstrictor in the blood. By inhibiting the conversion of angiotensin I to angiotensin II, constriction of the vessel is limited. Dry cough, headache, and hypotension are all common adverse effects of lisinopril and other ACE inhibitors. Lisinopril may cause diarrhea, not constipation; it is not known to cause hyperglycemia or indigestion.

Test-taking strategy: Analyze to determine what information the question asks for, which is adverse effects of ACE inhibitors. When considering adverse effects of medications, always consider an exaggerated effect of the therapeutic response. If the therapeutic response of ACE inhibitors is to lower blood pressure, the exaggerated response would be hypotension or conditions associated with hypotension. Another key to remember is what angiotensin does in the bloodstream and the response of bradykinin. Review the pharmacological class of ACE inhibitors and focus on the common adverse effects if you had difficulty answering this question.

Client needs category: Physiological integrity

Client needs subcategory: Pharmacological therapies

Cognitive level: Applying

---

9. A nurse is caring for a client who states crushing chest pressure over the sternum. The nurse places the client on oxygen and performs a 12-lead ECG. Identify the site where lead V$_6$ should be placed?

Answer

Rationale: The standard 12-lead ECG tracing is a representation of the heart's electrical activity recorded from electrodes on the body surface. The V$_6$ lead should be placed at the fifth intercostal space, at the midaxillary line. Correct lead placement is essential when performing a 12-lead ECG in order to accurately document the electrical potential of the heart. V$_6$ is one of the precordial leads and, combined with the other leads, records potential in the horizontal plane.

Test-taking strategy: Analyze to determine what information the question asks for, which is the location of an ECG lead. Review the placement of electrodes, keeping in mind that V_1 is placed medially and, as the numbers progress higher, the electrodes are placed more laterally. Visualize the placement of the leads using anatomical locations. Review ECG placement if you had difficulty answering this question.

Client needs category: Physiological integrity

Client needs subcategory: Reduction of risk potential

Cognitive level: Applying

---

10. A nurse is counseling a client about risk factors for hypertension. Which risk factors should the nurse list for primary hypertension? Select all that apply.

☐ **1.** Obesity
☐ **2.** Glomerulonephritis
☐ **3.** Head injury
☐ **4.** Stress
☐ **5.** Hormonal contraceptive use
☐ **6.** High intake of sodium or saturated fat

Answer: 1, 4, 6

Rationale: Primary or essential hypertension has no identifiable cause and tends to develop gradually over years. Obesity, stress, high intake of sodium or saturated fat, and family history are all risk factors for primary hypertension. Diabetes mellitus, head injury, and hormonal contraceptive use are risk factors for secondary hypertension.

Test-taking strategy: Analyze to determine what information the question asks for, which is the risk factors associated with primary hypertension. Note the key word "primary" inferring original cause. Consider any cause which alone can elevate blood pressure. Review the risk factors and types of hypertension if you had difficulty answering this question.

Client needs category: Health promotion and maintenance

Client needs subcategory: None

Cognitive level: Applying

11. A client is brought to the emergency department and diagnosed with first-degree AV block. When instructing the spouse using a diagram, identify the area in the conduction cycle where this block occurs.

Answer:

Rationale: An X is placed at the AV node located on the interatrial septum close to the tricuspid valve. First-degree AV block is a conduction disturbance in which electrical impulses flow normally from the sinoatrial node through the atria but are delayed at the AV node, thus prolonging the PR interval on an ECG. Although the conduction is slowed, there are no missed beats.

Test-taking strategy: Analyze to determine what information the question asks for, which is the site of specific blockage in the conduction cycle. Use the information of "AV" to narrow the location. Also consider the electrical conduction pathway at the AV site. Review first-degree AV block and the anatomy of the heart and how it relates to cardiac electrical activity if you had difficulty answering this question.

Client needs category: Physiological integrity

Client needs subcategory: Physiological adaptation

Cognitive level: Applying

---

12. A nurse is caring for a client in the immediate post-cardiac catheterization period. Which interventions should the nurse include in the client's care? Select all that apply.

☐ **1.** Monitor vital signs every 15 minutes for the first hour.

☐ **2.** Assess all peripheral pulses frequently.

☐ **3.** Restrict the client to bed rest for 2 to 6 hours.

☐ **4.** Assess the insertion site.

☐ **5.** Perform range-of-motion (ROM) exercises.

Answer: 1, 3, 4

Rationale: The key word is "immediate," indicating that care may be different throughout the recovery period. In the immediate period, the client's vital signs are typically monitored every 15 minutes for the first hour, then every 30 minutes for 2 hours or until vital signs are stable, and then every 4 hours or according to facility policy. All peripheral pulses do not require frequent assessment. (Always reflect on the word "all" in the selection.) The pulses in the affected extremity are usually assessed with every vital signs check. Clients typically remain in bed for 2 to 6 hours unless a special closure is used. The insertion site extremity is kept straight following the procedure, so ROM exercises would not be performed.

Test-taking strategy: Analyze to determine what information the question asks for, which is care of a client at a specific time. "Select all that apply" questions require considering each option to decide its merit. Focus on immediate assessment and postcatheterization care, which would include the recovery period. Consider anesthetic administered, medications, lab values, I.V.s, or incisions. Review post cardiac catheterization interventions if you had difficulty answering this question.

Client needs category: Safe and effective care environment

Client needs subcategory: Coordinated care

Cognitive level: Applying

---

13. A nurse is caring for a client with a new prescription of digoxin (Lanoxin). Which client statement would require further teaching about digoxin? Select all that apply.

- ☐ **1.** "I will take the digoxin at 9 a.m. daily."
- ☐ **2.** "I will take the digoxin with my antacids at night."
- ☐ **3.** "I will take my pulse before each dose of digoxin."
- ☐ **4.** "If I forget a dose, I will catch-up by doubling the next dose."
- ☐ **5.** "I will notify my doctor if experiencing increased fatigue or muscle weakness."
- ☐ **6.** "I understand that I will need annual blood work to check therapeutic levels."

Answer: 2, 4, 6

Rationale: Digoxin is a cardiac glycoside which slows and strengthens the heart providing a more regular rhythm. Digoxin has a narrowed therapeutic window requiring every 2 weeks–monthly serum blood level monitoring initially. It is usually helpful for a client to take digoxin at a specific time each day to establish its blood level and routine for administration. The nurse should teach the client to take the pulse before each dose of digoxin and to notify the practitioner if the rate or rhythm changes, specifically if the rate drops to less than 60 beats/minute. The client should also be instructed to report increasing fatigue or muscle weakness immediately, as these are signs of digitalis (digoxin) toxicity. Antacids inhibit the absorption of digoxin, so digoxin should not be taken with these drugs. If the client forgets to take a dose of digoxin, he/she may take the missed dose only up to 12 hours later.

Test-taking strategy: Analyze to determine what information the question asks for, which is a client statement that would be incorrect or need further teaching/clarification. "Select all that apply" questions require considering each option to decide its merit. When teaching about a new medication, consider basic knowledge of therapeutic regimen, side effects, and unique considerations related to medication management. Consider factors effecting safe administration of digoxin and review cardiac glycosides side effects if you had difficulty answering this question.

Client needs category: Health promotion and maintenance

Client needs subcategory: None

Cognitive level: Analyzing

14. A nurse is caring for a monitored client on the telemetry unit. When analyzing a cardiac monitor strip, the nurse notes an abnormality in the QRS wave on lead II. Identify the area in the conduction cycle of the heart where this abnormality occurs.

Answer:

Rationale: An X is placed on the left ventricle. The electrocardiography (ECG) shows the electrical activity of the heart over time as detected by electrodes attached to the body surface. Lead II is noted as a limb lead. The QRS complex reflects the rapid depolarization of the right and left ventricles, thus an abnormality in the ventricular conduction will be reflected in the QRS wave.

Test-taking strategy: Analyze to determine what information the question asks for, which is the area in the conduction cycle reflected with an abnormality in the QRS wave. If unsure, remember that the QRS reflects large heart muscle activity of the ventricles and encompasses a large amount of the ECG tracing. Review the anatomy and electrical activity of the heart, and focus on the QRS wave of the cardiac cycle if you had difficulty answering this question.

Client needs category: Physiological integrity

Client needs subcategory: Physiological adaptation

Cognitive level: Analyzing

15. A nurse places electrodes on a collapsed individual who was visiting a hospitalized family member, the monitor exhibits the following. Which intervention should the nurse do first?

Progress Notes

□ **1.** Place the client on oxygen.
□ **2.** Confirm the rhythm with a 12-lead ECG.
□ **3.** Begin chest compressions.
□ **4.** Assess the client's airway, breathing, and circulation.

Answer: 4

Rationale: The rhythm the client is experiencing is ventricular tachycardia (VT). The nurse must first assess the airway, breathing, and circulation, and level of consciousness to establish the client's stability and obtain further help from nursing staff. Different actions are required if the client's VT is unstable or pulseless.

Test-taking strategy: Analyze to determine what information the question asks for, which is what intervention should be done first following rhythm/waveform analysis. Note the key word "first" indicating a priority response. Consider that assessment comes before implementation in the nursing process. Recall the unusual waveform pattern and interpret as an emergency due to the inability of the heart to perfuse. Remember to treat the client, not the rhythm strip. Review ECG waveforms and nursing action if you had difficulty answering this question.

Client needs category: Physiological integrity

Client needs subcategory: Reduction of risk potential

Cognitive level: Analyzing

---

16. The nurse is mentoring a graduate practical nurse. When reviewing the steps needed to analyze an ECG rhythm strip, place the ECG analysis steps in order from first to last. Use all of the options.

| **1.** Measure the QRS duration. |
| **2.** Interpret the rhythm. |
| **3.** Analyze the P waves. |
| **4.** Determine the rate and rhythm. |
| **5** Measure the P-R interval. |

Answer: 4, 3, 5, 1, 2

Rationale: ECG rhythm strip analysis requires a systematic approach using a five-step method. First, determine the rate and rhythm of both the atria and the ventricles. Then, analyze the P waves for consistency. Next, measure the P-R interval and then the QRS duration. Finally, you can interpret the rhythm with all of the information that has been collected. If the nurse has answered all five steps within normal limits, the client is in sinus rhythm. The greater number of questions that the nurse notes inconsistent with normal limits, the greater the abnormal conduction through the heart.

Test-taking strategy: Analyze to determine what information the question asks for, which is rhythm strip analysis. Recall the above method of analysis. Note that the analysis notes deviations from normal, thus understanding the heart's conduction is essential. Review the analysis of rhythm strips using the five-step method if you had difficulty answering this question.

Client needs category: Safe and effective care environment

Client needs subcategory: Coordinated care

Cognitive level: Analyzing

17. A nurse is presenting health information at a community organization when one of the attendees passes out. The nurse assesses the attendee as being unresponsive. Indicate how the nurse should respond by placing the following actions in chronological order. Use all of the options.

1.	Appoint a person to call 911.

2.	Check for a pulse.

3.	Deliver two rescue breaths.

4.	Check for normal breathing.

5.	Perform chest compressions.

6.	Perform a head tilt-chin lift maneuver.

Answer: 1, 2, 5, 6, 4, 3

Rationale: Following the 2010 American Heart Association (AHA) guidelines for cardiopulmonary resuscitation (CPR), the rescuer should activate the emergency response system and get an automatic external defibrillator (AED) or appoint another person to do this. The next step is to check the pulse for no more than 10 seconds. If no pulse is detected, the rescuer gives 30 chest compressions. Next, the rescuer opens the airway with the head tilt-chin lift or jaw thrust maneuver and checks for breathing. If breathing is not detected, the rescuer gives two rescue breaths and immediately resumes chest compressions. The rescuer should use the AED as soon as it arrives.

Test-taking strategy: Analyze to determine what information the question asks for, which is arranging the options in an order in which they should be performed during resuscitation. Note the above sequence. The 2010 AHA guidelines for CPR stress administering compressions for restoring circulation in a pulseless victim. Review the guidelines if you had difficulty answering this question.

Client needs category: Physiological integrity

Client needs subcategory: Physiological adaptation

Cognitive level: Analyzing

Respiratory Disorders

1. A nurse is caring for a client with pneumonia who was prescribed ceftriaxone (Rocephin) oral suspension 600 mg once daily. The medication label indicates that the strength is 125 mg/5 mL. How many milliliters of medication should the nurse pour to administer the correct dose? Record your answer as a whole number.

_____ mL

Answer: 24

Rationale: Use the following formula to calculate the drug dosage:

Dose on hand/quantity on hand = dose desired/X.

Plug in the values for this equation and solve for X:

$$125 \text{ mg}/5 \text{ mL} = 600 \text{ mg}/X$$

$$X = 24 \text{ mL}.$$

Test-taking strategy: Analyze to determine what information the question asks for, which is the total amount of milliliters to be administered for the prescribed dose. Review dosage calculations using the ratio-and-proportion method. Recall that this method uses all known factors to determine the unknown (milliliter to be administered). Proofread your math calculations for accuracy. Review drug dosage calculations if you had difficulty answering this question.

Client needs category: Physiological integrity

Client needs subcategory: Pharmacological therapies

Cognitive level: Applying

2. A nurse is caring for a client with a chest tube connected to a three-chamber drainage system without suction. On the illustration below, identify which chamber that the nurse will mark to record the current drainage level.

Answer:

Rationale: A chest tube drains blood, fluid, and air from around the lungs. The drainage system, which the nurse measures each shift, is on the right. It has three calibrated chambers that show the amount of drainage collected. When the first chamber fills, drainage empties into the second; when the second chamber fills, drainage flows into the third. The water seal chamber is located in the center. The suction control chamber is on the left.

Test-taking strategy: Analyze to determine what information the question asks for, which is where drainage is collected in a chest drainage system. Recall that at the beginning of each shift, the nurse should assess the color, consistency, and amount of drainage present. The previous nurse marks the level of drainage on the collection chamber with the date and time. Review the care and components of chest tube drainage systems if you had difficulty answering this question.

Client needs category: Physiological integrity

Client needs subcategory: Reduction of risk potential

Cognitive level: Applying

3. A client comes to the emergency department with status asthmaticus. Based on the documentation note below, the nurse suspects that the client has what abnormality?

Progress Notes

2/1/10	Pt. wheezing. RR 44, BP 140/90, P 104,
1830	T 98.4°F. ABG results show pH 7.52, PaCO₂
	30 mm Hg, HCO₃⁻ 26 mEq/L, and PO₂
	77 mm Hg. ————————— C. Wynn, LPN

☐ **1.** Respiratory acidosis.
☐ **2.** Respiratory alkalosis.
☐ **3.** Metabolic acidosis.
☐ **4.** Metabolic alkalosis.

Answer: 2

Rationale: Following review of the nursing documentation, the nurse notes respiratory alkalosis related to alveolar hyperventilation. Respiratory alkalosis is marked by an increase in pH to more than 7.45 and a concurrent decrease in partial pressure of arterial carbon dioxide ($PaCO_2$) to less than 35 mm Hg. Metabolic alkalosis shows the same increase in pH but also an increased bicarbonate level and normal $PaCO_2$ (may be elevated also if compensatory mechanisms are working). Acidosis of any type means a low pH (below 7.35). Respiratory acidosis shows an elevated $PaCO_2$ and a normal to high bicarbonate level. Metabolic acidosis is characterized by a decreased bicarbonate level and a normal to low $PaCO_2$.

Test-taking strategy: Analyze to determine what information the question asks for, which is identification of a client's condition using data. First, consider the disease process and note abnormalities in assessment and lab data, which points to a respiratory complication. Next, evaluate lab results. Review criteria for blood gas values, acid–base disturbances, and compensation and the disease process of status asthmaticus if you had difficulty answering this question.

Client needs category: Physiological integrity

Client needs subcategory: Physiological adaptation

Cognitive level: Analyzing

---

4. A nurse is preparing a staff education program on innovative devices in pulmonary circulation. Beginning with basic concepts, place the following structures in chronological order to trace the pathway of normal pulmonary circulation. Use all of the options.

1. Pulmonary vein
2. Right ventricle
3. Pulmonary artery
4. Arterioles
5. Alveoli
6. Left atrium

Answer: 2, 3, 4, 5, 1, 6

Rationale: Pulmonary circulation is the movement of blood from the heart, to the lungs, and back to the heart again. Deoxygenated blood is ejected from the right ventricle into the pulmonary artery and then into the lungs via the arterioles and alveoli. The pulmonary vein then carries oxygenated blood back to the left atrium for circulation throughout the body.

Test-taking strategy: Analyze to determine what information the question asks for, which is the path of pulmonary circulation. Of the choices, select the right ventricle as a point of origin with deoxygenated blood. Continue through the process until oxygen-rich blood is pumped from the heart to the body systems. Review the cardiopulmonary system and pulmonary circulation if you had difficulty answering this question.

Client needs category: Physiological integrity

Client needs subcategory: Physiological adaptation

Cognitive level: Understanding

5. A client with a suspected pulmonary embolus is brought to the emergency department complaining of shortness of breath and chest pain. Which additional signs and symptoms are anticipated? Select all that apply.

- ☐ **1.** Low-grade fever
- ☐ **2.** Thick green sputum
- ☐ **3.** Bradycardia
- ☐ **4.** Frothy sputum
- ☐ **5.** Tachycardia
- ☐ **6.** Blood-tinged sputum

Answer: 1, 5, 6

Rationale: A pulmonary embolism (PE) is a blockage to one or more arteries in the lungs. In addition to pleuritic chest pain and dyspnea, a client with a pulmonary embolus may present with a low-grade fever, tachycardia, and blood-tinged sputum. Thick green sputum would indicate infection, and frothy sputum would indicate pulmonary edema. A client with a pulmonary embolus is tachycardic (to compensate for decreased oxygen supply), not bradycardic.

Test-taking strategy: Analyze to determine what information the question asks for, which is signs and symptoms of a PE. "Select all that apply" questions require considering each option to decide its merit. Recall that a PE is a medical emergency with symptoms of respiratory compromise. Review the pathophysiology and clinical manifestations of a PE if you had difficulty answering this question.

Client needs category: Physiological integrity

Client needs subcategory: Physiological adaptation

Cognitive level: Analyzing

---

6. A client with chronic obstructive pulmonary disease (COPD) is being evaluated for a lung transplant. Which initial assessment data would the nurse anticipate? Select all that apply.

- ☐ **1.** Decreased respiratory rate
- ☐ **2.** Dyspnea on exertion
- ☐ **3.** Barrel chest
- ☐ **4.** Shortened expiratory phase
- ☐ **5.** Clubbed fingers and toes
- ☐ **6.** Fever

Answer: 2, 3, 5

Rationale: COPD is one of the most common lung diseases making it difficult to breathe. Severity of the illness varies. Typical findings for clients with COPD include dyspnea on exertion, a barrel chest, and clubbed fingers and toes. Clients with COPD are usually tachypneic with a prolonged expiratory phase. Fever is not associated with COPD, unless an infection is also present.

Test-taking strategy: Analyze to determine what information the question asks for, which is common symptoms of a client with severe COPD needing a lung transplant. Consider symptoms associated with severe respiratory compromise. "Select all that apply" questions require considering each option to decide its merit. Review the anatomy and physiology of the respiratory system and focus on the pathophysiology and clinical manifestations of COPD if you had difficulty answering this question.

Client needs category: Physiological integrity

Client needs subcategory: Physiological adaptation

Cognitive level: Analyzing

7. A nurse is caring for a client with a traumatic injury and developing tension pneumothorax. Which assessment data would be of concern? Select all that apply.

☐ **1.** Decreased cardiac output.
☐ **2.** Flattened neck veins.
☐ **3.** Tracheal deviation to the affected side.
☐ **4.** Hypotension.
☐ **5.** Tracheal deviation to the opposite side.
☐ **6.** Bradypnea.

Answer: 1, 4, 5

Rationale: Tension pneumothorax results when air in the pleural space is under higher pressure than air in the adjacent lung. The site of the rupture of the pleural space acts as a one-way valve, allowing the air to enter on inspiration but not to escape on expiration. The air presses against the mediastinum, causing a tracheal shift to the opposite side and decreased venous return (reflected by decreased cardiac output and hypotension). Neck veins bulge with tension pneumothorax. This also leads to compensatory tachycardia and tachypnea.

Test-taking strategy: Analyze to determine what information the question asks for, which is signs of a developing tension pneumothorax. "Select all that apply" questions require considering each option to decide its merit. Recall the pathophysiology of the tension pneumothorax producing tension in the thoracic cavity and relate clinical manifestations of a high pressure environment. Review respiratory system physiology and assessment data if you had difficulty answering this question.

Client needs category: Physiological integrity
Client needs subcategory: Physiological adaptation
Cognitive level: Analyzing

---

8. A nurse is caring for a client with right-middle-lobe pneumonia. On the anterior view of the lungs below, identify the area where the nurse anticipates adventitious breath sounds such as crackles.

Answer:

Rationale: Note the placement of the X. The right lung is composed of three lobes: the right upper lobe, right middle lobe, and right lower lobe. The left lung is made up of only two lobes: the left upper lobe and left lower lobe. When assessing the anterior chest, the right lung is on the examiner's left.

Test-taking strategy: Analyze to determine what information the question asks for, which is identifying the area of pneumonia/area of adventitious breath sounds. The key is to recall which lung (right) has three lobes. Review the anatomy of the respiratory system and breath sound assessment techniques if you had difficulty answering this question.

Client needs category: Health promotion and maintenance

Client needs subcategory: None

Cognitive level: Applying

---

9. A client is prescribed continuous positive airway pressure (CPAP) therapy for sleep apnea. Identify on the illustration below where the mechanism maintaining the positive end-expiratory pressure is located.

Answer:

Rationale: The X is placed on the valve below the location of the oxygen tubing connecting to the face mask. CPAP ventilation maintains positive pressure in the airways throughout the respiratory cycle. The inlet valve attaches the oxygen tubing to the face mask, and the positive end-expiratory pressure valve, located below, maintains the pressure. CPAP can be used with or without a ventilator in intubated and nonintubated clients and can be administered just nasally for a less constrictive feeling. In addition to sleep apnea, CPAP is used to treat respiratory distress syndrome, pulmonary edema, pulmonary emboli, bronchiolitis, pneumonitis, viral pneumonia, and post-operative atelectasis.

Test-taking strategy: Analyze to determine what information the question asks for, which is location of the positive pressure mechanism. If unsure, review the structure of the mask. Consider attachments for the incoming air and look for a structure maintaining the pressure in the system and not allowing the air to escape. Review the structure and function of a CPAP machine if you had difficulty answering this question.

Client needs category: Physiological integrity

Client needs subcategory: Physiological adaptation

Cognitive level: Applying

10. A nurse is evaluating a client with primary pulmonary hypertension for a heart–lung transplant. Which medication treatment would the nurse anticipate to be included in the plan of care? Select all that apply.

- ☐ **1.** Oxygen therapy
- ☐ **2.** Aminoglycosides
- ☐ **3.** Diuretics
- ☐ **4.** Vasodilators
- ☐ **5.** Antihistamines
- ☐ **6.** Sulfonamides

Answer: 1, 3, 4

Rationale: Pulmonary hypertension is an increase in blood pressure in the pulmonary arteries, pulmonary vein, or pulmonary capillary. This increase in pressure makes it more difficult for the blood to flow through the lungs. Oxygen, diuretics, and vasodilators are among the common medication therapies used to treat pulmonary hypertension. Other treatments include fluid restriction, digoxin, calcium channel blockers, β-adrenergic blockers, and bronchodilators. Aminoglycosides and sulfonamides are antibiotics used to treat infections. Antihistamines are indicated to treat allergies, pruritus, vertigo, nausea, and vomiting; to promote sedation; and to suppress cough.

Test-taking strategy: Analyze to determine what information the question asks for, which is medication regimens for pulmonary hypertension. "Select all that apply" questions require considering each option to decide its merit. Consider the pathophysiology of pulmonary hypertension and focus on the benefits of each treatment. Since pulmonary hypertension decreases pulmonary blood flow, oxygen therapy is helpful. Next, focus on each medication classification and their ability to decrease hypertension. Review anticipated medical treatments for pulmonary hypertension if you had difficulty answering this question.

Client needs category: Physiological integrity

Client needs subcategory: Pharmacological therapies

Cognitive level: Applying

11. A nurse notes crackles on a client diagnosed with right-lower-lobe atelectasis. In which area would the nurse place the stethoscope to assess the adventitious breath sounds?

Answer:

Rationale: Note the placement of the X. To auscultate the right lower lobe from the anterior chest, the nurse should place the stethoscope between the fifth and sixth intercostal spaces to the left of the anterior axillary line.

Test-taking strategy: Analyze to determine what information the question asks for, which is site of the right lower lobe as that is the location of the crackles. Recall the position of the lobes in the thoracic cavity. Note the markings on the diagram to indicate the intercostals. Review the thoracic cavity landmarks associated with lung/lobe positions if you had difficulty answering this question.

Client needs category: Physiological integrity
Client needs subcategory: Reduction of risk potential
Cognitive level: Applying

---

12. A fireman is admitted with superficial skin wounds and a sprained back following an intense fire. No respiratory complaints are verbalized. Nearly 24 hours after admission, the fireman reports dyspnea, a harsh cough, and hoarseness. Which nursing interventions should the nurse add to the plan of care? Select all that apply.

☐ **1.** Monitor for fever.
☐ **2.** Make sure the client's oxygen saturation level remains below 98%.
☐ **3.** Auscultate the lungs for adventitious breath sounds.
☐ **4.** Assess for increased pulse rate.
☐ **5.** Monitor for increased anxiety levels.

Answer: 3, 4, 5

Rationale: More than half of all clients with pulmonary involvement following inhalation injury do not immediately demonstrate pulmonary signs. Any client with possible inhalation injury must be observed for at least 24 hours for possible respiratory complications. Maintaining increased oxygen saturation levels is essential, especially following a carbon monoxide inhalation injury, to prevent the development of carboxyhemoglobin, which competes with oxygen for available hemoglobin. The client does not typically develop a fever with inhalation injury, but may progress to acute respiratory syndrome with bilateral lung infiltrates, cardiac involvement with tachycardia, and increasing anxiety due to oxygen starvation.

Test-taking strategy: Analyze to determine what information the question asks for, which is nursing interventions for an inhalation injury. "Select all that apply" questions require considering each option to decide its merit. Focus on the information gathered during the nursing assessment and relate to clinical manifestations of inhalation injury. Keep in mind signs of respiratory compromise as priority nursing interventions. Review inhalation injury and respiratory interventions if you had difficulty answering this question.

Client needs category: Physiological integrity
Client needs subcategory: Physiological adaptation
Cognitive level: Analyzing

13. A nurse is caring for a client with history of heart failure and presenting with a pulmonary embolism (PE). The nurse documents admission findings of sudden shortness of breath, chest pain, and immobility. Which nursing diagnoses are admission priorities? Select all that apply.

☐ **1.** Activity intolerance related to inadequate oxygenation.
☐ **2.** Anxiety related to breathlessness.
☐ **3.** Disturbed sleep pattern related to inability to assume recumbent position.
☐ **4.** Ineffective breathing pattern related to hypoxia.
☐ **5.** Risk for decreased cardiac output related to failure of the left ventricle.
☐ **6.** Social isolation related to hospitalization.

Answer: 1, 2, 4, 5

Rationale: When planning care, the nurse should select nursing diagnoses that anticipate pulmonary compromise secondary to reduction of air, blood, and gas exchange because these are ensuing complications that can develop from a PE, particularly in a client with a history of heart failure. The prudent nurse should analyze the client's condition and anticipate the need for safe, supportive nursing interventions related to the client's activity intolerance, anxiety, ineffective breathing, and risk for decreased oxygen output. The client history does not indicate that this client has difficulty sleeping, and although social isolation is important to consider, it is not a priority.

Test-taking strategy: Analyze to determine what information the question asks for, which is priority admission nursing diagnosis. "Select all that apply" questions require considering each option to decide its merit. The key word is "admission" which focuses on the client's documented current symptoms. Review the pathophysiology and clinical manifestations of PE as it relates to applicable nursing diagnoses if you had difficulty answering this question.

Client needs category: Physiological integrity
Client needs subcategory: Basic care and comfort
Cognitive level: Evaluating

---

14. The nurse is caring for a senior citizen who lives alone. When evaluating the effectiveness of adding Advair Diskus (fluticasone propionate and salmeterol) to the chronic obstructive airway disease (COPD) client's medication regimen, which client statements would support symptom improvement? Select all that apply?

☐ **1.** "I have noted an increase in sputum production."
☐ **2.** "I have begun walking to the mailbox each morning for my newspaper."
☐ **3.** "I can rely on the medication when I have an exacerbation of symptoms."
☐ **4.** "I seem to cough more in the morning hours."
☐ **5.** "I can now push my granddaughter on the swings when she visits."
☐ **6.** "The nurse aide no longer comes to the house to help me bathe."

Answer: 2, 5, 6

Rationale: Advair Diskus is a combination of steroid and bronchodilator used in the treatment of chronic asthma and chronic obstructive airway disease. The medication is intended to be used daily. It is not a rescue inhaler, and additional doses do not improve respiratory function. Evaluation of effectiveness includes improvement in respiratory status and ability to perform activities of daily living/quality of life activities such as walking and playing. Side effects of the medication include an increase in cough and sputum production.

Test-taking strategy: Analyze to determine what information the question asks for, which is information that would indicate improvement in respiratory status. "Select all that apply" questions require considering each option to decide its merit. Evaluate each client statement for evidence of symptom improvement or overall client activity (ADL) improvement. Review the pathophysiology and symptoms of COPD if you had difficulty answering this question.

Client needs category: Physiological integrity
Client needs subcategory: Pharmacological therapies
Cognitive level: Evaluating

15. The nurse has been assigned to care for the following six clients. Which clients would the nurse expect to be at risk for the development of pulmonary embolism (PE)? Select all that apply.

☐ **1.** A client who is on complete bed rest following extensive spinal surgery.

☐ **2.** A client who has a large venous stasis ulcer on the right ankle area.

☐ **3.** A client who has recently been admitted with a broken femur and is awaiting surgery.

☐ **4.** A client who has a pleural effusion secondary to lung cancer.

☐ **5.** A client who is receiving supplemental oxygen following shoulder surgery.

☐ **6.** A client who has undergone a total vaginal hysterectomy and is now on estrogen replacement therapy.

Answer: 1, 2, 3, 6

Rationale: Bed rest, poor venous circulation, fractures, and hormone replacement therapy can cause formation of a thromboembolus, placing these clients at risk for developing a PE. A deep vein thrombosis could break loose in the leg and travel to the lungs as a pulmonary embolus. The clot would then lodge in the pulmonary arteries or arterioles and impede blood flow. The client who is on complete bed rest is at risk for venous stasis, and the client who has a venous stasis ulcer is already demonstrating this condition. The client with a broken femur is at risk for a fat embolus, another form of PE. The client on estrogen replacement therapy is at increased risk for thromboembolic disorders. Pleural effusion and lung cancer usually have no effect on thrombus formation, and oxygen therapy does not cause venous stasis or increase the risk of a PE.

Test-taking strategy: Analyze to determine what information the question asks for, which is identifying a client population who are at risk for developing a PE. "Select all that apply" questions require considering each option to decide its merit. Review the pathophysiology of thromboembolic disorders and consider the factors that lead to blood stasis and clotting if you had difficulty answering this question.

Client needs category: Physiological integrity

Client needs subcategory: Physiological adaptation

Cognitive level: Evaluating

16. The nurse is caring for several clients on the respiratory unit who are receiving the β-adrenergic agonist bronchodilator albuterol (Accuneb) in the prescribed nebulizer treatments. Which side effects would the nurse expect to assess following administration? Select all that apply.

☐ **1.** Increased tachypnea.
☐ **2.** Irritability and nervousness.
☐ **3.** Tachycardia.
☐ **4.** Increased somnolence.
☐ **5.** Insomnia.
☐ **6.** Anxiety.

Answer: 2, 3, 5, 6

Rationale: Albuterol (Accuneb) is prescribed to prevent and treat wheezing, difficulty breathing, and chest tightness caused by lung diseases such as asthma and chronic obstructive lung disease (COPD). Irritability, nervousness, tachycardia, insomnia, and anxiety are common side effects of β-adrenergic agonist bronchodilators that result from sympathetic nervous system stimulation. The expected therapeutic effect of a bronchodilator is decreased dyspnea and slower (not increased) breathing. Increased somnolence does not occur with sympathetic nervous system stimulation.

Test-taking strategy: Analyze to determine what information the question asks for, which is expected side effects following albuterol administration. "Select all that apply" questions require considering each option to decide its merit. Break down the classification of adrenergics (adrenaline) and agonists (mimic the action of the naturally occurring substance) and relate to sympathetic nervous system stimulation. Review the action and side effects of β-adrenergic agonists if you had difficulty answering this question.

Client needs category: Physiological integrity

Client needs subcategory: Pharmacological therapies

Cognitive level: Applying

---

17. A nurse is caring for a client with pulmonary edema whose respiratory status is declining. Chronologically arrange the nursing interventions to prioritize care. Use all the options.

| 1. Administer oxygen via nasal cannula at 2 L/minute. |
| 2. Call the physician. |
| 3. Position the client upright at a 45° angle. |
| 4. Prepare suctioning equipment at the bedside. |
| 5. Notify RN to administer furosemide (Lasix) 40 mg I.V. STAT. |
| 6. Insert an indwelling urinary catheter. |

Answer: 3, 1, 4, 2, 5, 6

Rationale: The order of priority moves from the simple to the complex for bedside interventions when a client is in respiratory distress. The nurse should first attempt to maximize respiratory excursion as much as possible by sitting the client up, and then provide supplemental oxygen to minimize impending hypoxia. It is also important to have suction equipment readily available because the client may choke on oral secretions due to the pulmonary edema. After performing these interventions, the nurse should notify the physician and anticipate orders for administration of a diuretic (such as Lasix) and insertion of an indwelling urinary catheter to measure eventual output.

Test-taking strategy: Analyze to determine what information the question asks for, which is arranging nursing actions when caring for a client with a declining respiratory status. First, assess the client and determine nursing actions to improve the respiratory status and prepare for any potential emergency. Next, move from the client to notify the physician and anticipate medical orders. Review priority care of individuals with pulmonary edema if you had difficulty answering this question.

Client needs category: Physiological integrity

Client needs subcategory: Reduction of risk potential

Cognitive level: Analyzing

---

18. A nurse is caring for a client diagnosed with pneumonia, a urinary tract infection, dehydration, and temperature of 101.4°F (38.6°C). The physician orders 1,000 mL of D_5W to infuse over 8 hours. The available drop factor is 20 gtt/mL. The nurse should regulate the I.V. flow rate to deliver how many drops per minute? Round your answer to the nearest whole number.

_____ gtt/min

Answer: 42

Rationale: Calculate the flow rate using the formula below:

$$\frac{\text{Total volume ordered}}{\text{Number of hours}} = \text{Flow rate}$$

$$\frac{1,000 \text{ mL}}{8 \text{ hours}} = 125 \text{ mL/hour}$$

Change from mL/hour to drops/minute using the provided drop factor.

$$\frac{125 \text{ mL}}{60 \text{ min}} \times \frac{20 \text{ gtt}}{1 \text{ mL}} = 41.66$$

Rounded off, this is 42 gtt/min.

Test-taking strategy: Analyze to determine what information the question asks for, which is drops per minute. Always refer to the dosage/time or quantity that the question requires the final answer to be calculated to, which, in this case, is drops/minute. Follow the formula, setting up the equation to end with the desired dosage. Proofread your math calculations. Review the calculation of I.V. drip rates if you had difficulty answering this question.

Client needs category: Physiological integrity

Client needs subcategory: Pharmacological therapies

Cognitive level: Applying

---

19. The licensed practical nurse (LPN) is performing a purified protein derivative (PPD) test on a nursing home resident. Which statements about this test are correct? Select all that apply.

- ☐ **1.** A PPD test is done to test for allergies.
- ☐ **2.** Always aspirate before injecting the PPD solution.
- ☐ **3.** The PPD test is an intradermal test.
- ☐ **4.** Hold the syringe at a 45° angle to the skin.
- ☐ **5.** The preferred injection site is the ventral surface of the forearm.
- ☐ **6.** No wheal should appear at the site following injection.

Answer: 3, 5

Rationale: The PPD test is used to determine whether a person has been exposed/infected with the _Tuberculosis_ bacillus. PPD tests should be injected intradermally in the ventral forearm, unless contraindicated, without aspiration prior to injecting. The syringe should be held at a 10° to 15° angle from the site so the needle enters the dermis as nearly parallel to the skin as possible. A small wheal should appear; this indicates that the medication has been injected into the dermis.

Test-taking strategy: Analyze to determine what information the question asks for, which is correct statements related to the administration of a PPD. "Select all that apply" questions require considering each option to decide its merit. First, visualize the technique to place medication in the intradermal layer of the skin. Also, recall that no allergy is being tested. Review the rationale and procedure for administering a PPD test if you had difficulty answering this question.

Client needs category: Physiological integrity

Client needs subcategory: Pharmacological therapies

Cognitive level: Applying

1. A nurse is providing discharge instructions on phenytoin (Dilantin) to a female client with tonic-clonic seizure disorder. Which instructions should the nurse include? Select all that apply.

☐ **1.** Monitor the body for any skin rash.
☐ **2.** Maintain adequate amounts of fluid and fiber in the diet.
☐ **3.** Perform good oral hygiene, including daily brushing and flossing.
☐ **4.** Receive necessary periodic blood work.
☐ **5.** Report any problems with walking or coordination, slurred speech, or nausea.
☐ **6.** Feel safe about taking this drug, even during pregnancy.

Answer: 1, 3, 4, 5

Rationale: If a rash appears 10 to 14 days after starting phenytoin, the client should notify the physician who may discontinue the medication. Because it may cause gingival hyperplasia, the client must practice good oral hygiene and see a dentist regularly. Periodic blood work is necessary to monitor complete blood counts, platelet count, hepatic function, and drug levels. Signs and symptoms of phenytoin toxicity include problems with walking or coordination, slurred speech, and nausea. Other signs are lethargy, diplopia, and nystagmus. These must be reported to the physician immediately. Although adequate amounts of fluid and fiber are part of a healthy diet, they are not required for a client taking phenytoin. Phenytoin must be used cautiously during pregnancy because it poses an increased risk of birth defects; phenobarbital is safer to take during pregnancy.

Test-taking strategy: Analyze to determine what information the question asks for, which is discharge instructions for phenytoin. "Select all that apply" questions require considering each option to decide its merit. Critically think through the distractors considering the common side effects of phenytoin and review the adverse and toxic effects of this classification of medications. Review the therapeutic action of phenytoin with common side effects if you had difficulty answering this question.

Client needs category: Physiological integrity

Client needs subcategory: Pharmacological therapies

Cognitive level: Applying

2. A nurse assesses a client with suspected bacterial meningitis. Which documented finding of meningeal irritation suggests this diagnosis? Select all that apply.

☐ **1.** Generalized seizures
☐ **2.** Nuchal rigidity
☐ **3.** Positive Brudzinski's sign
☐ **4.** Positive Kernig's sign
☐ **5.** Babinski's reflex
☐ **6.** Photophobia

Answer: 2, 3, 4, 6

Rationale: Irritation of the meninges of the brain can be caused by a virus or bacteria. Signs of meningeal irritation include nuchal rigidity, positive Brudzinski's and Kernig's signs, and photophobia. Other signs of meningeal irritation are exaggerated and symmetrical deep tendon reflexes as well as opisthotonos (a spasm in which the back and extremities arch backward so that the body rests on the head and heels). Generalized seizures may accompany meningitis, but they are caused by irritation to the cerebral cortex, not the meninges. Babinski's reflex is a reflex action of the toes that reflects corticospinal tract disease in adults.

Test-taking strategy: Analyze to determine what information the question asks for, which is documented assessment findings which suggest bacterial meningitis. "Select all that apply" questions require considering each option to decide its merit. Review the pathophysiology and clinical manifestations of bacterial meningitis if you had difficulty answering this question.

Client needs category: Physiological integrity

Client needs subcategory: Physiological adaptation

Cognitive level: Applying

---

3. A nurse is preparing to administer phenytoin (Dilantin) to a 99 lb client with a seizure disorder. The medication administration record documents phenytoin 5 mg/kg/day to be administered in three divided doses. How many milligrams of phenytoin should be administered in the first dose? Record your answer as a whole number.

_____ mg

Answer: 75

Rationale: First, convert the client's weight to kilograms:

$$1 \text{ kg} = 2.2 \text{ lb}$$
$$99 \text{ lb} \div 2.2 \text{ lb/kg} = 44 \text{ kg}.$$

Then calculate the total daily dosage:

$$44 \text{ kg} \times 5 \text{ mg/kg} = 220 \text{ mg/day}.$$

Finally, divide the total daily dosage into three parts:

$$220 \text{ mg} \div 3 \text{ doses} = 75 \text{ mg/dose}.$$

Test-taking strategy: Analyze to determine what information the question asks for, which is the dose (mg) of phenytoin to be administered. First, change the weight from pounds to kilograms to be able to fit into the equation (mg/kg). Calculate using the formula above. Note that the first dose is the same as the third dose of the day because the daily dose is divided evenly. Proofread the math calculation. Review dosage in milligrams according to body weight if you had difficulty answering this question.

Client needs category: Physiological integrity

Client needs subcategory: Pharmacological therapies

Cognitive level: Applying

4. A nurse is assessing a client's extraocular eye movements as part of evaluating neurological functioning. Which cranial nerve status is documented? Select all that apply.

☐ **1.** Optic (II).
☐ **2.** Oculomotor (III).
☐ **3.** Trochlear (IV).
☐ **4.** Trigeminal (V).
☐ **5.** Abducens (VI).
☐ **6.** Acoustic (VIII).

Answer: 2, 3, 5

Rationale: Assessing extraocular eye movements helps evaluate the function of cranial nerves III (oculomotor), IV (trochlear), and VI (abducens). The oculomotor nerve originates in the brain stem and controls the movement of the eyeball up, down, and inward; raises the eyelid; and constricts the pupil. The trochlear nerve rotates the eyeball downward and outward. The abducens nerve originates in the pons and rotates the eyeball laterally. Assessing the client's vision helps evaluate cranial nerve II (optic). Cranial nerve V (trigeminal) has three branches: assessing the corneal reflex helps the nurse evaluate the ophthalmic branch functions; assessing sensation to the cheek, upper jaw, teeth, lips, hard palate, maxillary sinus, and part of the nasal mucosa helps evaluate the maxillary branch functions; and assessing sensation to the lower lip, chin, ear, mucous membrane, lower teeth, and tongue helps evaluate the mandibular branch functions. Assessing hearing and balance helps evaluate the cochlear and vestibular branches of cranial nerve VIII (acoustic).

Test-taking strategy: Analyze to determine what information the question asks for, which is assessing the cranial nerves involved in extraocular movements. "Select all that apply" questions require considering each option to decide its merit. Simple recall of the 12 cranial nerves is essential in completing a neurological examination. Use of pneumonic phrases such as "On Old Olympus Towering Top, A Fin and German Viewed Some Hops" can be helpful to recall the cranial nerves and select the correct options to answer the question. Review the cranial nerves and, specifically, those involved with extraocular movements if you had difficulty answering this question.

Client needs category: Physiological integrity
Client needs subcategory: Physiological adaptation
Cognitive level: Analyzing

5. A nurse is comparing the neurological status of a client who suffered a head injury with the status on the previous shift. Using the Glasgow Coma Scale, the nurse determines that the client's score has changed from 11 to 15. Which of the following responses did the nurse assess in this client? Select all that apply.

☐ **1.** Spontaneous eye opening.
☐ **2.** Tachypnea, bradycardia, and hypotension.
☐ **3.** Unequal pupil size.
☐ **4.** Orientation to person, place, and time.
☐ **5.** Pain localization.
☐ **6.** Incomprehensible sounds.

Answer: 1, 4

Rationale: The Glasgow Coma Scale is a tool to assess a client's response to stimuli. To achieve a perfect score of 15 on the Glasgow Coma Scale, the client would have to open his eyes spontaneously (4), obey verbal commands (6), and be oriented to person, place, and time (5). Vital signs and pupil size are not assessed with the Glasgow Coma Scale. The ability to localize pain earns a motor response score of 5, not the top score of 6. Making incomprehensible sounds earns a verbal response score of 2, not a 5.

Test-taking strategy: Analyze to determine what information the question asks for, which is change or improvement in the client's neurological status. "Select all that apply" questions require considering each option to decide its merit. Recall that a perfect score of 15 would indicate normal neurological function. Review the Glasgow Coma Scale and neurological assessment techniques if you had difficulty answering this question.

Client needs category: Physiological integrity

Client needs subcategory: Physiological adaptation

Cognitive level: Analyzing

---

6. The nurse is educating a client and family about macular degeneration. Which photo would be utilized to best illustrate what these clients typically see?

☐ **1.**

☐ **2.**

☐ **3.**

☐ **4.**

Answer: 2

Rationale: Macular degeneration is a medical condition that typically affects the eyesight of older adults. The central vision is most affected in clients, thus revealing a blurred or distorted image in the middle of the visual field. Peripheral vision is usually maintained. The visual field is neither totally blurred nor completely clear.

Test-taking strategy: Analyze to determine what information the question asks for, which is the illustration that depicts a client's visual field. Recall that the macula is the center area of the retina, which provides the most detailed central vision. Degeneration in this area would compromise the center of the visual field. Review the symptoms of macular degeneration if you had difficulty answering this question.

Client needs category: Physiological integrity

Client needs subcategory: Physiological adaptation

Cognitive level: Analyzing

7. A nurse is caring for a client with a T5 complete spinal cord injury. Upon assessment, the nurse notes flushed skin, diaphoresis above T5, and blood pressure of 162/96 mm Hg. The client reports a severe, pounding headache. Which nursing interventions would be appropriate for this client? Select all that apply.

☐ **1.** Elevate the head of the bed to 90°.
☐ **2.** Loosen constrictive clothing.
☐ **3.** Use a fan to reduce diaphoresis.
☐ **4.** Assess for bladder distention and bowel impaction.
☐ **5.** Administer antihypertensive medication.
☐ **6.** Place the client in a supine position with legs elevated.

Answer: 1, 2, 4, 5

Rationale: The client is exhibiting signs and symptoms of autonomic dysreflexia, a potentially life-threatening emergency caused by an uninhibited response from the sympathetic nervous system resulting from a lack of control over the autonomic nervous system. The nurse should immediately elevate the head of the bed to 90° and place the legs in a dependent position to decrease venous return to the heart and increase venous return from the brain. Because tactile stimuli can trigger autonomic dysreflexia, any constrictive clothing should be loosened. The nurse should also assess for distended bladder and bowel impaction—which may trigger autonomic dysreflexia—and correct any problems. Elevated blood pressure is the most life-threatening complication of autonomic dysreflexia because it can cause stroke, MI, or seizure activity. If removing the triggering event does not reduce the client's blood pressure, I.V. antihypertensives should be administered. A fan should not be used because a cold draft may trigger autonomic dysreflexia.

Test-taking strategy: Analyze to determine what information the question asks for, which is nursing interventions for a client exhibiting signs of autonomic dysreflexia. "Select all that apply" questions require considering each option to decide its merit. Recall that this syndrome particularly occurs in individuals with spinal cord injuries at the splanchnic sympathetic outflow (T5-T6) level. Review the pathophysiology of spinal cord injury and the clinical manifestations of complications such as autonomic dysreflexia if you had difficulty answering this question.

Client needs category: Physiological integrity

Client needs subcategory: Reduction of risk potential

Cognitive level: Analyzing

8. A nurse is preparing to teach students in a health class about hearing pathways. Place the following steps in chronological order to match how the nurse should describe the normal pathway of sound wave transmission and hearing to the class. Use all of the options.

1.	Interpretation of sound by the cerebral cortex.

2.	Transmission of vibrations through the hammer, anvil, and stirrup.

3.	Stimulation of nerve impulses in the inner ear.

4.	Transmission of vibrations to the auditory area of the cerebral cortex.

5.	Collection of the sound waves in the pinna.

Answer: 5, 2, 3, 4, 1

Rationale: Sound waves travel through the air and are collected by the pinna which is the visible portion of the outer ear. Vibrations transmit through the canal and bones of the hammer, anvil, and stirrup. Next, there is stimulation sending nerve impulses to the inner ear. The cochlear branch of the acoustic nerve transmits these vibrations to the auditory area of the cerebral cortex. The cerebral cortex then interprets the sound.

Test-taking strategy: Analyze to determine what information the question asks for, which is pathway of sound wave transmission. Critically think through movement of the sound waves from outside the body to the inner ear and then to the brain. Review the anatomy and physiology of the ear and the physiology of the nervous system related to hearing if you had difficulty answering this question.

Client needs category: Health promotion and maintenance

Client needs subcategory: None

Cognitive level: Understanding

9. A community nurse is leading a support group discussion on the progressive nature of multiple sclerosis (MS). Arrange the following degenerative changes in the order in which they occur. Use all of the options.

1.	Degeneration of axons.

2.	Demyelination throughout the central nervous system.

3.	Periodic and unpredictable exacerbations and remissions.

4.	Plaque formation that interrupts nerve impulses.

5.	The immune system attacks myelin.

Answer: 5, 2, 1, 4, 3

Rationale: MS is believed to be an autoimmune disease where the body perceives myelin to be a foreign agent and attacks it. MS produces patches of demyelination throughout the central nervous system, resulting in myelin loss from the axis cylinders and degeneration of the axons. Plaques form in the involved area and become sclerosed, interrupting the flow of nerve impulses and resulting in a variety of symptoms. Periodic and unpredictable exacerbations and remissions occur. The prognosis varies.

Test-taking strategy: Analyze to determine what information the question asks for, which is progressive changes in clients with MS. Consider how the disease originates and then progresses. If unsure, select the first and last in the sequence which leaves three selections to order. Review the pathophysiology of MS progression if you had difficulty answering this question.

Client needs category: Physiological integrity

Client needs subcategory: Physiological adaptation

Cognitive level: Applying

10. A nurse is monitoring a client's intracranial pressure (ICP) after a traumatic head injury. The physician calls and asks for a report on the client's condition. Based on the documentation below, how should the nurse respond?

Flow Sheet				
	0800	0805	0810	0815
ICP	20	18	18	16

☐ **1.** "The client's ICP remains elevated."
☐ **2.** "The client's ICP has decreased to lower than normal limits."
☐ **3.** "The client's ICP is within normal limits."
☐ **4.** "The client's ICP was elevated but now has returned to normal."

Answer: 1

Rationale: A normal ICP is between 0 and 15 mm Hg. The documentation shows pressures greater than 15 mm Hg.

Test-taking strategy: Analyze to determine what information the question asks for, which is interpretation of ICP data. Recall that ICP can normally be at 0 and then as high as 15. Memorization of the ICP parameter is essential for interpretation. Review normal values of ICP if you had difficulty answering this question.

Client needs category: Physiological integrity

Client needs subcategory: Reduction of risk potential

Cognitive level: Analyzing

---

11. A nurse is documenting a health assessment when the client states having problems with balance, as well as, fine and gross motor function. When collaborating with the health team, in which area on the illustration of the brain would the nurse highlight as an area of concern?

Answer:

Rationale: Note the placement of the X. The cerebellum is the portion of the brain that controls balance and fine and gross motor function. The cerebellum is located at the base of the skull and above the brain stem.

Test-taking strategy: Analyze to determine what information the question asks for, which is the area of the brain responsible for motor function. Once determined, locate the area on the illustration. Knowledge of anatomy and physiology of the brain is essential. Review the location and function of the lobes of the brain if you had difficulty answering this question.

Client needs category: Physiological integrity

Client needs subcategory: Physiological adaptation

Cognitive level: Analyzing

12. A nurse is performing a neurological assessment during a client's routine physical examination. To assess for a Babinski reflex, indicate the point where the nurse places the tongue blade to begin stroking the foot.

Answer:

Rationale: To test for a Babinski reflex, use a tongue blade to slowly stroke the side of the sole of the foot. Start at the heel and move toward the great toe. The normal response in an adult is plantar flexion of the toes. Upward movement of the great toe and fanning of the little toes—Babinski's reflex—is abnormal in clients over the age of 12 to 18 months.

Test-taking strategy: Analyze to determine what information the question asks for, which is the correct procedure to assess a Babinski reflex. Recall that reflexes are predictable, uncontrolled responses to stimuli which, in this case, are stroking the sole of the foot. Review the procedure to elicit a Babinski reflex if you had difficulty answering this question.

Client needs category: Health promotion and maintenance

Client needs subcategory: None

Cognitive level: Understanding

---

13. The nurse is caring for a client who is experiencing an exacerbation of gout. When providing instruction, which dietary modifications are stressed? Select all that apply.

- ☐ **1.** Eat a low-purine diet.
- ☐ **2.** Limit fluid intake to no more than 1 L/day.
- ☐ **3.** Eat a high-protein diet, with at least two servings of lean meat per day.
- ☐ **4.** Eat a high-purine diet.
- ☐ **5.** Limit alcohol intake.

Answer: 1, 5

Rationale: Gout is characterized by an abnormal metabolism of uric acid. Individuals either produce too much uric acid or their body is unable to metabolize and excrete it. Purines are metabolized into uric acid. The client who suffers from gout should be placed on a low-purine diet with foods such as peanut butter, cherries, rice, pasta, fruits, and vegetables. Fluids do not have to be limited. Alcohol intake should be limited as it is thought to trigger an exacerbation.

Test-taking strategy: Analyze to determine what information the question asks for, which is dietary modifications for a client with gout. "Select all that apply" questions require considering each option to decide its merit. Consider dietary modifications that relate to the production of uric acid and relate to a low-purine diet. Review dietary modifications, especially purines, if you had difficulty answering this question.

Client needs category: Physiological integrity

Client needs subcategory: Basic care and comfort

Cognitive level: Applying

14. The nurse is caring for a client who is scheduled to undergo a computerized tomography (CT) scan to assess recent symptoms of muscle weakness and tingling in the extremities. Which information should the nurse include in a preprocedural teaching plan? Select all that apply.

- ☐ **1.** The test requires standing alone without assistance.
- ☐ **2.** A contrast dye may be given before the test.
- ☐ **3.** Throat irritation and facial flushing may occur if contrast dye is used.
- ☐ **4.** All medications must be withheld for 12 hours prior to the procedure.
- ☐ **5.** The CT scan is considered an invasive procedure, but not dangerous.
- ☐ **6.** It is necessary to report any known allergies to iodine or seafood prior to the procedure.

Answer: 2, 3, 6

Rationale: The nurse should inform the client who is scheduled to undergo a CT scan that a contrast medium may be administered before the procedure and that the dye can cause throat irritation and facial flushing. Because the dye is iodine based, it is essential for the client to report any known allergies to iodine or seafood before testing begins. The CT scan is not invasive or dangerous. The client will need to lie still (not stand) during the procedure and will not be able to take routine medications for 24 hours beforehand.

Test-taking strategies: Analyze to determine what information the question asks for, which is teaching prior to a CT scan. "Select all that apply" questions require considering each option to decide its merit. The key word is "preprocedural" meaning preparation/teaching for the CT scan. Review procedure guidelines for a CT scan if you had difficulty answering this question.

Client needs category: Physiological integrity

Client needs subcategory: Reduction of risk potential

Cognitive level: Applying

---

15. A nurse is caring for a client, diagnosed with Alzheimer's disease, who scored a 7 (High risk) on the Hendrich II Fall Risk Model. Which nursing interventions should the nurse implement? Select all that apply.

1. Implement a bed alarm.
2. Request a low-dose sedative.
3. Instruct the client to ask for help before ambulating.
4. Maintain the bed in the lowest position.
5. Offer toileting every 2 to 3 hours.
6. Advise family to notify staff when leaving.

Answer: 1, 4, 5, 6

Rationale: Preventing a client from falling and causing further illness or injury is a role of the nurse. The Hendrich II Fall Risk Model is used in some acute care facilities to determine the potential for a fall. Assessment of a client's fall risk is a National Patient Safety Goal set by the Joint Commission and should be completed on admission. Nursing interventions such as implementing a bed alarm, maintaining the bed in the lowest position, offering toileting, and having the family notify staff when leaving are all appropriate nursing interventions to prevent falls. Sedating a client using chemical restraints is a last resort. Instructing a client to ask for help before ambulating is not effective in a client with Alzheimer's disease who will have difficulty remembering the instructions.

Test-taking strategy: Analyze to determine what information the question asks for, which is nursing interventions to prevent falls. "Select all that apply" questions require considering each option to decide its merit. When considering fall risk, think "safety." Always consider client-specific interventions when developing a plan of care. Due to this client diagnosis, following instructions will be limited. Review fall precautions if you had difficulty answering this question.

Client needs category: Physiological integrity

Client needs subcategory: Reduction of risk potential

Cognitive level: Applying

16. A client is scheduled to undergo cerebral angiography to allow for examination of the cerebral arteries. Place the following interventions in the order in which the nurse would perform them. Use all of the options.

1. Administer antianxiety medication if ordered.

2. Ask the client about allergies to iodine, seafood, or radiopaque dyes.

3. Make sure the client has signed an informed consent form.

4. Maintain the affected extremity in straight alignment for 6 hours as ordered.

5. Encourage the client to verbalize questions about the procedure.

Answer: 5, 3, 2, 1, 4

Rationale: It is important to provide the client with an opportunity to ask questions about the procedure before obtaining informed consent. The nurse should ask about allergies to iodine, seafood, or radiopaque dyes because the procedure uses an iodine-based contrast medium. This should be done before administering antianxiety medication to the client. After the procedure, the affected extremity should be maintained in straight alignment for 6 hours.

Test-taking strategy: Analyze to determine what information the question asks for, which is ordered nursing actions before and after a cerebral angiography. When caring for a client prior to a procedure think "consent and special preparation" and after the procedure think "assessment and special considerations." Consider which interventions would be completed before others. Review the nursing interventions related to cerebral angiography if you had difficulty answering this question.

Client needs category: Physiological integrity

Client needs subcategory: Reduction of risk potential

Cognitive level: Applying

Gastrointestinal Disorders

1. A nurse is reviewing the function of the gastrointestinal (GI) tract and causes of gastroesophageal reflux disease with a client. Illustrate on the diagram the location of the structure that prevents the food from moving backward up the esophagus.

Answer:

Rationale: An X is placed on the lower esophageal sphincter which is a ring of muscle fibers that prevents food from moving backward from the stomach into the esophagus. If this sphincter does not close well, food, fluids, and stomach contents can irritate and even damage the esophagus.

Test-taking strategy: Analyze to determine what information the question asks for, which is the location of the structure preventing stomach backflow. Consider that this structure would need to be located at the junction between the stomach and the esophagus. Review the anatomy of the GI system and the pathophysiology of the disorder if you had difficulty answering this question.

Client needs category: Health promotion and maintenance

Client needs subcategory: None

Cognitive level: Understanding

2. As part of a routine screening for colorectal cancer, a client must undergo fecal occult blood testing. Which foods should the nurse instruct the client to avoid for 48 to 72 hours before the test and throughout the collection period? Select all that apply.

☐ **1.** High-fiber foods.
☐ **2.** Red meat.
☐ **3.** Turnips.
☐ **4.** Cantaloupe.
☐ **5.** Tomatoes.
☐ **6.** Peas.

Answer: 2, 3, 4

Rationale: The client should avoid red meat, poultry, and fish as well as beets, broccoli, cauliflower, horseradish, mushrooms, and turnips. Such fruits as cantaloupe, melons, and grapefruit are also prohibited. Tomatoes and peas are acceptable. The client should be taught to maintain a high-fiber diet in order to promote colonic emptying time and fecal bulk, which aid in obtaining specimens.

Test-taking strategy: Analyze to determine what information the question asks for, which is food to avoid when having fecal occult blood testing. "Select all that apply" questions require considering each option to decide its merit. Consider that the examination tests for blood in the stool so any introduction of the blood into the GI system or irritation could cause a positive result. Also, certain food alters the test, so an understanding of the diet is essential. Review the preparation for fecal occult blood test and the role of foods in the digestive tract if you had difficulty answering the question.

Client needs category: Health promotion and maintenance

Client needs subcategory: None

Cognitive level: Applying

---

3. A client returns from the operating room after undergoing extensive abdominal surgery. The client is receiving 1,000 mL of lactated Ringer's solution via a central line infusion. The physician orders the I.V. fluid to be infused at 125 mL/hour plus the total output of the previous hour. The drip factor of the tubing is 15 gtt/mL and the output for the previous hour was 75 mL via Foley catheter, 50 mL via nasogastric tube, and 10 mL via Jackson Pratt tube. For how many drops (gtt) per minute should the nurse set the I.V. flow rate to deliver the correct amount of fluid? Record your answer as a whole number.

_____ gtt/minute

Answer: 65

Rationale: First, calculate the volume to be infused (in milliliters):

75 mL + 50 mL + 10 mL = 135 mL total output for the previous hour

135 mL + 125 mL ordered as a constant flow = 260 mL to be infused over the next hour.

Next, use the formula:

Volume to be infused/total minutes to be infused × drop factor = drops/minute.

In this case:

260 mL/60 minutes × 15 gtt/mL = 65 gtt/minute.

Test-taking strategy: Analyze to determine what information the question asks for, which is I.V. flow rate in drops/minute. Carefully read and calculate the volume to be infused per physician's order. Proofread your work. Next, use the standard formula calculating drip factors. Review calculation of drip rates if you had difficulty answering this question.

Client needs category: Physiological integrity

Client needs subcategory: Pharmacological therapies

Cognitive level: Analyzing

4. A nurse is caring for a client with a retroperitoneal abscess who is receiving gentamicin 300 mg I.V. every 8 hours. Which client data should the nurse monitor? Select all that apply.

☐ **1.** Hearing.
☐ **2.** Urine output.
☐ **3.** HCT.
☐ **4.** BUN and serum creatinine levels.
☐ **5.** Serum calcium level.
☐ **6.** Muscle tone.

Answer: 1, 2, 4

Rationale: Adverse effects of gentamicin include ototoxicity and nephrotoxicity; consequently, the nurse must monitor the client's hearing and instruct to report any hearing loss or tinnitus. Signs of nephrotoxicity include decreased urine output and elevated BUN and serum creatinine levels. Gentamicin does not affect the serum calcium level, HCT, or muscle tone.

Test-taking strategy: Analyze to determine what information the question asks for, which is client data which could indicate a concern. "Select all that apply" questions require considering each option to decide its merit. Recall that a peak and trough is needed to monitor therapeutic drug levels as the medication has a narrow drug index. Consider what information could be obtained from each option. Review common side effects and potential toxicity of the classification of aminoglycosides if you had difficulty answering this question.

Client needs category: Physiological integrity
Client needs subcategory: Pharmacological therapies
Cognitive level: Analyzing

---

5. A nurse is assessing the abdomen of a client who was admitted to the emergency department with suspected appendicitis. Identify the area of the abdomen that the nurse should palpate last.

Answer:

Rationale: An acute attack of appendicitis localizes as pain and tenderness in the lower right quadrant, midway between the umbilicus and the crest of the ilium. This area should be palpated last in order to determine if pain is also present in other areas of the abdomen.

Test-taking strategy: Analyze to determine what information the question asks for, which is area of the abdomen to palpate last when appendicitis is suspected. Recall that the classic sign of appendicitis is a pain when palpation and release (rebound tenderness) occurs over McBurney's point in the right lower quadrant. Since this is the classic sign, palpate last to differentiate between the other areas of the abdomen. Review the anatomy of the abdomen and review abdominal assessment techniques, if you had difficulty answering this question.

Client needs category: Physiological integrity
Client needs subcategory: Physiological adaptation
Cognitive level: Applying

6. While preparing a client for an upper GI endoscopy (esophagogastroduodenoscopy), the nurse would be correct to implement which intervention? Select all that apply.

☐ **1.** Administer a preparation to cleanse the GI tract, such as Golytely or Fleets Phospho-Soda.

☐ **2.** Instruct not to eat or drink for 6 to 12 hours before the procedure.

☐ **3.** Teach only to ingest a clear liquid diet for 24 hours before the procedure.

☐ **4.** Inform the client of receiving a sedative before the procedure.

☐ **5.** Encourage the client to eat and drink immediately after the procedure.

Answer: 2, 4

Rationale: The client should not eat or drink for 6 to 12 hours before the procedure to ensure that the upper GI tract is clear for viewing. Before the endoscope is inserted, the client will receive a sedative that will help in relaxation, but leave conscious. GI tract cleansing and a clear liquid diet are interventions for a client having a lower GI tract procedure, such as a colonoscopy. Food and fluids must be withheld until the gag reflex returns after the procedure.

Test-taking strategy: Analyze to determine what information the question asks for, which is nursing interventions prior to an upper GI endoscopy. "Select all that apply" questions require considering each option to decide its merit. When caring for a client prior to a procedure think "special preparation" or protocol to be followed. Review client safety and GI tract preparation, and review pre- and postendoscopy nursing interventions if you had difficulty answering this question.

Client needs category: Physiological integrity

Client needs subcategory: Reduction of risk potential

Cognitive level: Applying

---

7. A nurse is caring for a client who recently had a bowel resection. The client has a hemoglobin level of 8 g/dL and HCT of 30%. Dextrose 5% in half-normal saline solution ($D_5\frac{1}{2}NS$) is infusing through a triple-lumen central catheter at 125 mL/hour. The physician's orders include:

- gentamicin 80 mg I.V. piggyback in 50 mL D_5W over 30 minutes
- ranitidine (Zantac) 50 mg I.V. in 50 mL D_5W piggyback over 30 minutes
- one unit of 250 mL of packed red blood cells (RBCs) over 3 hours
- nasogastric tube flushes with 30 mL of normal saline solution every 2 hours.

How many milliliters should the nurse document as the total intake for the 8-hour shift? Record your answer as a whole number.

_____ mL

Answer: 1,470

Rationale: Add up the total intake as follows:

I.V. of $D_5\frac{1}{2}NS$ at 125 mL × 8 hours = 1,000 mL

gentamicin piggyback = 50 mL

ranitidine piggyback = 50 mL

packed RBCs = 250 mL

+ nasogastric flushes 30 mL × 4 = 120 mL
_____
Total = 1,470 mL.

Test-taking strategy: Analyze to determine what information the question asks for, which is total intake in milliliters for an 8-hour shift. Carefully read all information provided and align in columns the addition equation to decrease the chance of a calculation error. Proofread your calculation.

Client needs category: Physiological integrity

Client needs subcategory: Physiological adaptation

Cognitive level: Analyzing

8. A nurse is caring for a client with history of chronic intestinal irritation. The client asks, "Is there any type of colostomy where I would not need a continuous colostomy bag?" Indicate the location where a client could have an ostomy that eventually might not require wearing an ostomy bag.

Answer:

Rationale: With a sigmoid colostomy, the feces are solid; therefore, the client might eventually gain enough control and not need to wear a colostomy bag. With a descending colostomy, the feces are semi-soft. With a transverse colostomy, the feces are soft. With an ascending colostomy, the feces are fluid. In these three latter cases, the client would be unlikely to gain control of elimination and consequently would need to continue wearing an ostomy bag.

Test-taking strategy: Analyze to determine what information the question asks for, which is site where a client may not continuously need to wear an ostomy bag. Think of how a person with a colostomy could mimic a normal bowel movement. Consider the path and contents of the colon to determine proper placement. Review the anatomy of the GI system and review ostomy care if you had difficulty answering this question.

Client needs category: Physiological integrity

Client needs subcategory: Basic care and comfort

Cognitive level: Applying

9. A nurse is calling report to the medical–surgical (med-surge) floor staff regarding a client with acute diverticulitis. Which symptoms does the med-surge nurse anticipate? Select all that apply.

- ☐ **1.** Vomiting.
- ☐ **2.** Cramping pain in the left lower abdominal quadrant.
- ☐ **3.** Bowel irregularity.
- ☐ **4.** Heartburn.
- ☐ **5.** Intervals of diarrhea.
- ☐ **6.** Hiccuping.

Answer: 2, 3, 5

Rationale: Acute diverticulitis is a common digestive disease typically found in the large intestine. Signs and symptoms of acute diverticulitis include bowel irregularity, intervals of diarrhea, abrupt onset of cramping pain in the left lower abdomen, and a low-grade fever. Vomiting, heartburn, and hiccuping are not signs of the disorder.

Test-taking strategy: Analyze to determine what information the question asks for, which is signs of acute diverticulitis. "Select all that apply" questions require considering each option to decide its merit. Recall that diverticulitis occurs from an outpouching on the colon which becomes inflamed and symptoms correspond. Review the pathophysiology of diverticulitis and related signs and symptoms if you had difficulty answering this question.

Client needs category: Physiological integrity

Client needs subcategory: Physiological adaptation

Cognitive level: Applying

---

10. A client is admitted with inflammatory bowel syndrome (Crohn's disease). Which nursing measures would be included in the client's care plan? Select all that apply.

- ☐ **1.** Lactulose therapy.
- ☐ **2.** High-fiber diet.
- ☐ **3.** High-protein milkshakes.
- ☐ **4.** Corticosteroid therapy.
- ☐ **5.** Antidiarrheal medications.

Answer: 4, 5

Rationale: Inflammatory bowel syndrome (Crohn's disease) is an inflammatory bowel disease caused by inflammation to the lining of the digestive tract which can lead to abdominal pain, severe diarrhea, and even malnutrition. Corticosteroids such as prednisone reduce the signs and symptoms of diarrhea, pain, and bleeding by decreasing inflammation. Antidiarrheals such as diphenoxylate (Lomotil) combat diarrhea by decreasing peristalsis. Lactulose is used to treat chronic constipation and would aggravate the symptoms of Crohn's disease. A high-fiber diet and milk and milk products are contraindicated in clients with Crohn's disease because they may promote diarrhea.

Test-taking strategy: Analyze to determine what information the question asks for, which is nursing measures in the plan of care. First, consider measures to decrease inflammation in the bowel. Next, consider nursing measures to treat the symptoms. "Select all that apply" questions require considering each option to decide its merit. Review the pathophysiology and treatment of Crohn's disease and focus on clinical manifestations and nursing interventions if you had difficulty answering this question.

Client needs category: Safe and effective care environment

Client needs subcategory: Coordinated care

Cognitive level: Applying

11. The nurse is caring for a client admitted with cirrhosis of the liver. Which laboratory results are consistent with the disease process? Select all that apply.

- ☐ **1.** Prothrombin time 22 seconds.
- ☐ **2.** Potassium 4.0 mEq/L
- ☐ **3.** Albumin 7.2 g/dL.
- ☐ **4.** Ammonia 96 μg/dL.
- ☐ **5.** Platelets 75,000 cells/mm³.
- ☐ **6.** Amylase 250 units/L.

Answer: 1, 4, 5

Rationale: The client with cirrhosis has liver dysfunction and impaired coagulation and rising ammonia levels. The prothrombin time is prolonged (normal is 9.5 to 11.0 seconds), and the platelet count is low (normal is 150,000 to 450,000 cells/mm³). A normal ammonia level is 35 to 65 μg/dL, and this client's level is elevated, placing the client at risk for hepatic encephalopathy. A client with cirrhosis typically has hypokalemia because of the diuretic therapy used to treat the fluid retention associated with the disease. Here, the potassium level is within normal limits (3.8 to 5.5 mEq/L). In cirrhosis, the albumin level is also typically low (normal is 3.4 to 5.0 g/dL) due to alterations in protein metabolism in the liver. Levels of amylase, a pancreatic enzyme, typically increase with pancreatitis, not cirrhosis (normal level is 25 to 151 units/L).

Test-taking strategy: Analyze to determine what information the question asks for, which is laboratory values consistent with a diagnosis of cirrhosis of the liver. "Select all that apply" questions require considering each option to decide its merit. First, consider that laboratory values would be elevated in the client with liver dysfunction. Next, consider the impact of other organs and the corresponding lab values. Review the pathophysiology of cirrhosis and focus on normal and abnormal laboratory values if you had difficulty answering this question.

Client needs category: Physiological integrity

Client needs subcategory: Reduction of risk potential

Cognitive level: Analyzing

12. The nurse is evaluating how a client with hepatitis A understands the discharge teaching given. Which client statements indicate that further teaching is needed? Select all that apply.

- ☐ **1.** "I can have an occasional glass of wine with my meal as I recover."
- ☐ **2.** "My family and I do not need to take any special precautions as long as I take my medication."
- ☐ **3.** "My bath towels shouldn't be used by any other family members."
- ☐ **4.** "My family members should receive the hepatitis A vaccine to prevent them from getting the disease."
- ☐ **5.** "My spouse and I can have intercourse and kiss."
- ☐ **6.** "I should wear a mask when visitors come."

Answer: 1, 2, 5, 6

Rationale: Hepatitis A is inflammation (irritation and swelling) of the liver from the hepatitis A virus. The hepatitis A virus is found mostly in the blood and stools of the infected person. Clients with hepatitis should abstain from alcohol to prevent exacerbation of the disease. Standard precautions and meticulous hand washing should be practiced by all family members. All family members should avoid close contact with the client; this includes avoiding intercourse, kissing, and the use of any personal items (such as bath towels and eating utensils) that may be contaminated with the client's feces. Because hepatitis A is transmitted by the oral–fecal route, not the respiratory route, wearing a mask is not necessary. The hepatitis A vaccine should be given prophylactically to all family members and close contacts to prevent disease transmission.

Test-taking strategy: Analyze to determine what information the question asks for, which is a client statement that indicates the need for further teaching. "Select all that apply" questions require considering each option to decide its merit. When appraising each option, look for an incorrect statement in need of further teaching. Consider the nature of the illness and mode of transmission. Review the pathophysiology and transmission route for hepatitis A if you had difficulty answering this question.

Client needs category: Health promotion and maintenance

Client needs subcategory: None

Cognitive level: Applying

13. At the beginning of the shift, the nurse is assigned a client with an ascending colostomy. Which picture identifies the correct placement where the nurse will assess the stoma?

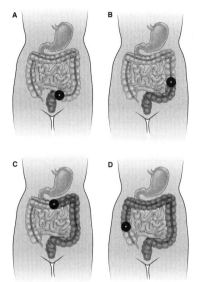

Answer: D

Rationale: A colostomy can be performed along any site of the colon. The location of an ascending colostomy is on the right side of the abdomen. An ostomy located in the ascending colon would likely produce continuous liquid output because feces in this section contain the most water and, therefore, have a liquid consistency. A sigmoid colostomy is located on the sigmoid colon and located close to the location of a descending colostomy in the left side of the abdomen. The transverse colostomy is horizontal across middle abdomen or toward the right side of the body across the abdomen.

Test-taking strategy: Analyze to determine what information the question asks for, which is the location of an ascending colostomy. Recall that a colostomy is a surgical procedure, which brings the colon out along various locations on the abdominal wall. Note that identifying the placement uses anatomical position when reporting right and left locations. Review information on various types of colostomies if you had difficulty answering this question.

Client needs category: Physiological integrity

Client needs subcategory: Physiological adaptation

Cognitive level: Applying

---

14. A client has been admitted to the emergency department with severe right upper quadrant pain. Based on the signs and symptoms and laboratory data documented in the chart below, the nurse would expect the client to have which diagnosis?

Progress Notes	
03/12/10 0730	Client admitted to the emergency department with severe right upper quadrant pain radiating to the back, nausea and vomiting, and fever. Laboratory results received via telephone as follows: glucose 462 mg/dL, WBC 14,000 cells/mm³, lipase 214 units/L, and calcium 6.5 mg/dL.————Andrea Nichols, LPN

☐ **1.** Peptic ulcer.
☐ **2.** Crohn's disease.
☐ **3.** Pancreatitis.
☐ **4.** Irritable bowel syndrome.

Answer: 3

Rationale: The assessment findings combined with the laboratory results suggest pancreatitis. Signs and symptoms of pancreatitis include severe right upper quadrant pain, fever, nausea, and vomiting. Inflammation of the pancreas results in leukocytosis. Injured β-cells are unable to produce insulin, leading to hyperglycemia, which may be as high as 500 to 900 mg/dL. Lipase and amylase levels become elevated as the pancreatic enzymes leak from injured pancreatic cells. Calcium becomes trapped as fat necrosis occurs, leading to hypocalcemia. Peptic ulcer, Crohn's disease, and irritable bowel syndrome do not cause amylase or lipase levels to increase.

Test-taking strategy: Analyze to determine what information the question asks for, which is a potential medical diagnosis obtained through assessment data. Utilize the data to provide clues to potential disorders. Begin with subjective data as reported by the client and next consider objective data such as laboratory values. Relate to signs and symptoms of options. Review various disorders with severe right upper quadrant pain if you had difficulty answering this question.

Client needs category: Physiological integrity

Client needs subcategory: Reduction of risk potential

Cognitive level: Analyzing

15. The nurse is preparing to administer a 75% strength tube-feeding formula. The full-strength formula is available. To prepare 500 mL of feeding, the nurse should plan to dilute how many milliliters of the full-strength formula with water? Record your answer as a whole number.

_____ mL

Answer: 375

Rationale: To determine the amount of formula to use, multiply the 500 mL of full-strength formula by 75% (0.75):

$$500 \text{ mL} \times 0.75 = 375 \text{ mL}.$$

Test-taking strategy: Analyze to determine what information the question asks for, which is the amount of formula to fluid ratio to administer a 75% concentration. Consider that a 75% concentration is less than 1; thus, multiplying by a 0.75 is correct. Review dosage calculations based on percentages if you had difficulty answering this question.

Client needs category: Physiological integrity

Client needs subcategory: Pharmacological therapies

Cognitive level: Applying

---

16. The nurse is assisting a client to ambulate following a bowel resection for diverticulitis. Suddenly, the client complains of sharp abdominal pain. The nurse assesses the client and determines the wound has eviscerated. Prioritize the following nursing actions in chronological order to show how the nurse should respond. Use all of the options.

1. Assess the client's response.
2. Call for assistance from other nursing personnel.
3. Cover the wound with sterile, nonadherent dressing moistened with sterile normal saline solution.
4. Document the incident, including the client's condition.
5. Place the client in low Fowler's position.

Answer: 2, 5, 3, 1, 4

Rationale: When evisceration of an abdominal wound occurs, the nurse should remain with the client and summon help to bring necessary supplies to the client's room. The client should be placed in low Fowler's position to lessen tension on the abdomen. The nurse should not attempt to reinsert protruding organs. Instead, the nurse should moisten sterile, nonadherent dressings with warm, sterile normal saline solution and cover the wound. It is important to conduct an ongoing client assessment until the surgeon arrives because the client is at risk for shock. Documentation of the incident and the client's condition should be completed immediately after the incident.

Test-taking strategy: Analyze to determine what information the question asks for, which is nursing care when an evisceration occurs. When prioritizing, think "safety" first. Next, focus on nursing interventions related to postoperative wound dehiscence. Lastly, document as soon as possible. Review emergency care protocols related to a wound evisceration if you had difficulty answering this question.

Client needs category: Physiological integrity

Client needs subcategory: Physiological adaptation

Cognitive level: Analyzing

Genitourinary Disorders

1. The licensed practical nurse is collaborating with the registered nurse validating a test dose of mannitol solution I.V. for a client with marked oliguria. The ordered test dose is 0.2 g/kg of 15% mannitol solution I.V. The client weighs 132 lb. How many grams should the nurse administered? Record your answer as a whole number.

_____ g

Answer: 12

Rationale: First, convert the client's weight from pounds to kilograms:

132 lb ÷ 2.2 kg/lb = 60 kg.

Then, to calculate the number of grams to administer, multiply the ordered number of grams by the client's weight in kilograms:

0.2 g/kg × 60 kg = 12 g.

Test-taking strategy: Analyze to determine what information the question asks for, which is the number of grams of mannitol to administer according to the client's weight. Recall that many doses are calculated according to unit dosage (mg, g, mL, etc.) per kilogram. Be careful that the unit dosage is consistent with what the question is asking. Review I.V. calculations and weight dosing if you had difficulty answering this question.

Client needs category: Physiological integrity

Client needs subcategory: Pharmacological therapies

Cognitive level: Applying

2. A nurse is obtaining a health history from a male senior citizen. The client states that he is having urinary hesitancy, slight dysuria, and dribbling. He denies complaints of hematuria. Identify the area where the nurse anticipates the primary cause of the urinary dysfunction.

Answer:

Rationale: Note that the X is over the prostate gland. The walnut-sized prostate gland lies beneath the bladder and surrounds the urethra. When the prostate gland becomes enlarged, which commonly occurs as a male ages, urination becomes affected as the prostate gland narrows the passage of urine through the urethra.

Test-taking strategy: Analyze to determine what information the question asks for, which is location of the cause of the urinary dysfunction. Look to the symptoms and note the age of the client for clues of the cause of the urinary problems. Review the anatomy of the male genitourinary system if you had difficulty answering this question.

Client needs category: Physiological integrity

Client needs subcategory: Physiological adaptation

Cognitive level: Applying

---

3. After a retropubic prostatectomy, a client needs continuous bladder irrigation. The client has an I.V. line with dextrose in 5% water infusing at 40 mL/hour and a triple-lumen urinary catheter with normal saline solution infusing at 200 mL/hour. The nurse empties the urinary catheter drainage bag three times during an 8-hour period for a total of 2,780 mL. How many milliliters should the nurse calculate as urine? Record your answer as a whole number.

_____ mL

Answer: 1,180

Rationale: During 8 hours, 1,600 mL of bladder irrigant has been infused (200 mL × 8 hours = 1,600 mL/8 hours). The nurse should subtract this amount from the total volume in the drainage bag to determine the urine output (2,780 mL – 1,600 mL = 1,180 mL).

Test-taking strategy: Analyze to determine what information the question asks for, which is the amount of urine production in an 8-hour shift. Focus on the output and disregard extraneous information of the I.V. Note that finding the urine amount comes from the total amount of urine minus the amount of bladder irrigation. Proofread your math calculation. Review the methods for calculating urinary elimination with bladder irrigation if you had difficulty answering this question.

Client needs category: Physiological integrity

Client needs subcategory: Basic care and comfort

Cognitive level: Applying

4. A nurse is caring for a client with chronic renal failure. The laboratory results indicate hypocalcemia and hyperphosphatemia. When assessing the client, the nurse should be alert for which occurrence? Select all that apply.

☐ **1.** Trousseau's sign.
☐ **2.** Cardiac arrhythmias.
☐ **3.** Constipation.
☐ **4.** Decreased clotting time.
☐ **5.** Drowsiness and lethargy.
☐ **6.** Fractures.

Answer: 1, 2, 6

Rationale: Chronic renal failure is the slow process of losing kidney function over time. At some point, the kidney will not be able to remove excess fluid and wastes from the body causing fluid and electrolyte complications. Hypocalcemia is a calcium deficit that causes nerve fiber irritability and repetitive muscle spasms. Signs and symptoms of hypocalcemia include Trousseau's sign, cardiac arrhythmias, diarrhea, increased clotting times, anxiety, and irritability. The calcium–phosphorus imbalance leads to brittle bones and pathologic fractures. Drowsiness and lethargy are not typically associated with hypercalcemia.

Test-taking strategy: Analyze to determine what information the question asks for, which is complications resulting from hypocalcemia and hyperphosphatemia. "Select all that apply" questions require considering each option to decide its merit. Consider the effects of calcium and phosphate in the system and relate complications when there is an alteration of too much or too little. Review the signs and symptoms of hypocalcemia and hyperphosphatemia, and review fluids and electrolyte imbalances if you had difficulty answering this question.

Client needs category: Physiological integrity

Client needs subcategory: Reduction of risk potential

Cognitive level: Applying

5. A nurse is explaining menstruation to a class of junior high girls. The nurse creates a fun activity to determine if the teaching was successful. Place the pathophysiologic steps of the menstrual cycle listed below in the correct sequential order. Use all of the options.

1. The level of estrogen in the blood peaks.
2. Peak endometrial thickening occurs.
3. Increased estrogen and progesterone levels inhibit luteinizing hormone.
4. The top layer of the endometrium breaks down and sloughs.
5. A follicle matures and ovulation occurs.
6. The endometrium begins thickening.

Answer: 4, 6, 1, 5, 2, 3

Rationale: The menstrual cycle begins with the first day of menstruation, when the top layer of endometrium breaks down and begins to slough off. As the endometrium thickens, the level of estrogen in the blood begins to rise and eventually peak. The follicle matures and ovulation occurs when estrogen levels peak. After ovulation, the endometrium continues to thicken to its peak level. Increased estrogen and progesterone levels inhibit follicle-stimulating hormone, which causes a feedback loop that then decreases estrogen and progesterone production. This causes the top layer of the endometrium to break down and slough, restarting the cycle in a nonpregnant female.

Test-taking strategy: Analyze to determine what information the question asks for, which is the order of events occurring during the menstrual cycle. Carefully read each option. It can be helpful to select the first in the series and last in the series allowing a narrowing of middle options. Also, it is important to recognize that the menstrual cycle begins with the first day of menstruation. Review normal growth and development and the menstrual cycle if you had difficulty answering this question.

Client needs category: Health promotion and maintenance

Client needs subcategory: None

Cognitive level: Applying

---

6. A client requires behavioral therapies to decrease or eliminate urinary incontinence. Which procedures would the nurse expect to include in the teaching plan for this client? Select all that apply.

☐ **1.** Kegel exercises.
☐ **2.** Prompted voiding.
☐ **3.** External catheters.
☐ **4.** Biofeedback.
☐ **5.** Self-catheterization devices.
☐ **6.** Post void residual monitoring.

Answer: 1, 2, 4

Rationale: Clients, particularly females, have conditions relating to alterations in urinary output. Kegel exercises, prompted voiding, and biofeedback are behavioral therapies used to decrease or eliminate urinary incontinence. Both external catheters and self-catheterization devices are used to collect urine. Post void residual monitoring assesses the ability to empty the bladder but does not decrease or eliminate urinary incontinence.

Test-taking strategy: Analyze to determine what information the question asks for, which is behavioral therapies to eliminate urinary incontinence. "Select all that apply" questions require considering each option to decide its merit. The key term is "behavioral therapies," providing a clue that it is teaching that provides the client control over the urinary condition. Review bladder training techniques if you had difficulty answering this question.

Client needs category: Health promotion and maintenance

Client needs subcategory: None

Cognitive level: Applying

7. A nurse is explaining self-catheterization to a female client who has been diagnosed with urogenic bladder. Which instructions should the nurse include in the teaching? Select all that apply.

☐ **1.** Tampons may remain in place during menstruation.

☐ **2.** The meatus should be cleaned with a towelette or soapy washcloth and then rinsed.

☐ **3.** Sterile technique is not required.

☐ **4.** A new intermittent catheterization set should be used each time.

☐ **5.** Finding the urinary meatus always requires visualization with a mirror.

Answer: 2, 3

Rationale: Cleaning the meatus with a towelette or soapy washcloth decreases the risk of introducing bacteria into the bladder. Sterile technique is not required during self-catheterization. Leaving a tampon in place can restrict the urethra and impede catheter insertion. It is not necessary to use a new intermittent catheter each time; washing the catheter and allowing it to air-dry after each use is usually sufficient. The urinary meatus can be found using visual or tactile techniques.

Test-taking strategy: Analyze to determine what information the question asks for, which is key points in self-catheterization. "Select all that apply" questions require considering each option to decide its merit. Focus on clean versus sterile technique during catheterization instruction. Review catheter care and self-catheterization technique if you had difficulty answering this question.

Client needs category: Health promotion and maintenance

Client needs subcategory: None

Cognitive level: Applying

8. The nurse is reviewing a client's urine culture and sensitivity test results. Which findings would the nurse expect to see in normal urine? Select all that apply.

☐ **1.** Ketones.

☐ **2.** Protein.

☐ **3.** White blood cells.

☐ **4.** Crystals.

☐ **5.** Nitrates.

☐ **6.** Bilirubin.

Answer: 2, 3

Rationale: A urine culture is a test to detect and identify organisms, such as bacteria and components, within the urine. Information obtained can identify a urinary tract infection, kidney disease, or high blood glucose. Small amounts of protein and white blood cells are normal. Ketones, crystals, nitrates, and bilirubin are all abnormal findings.

Test-taking strategy: Analyze to determine what information the question asks for, which is findings in normal urine. "Select all that apply" questions require considering each option to decide its merit. Recall what information is reported in a urine culture and what information reported would be abnormal. Note that white blood cells are found in even normal cultures such as they are in normal complete blood counts. Review normal urinalysis findings and other routine urinalysis and laboratory tests if you had difficulty answering this question.

Client needs category: Physiological integrity

Client needs subcategory: Physiological adaptation

Cognitive level: Understanding

9. A nurse is assessing a client with right flank pain, fever, and chills. A urine culture is obtained, and a diagnosis of suspected right pyelonephritis is documented. When instructing the client on the diagnosis, the nurse uses a diagram of the urinary structures. Identify with an X the area associated with the diagnosis.

Answer

Rationale: Pyelonephritis is a type of urinary tract infection that affects one or both kidneys. Right pyelonephritis is on the right side of the client's body but would be documented on the left in the anatomical position. Bacteria and viruses can move to the kidneys from the bladder or can be carried from other body systems through the blood stream causing the disease process.

Test-taking strategy: Analyze to determine what information the question asks for, which is the site of right pyelonephritis. If unsure, use medical terminology to determine the site (nephro = kidney). Review the names and locations of urinary structures if you had difficulty answering this question.

Client needs category: Physiological integrity

Client needs subcategory: Physiological adaptation

Cognitive level: Understanding

10. A nurse is providing health teaching on female sexuality and provides illustration for education on the female anatomy. When discussing problems with sexual excitation, the nurse is correct to indicate which site as the area of sexual stimulation?

Answer:

Rationale: Sexual excitement causes various physiological changes in the female body. The area associated with sexual stimulation is located near the vaginal entrance and behind the labia minora. The clitoris is directly associated with engorgement and climax.

Test-taking strategy: Analyze to determine what information the question asks for, which is a site of female sexual stimulation. Review the anatomy of the female reproductive system and female sexuality if you had difficulty answering this question.

Client needs category: Health promotion and maintenance

Client needs subcategory: None

Cognitive level: Remembering

---

11. The nurse caring for a client with stress incontinence who is ordered a cystometrography. The client inquires about the nature of the procedure. Place in chronological order the sequence of events for this procedure. Use all the options.

1. Client is asked to void normally.
2. Urinary catheter is inserted.
3. Any residual urine is noted.
4. Fluid is instilled into the urinary catheter.
5. Client is asked to void following instillation.
6. Urge to void is recorded.

Answer: 1, 2, 4, 6, 5, 3

Rationale: A cystometrography is a urological procedure that measures the amount of pressure exerted on the bladder at various bladder volumes. First, the client is asked to void normally. Then a urinary catheter is inserted, and fluid is instilled. The first urge to void is recorded. Following the procedure, the client is instructed to void and any residual urine is noted. Finally, the catheter is removed.

Test-taking strategy: Analyze to determine what information the question asks for, which is the procedure for completing a cystometrography. Recall that the procedure measures bladder volumes and the pressure associated; thus, various volumes of fluid must be present in the bladder. Volume begins with little urine in the bladder and then fluid volume increases. Review the physiology of the genitourinary system and the cystometrography procedure if you had difficulty answering this question.

Client needs category: Physiological integrity

Client needs subcategory: Reduction of risk potential

Cognitive level: Analyzing

1. A nurse is caring for a client newly diagnosed with osteoporosis. Which statements should the nurse include when teaching the client about the disease? Select all that apply.

- ☐ **1.** Osteoporosis is common in females after menopause.
- ☐ **2.** Osteoporosis is a degenerative disease characterized by a decrease in bone density.
- ☐ **3.** The disease is congenital, caused by poor dietary intake of milk products.
- ☐ **4.** Osteoporosis can cause pain and injury.
- ☐ **5.** Passive ROM exercises can promote bone growth.
- ☐ **6.** Weight-bearing exercise should be avoided.

Answer: 1, 2, 4

Rationale: Osteoporosis is a degenerative metabolic bone disorder in which the rate of bone resorption accelerates and the rate of bone formation decelerates, thus decreasing bone density. Postmenopausal women are at increased risk for this disorder because of their loss of estrogen. The decrease in bone density can cause pain and injury. Osteoporosis is not a congenital disorder; however, low calcium intake does contribute to it. Passive ROM exercises may be performed, but they will not promote bone growth. The client should be encouraged to participate in weight-bearing exercise because it promotes bone growth.

Test-taking strategy: Analyze to determine what information the question asks for, which is key points in osteoporosis teaching. "Select all that apply" questions require considering each option to decide its merit. Recall that the bones of the spine become less dense causing skeletal changes. Consider factors that promote bone growth. Review key points and treatments for osteoporosis if you had difficulty answering this question.

Client needs category: Physiological integrity

Client needs subcategory: Physiological adaptation

Cognitive level: Applying

---

2. A nurse is preparing discharge instructions for an above-the-knee amputation client. Which instructions would be a priority? Select all that apply.

- ☐ **1.** Massage the residual limb in a motion away from the suture line.
- ☐ **2.** Avoid using heat application to ease pain.
- ☐ **3.** Immediately report twitching, spasms, or phantom limb pain.
- ☐ **4.** Avoid exposing the skin around the residual limb to excessive perspiration.
- ☐ **5.** Be sure to perform the prescribed exercises.
- ☐ **6.** Rub the residual limb with a dry washcloth for 4 minutes three times daily if the limb is sensitive to touch.

Answer: 4, 5, 6

Rationale: The nurse should advise the client that perspiration on the residual limb may cause irritation. The client should exercise as instructed to minimize complications. In addition, rubbing the limb as described with a dry washcloth helps desensitize the skin. The nurse should instruct the client to massage the residual limb toward the suture line—not away from it—to mobilize the scar and prevent its adherence to the bone. Twitching, spasms, or phantom limb pain are normal reactions to an amputation and do not need to be reported. The nurse should inform the client that these symptoms might be eased by heat, massage, or gentle pressure.

Test-taking strategy: Analyze to determine what information the question asks for, which are priority discharge instructions. "Select all that apply" questions require considering each option to decide its merit. When considering instruction think "surgical complications to watch for" and "amputation care" as priorities. Select the options that would increase the clients' ability to safely care for the new amputation. Review postoperative care to promote self-care and wound healing, and review postamputation rehabilitation if you had difficulty answering this question.

Client needs category: Safe and effective care environment

Client needs subcategory: Coordinated care

Cognitive level: Applying

---

3. A nurse is assigned a client with an acute exacerbation of rheumatoid arthritis (RA). Which medical facts about RA are essential in developing a plan of care? Select all that apply.

- ☐ **1.** Onset is acute and usually occurs between ages 20 and 40.
- ☐ **2.** The client experiences stiff, swollen joints bilaterally.
- ☐ **3.** The client may not exercise once the disease is diagnosed.
- ☐ **4.** Erythrocyte sedimentation rate (ESR) is elevated, and x-rays show erosions and decalcification of involved joints.
- ☐ **5.** Inflamed cartilage triggers complement activation, which stimulates the release of additional inflammatory mediators.
- ☐ **6.** The first-line treatment is gold salts and methotrexate.

Answer: 2, 4, 5

Rationale: RA is a chronic disorder where individuals experience stiff, swollen joints due to a severe inflammatory reaction. Elevated ESR and x-ray evidence of bony destruction are indicative of severe involvement. RA starts insidiously, with fatigue, persistent low-grade fever, anorexia, and vague skeletal symptoms, usually in middle age between the ages 35 and 50 years. Maintaining the ROM by a prescribed exercise program is essential, but clients must rest between activities. Salicylates and nonsteroidal anti-inflammatory drugs are considered the first-line treatments.

Test-taking strategy: Analyze to determine what information the question asks for, which is developing a care plan related to essential facts of RA. "Select all that apply" questions require considering each option to decide its merit. Consider that knowledge of a disease process and treatment is crucial in developing a plan of care. Understanding the severity allows for client-centered care. Review pathophysiology and treatment of RA if you had difficulty answering this question.

Client needs category: Physiological integrity

Client needs subcategory: Physiological adaptation

Cognitive level: Applying

4. A nurse is caring for a client who fell and fractured the neck of femur. When documenting the site for the family members, place an X on the area where the fracture occurred.

Answer:

Rationale: The neck of the femur is a flattened pyramidal process of bone, connecting the femoral head with the femoral shaft just below the ball and socket. When a femoral neck fracture occurs, the ball is disconnected from the rest of the thigh bone.

Test-taking strategy: Analyze to determine what information the question asks for, which is the site of the femoral neck fracture. If unsure, use the descriptive name (femoral-femur, neck-top of the femur before ball and socket) to direct to the fractured site. Review the anatomy of the upper leg if you had difficulty answering this question.

Client needs category: Physiological integrity

Client needs subcategory: Physiological adaptation

Cognitive level: Understanding

5. A nurse is putting groceries in the car when an elderly client falls off of a curb. The nurse assesses the client and has a bystander call for an ambulance. Which assessment findings provide data of a suspected right hip fracture? Select all that apply.

☐ **1.** The right leg is longer than the left leg.
☐ **2.** The right leg is shorter than the left leg.
☐ **3.** The right leg is abducted.
☐ **4.** The right leg is adducted.
☐ **5.** The right leg is externally rotated.
☐ **6.** The right leg is internally rotated.

Answer: 2, 4, 5

Rationale: A hip fracture is a serious injury, particularly if you are elderly. Subjective signs of a hip fracture include the inability to move after a fall, pain, and the inability to bear weight and stiffness. Objective signs of a hip fracture include the affected leg is shorter, adducted, and externally rotated.

Test-taking strategy: Analyze to determine what information the question asks for, which is assessment data of a suspected right hip fracture. "Select all that apply" questions require considering each option to decide its merit. Note that the options are opposites, thus there will be three correct answers. Change to review the clinical manifestations of fractures, specifically of the femur if you had difficulty answering this question.

Client needs category: Physiological integrity

Client needs subcategory: Physiological adaptation

Cognitive level: Applying

6. A nurse is admitting a client scheduled for a laminectomy of the L1 and L2 vertebrae. Upon returning from the surgical procedure, place an X where the nurse assesses the surgical incision?

Answer:

Rationale: Note the placement of the X in the lower back. In a laminectomy, one or more of the bony laminae that cover the vertebrae are removed. The incision for the surgery is at the site of the vertebrae. There are five lumbar vertebrae that are numbered from top to bottom. L5 is the closest to the sacrum. Count up from the sacrum to locate L1 and L2.

Test-taking strategy: Analyze to determine what information the question asks for, which is the site of the surgical procedure (L1 and L2). Recall that there are 7 cervical vertebrae, 12 thoracic vertebrae, and 5 lumbar vertebrae. Review the anatomy of the spinal column and the laminectomy surgical procedure if you had difficulty answering this question.

Client needs category: Physiological integrity

Client needs subcategory: Physiological adaptation

Cognitive level: Understanding

7. A client is being discharged to a transitional rehabilitation care facility following a hip replacement due to degenerative arthritis. When reporting to the nursing assistant, which nursing actions would the nurse stress as essential? Select all that apply.

- [ ] **1.** Place the client in high Fowler's position.
- [ ] **2.** Avoid any hip flexion exercises.
- [ ] **3.** Place two pillows between the client's knees.
- [ ] **4.** Place a raised toilet seat in the bathroom.
- [ ] **5.** Keep the client's feet elevated.
- [ ] **6.** Maintain the client on bed rest until the incision heals.

Answer: 2, 3, 4

Rationale: The hip is one of the body's largest joints. In a total hip replacement, the damaged bone and cartilage are removed and replaced with prosthetic components. Until healing occurs, the legs must be spread outward (abducted) away from the body by placing pillows or an abductor foam wedge between the legs. Adduction of the hip or flexion greater than 90° may dislocate the prosthesis from the joint. Raising the head of the bed 90° creates excessive hip flexion. Using a raised toilet seat is appropriate to avoid bending. The client will be out of bed for physical therapy once to twice daily. Keeping the feet elevated is not part of the hip replacement protocol.

Test-taking strategy: Analyze to determine what information the question asks for, which is nursing actions in the rehab setting. "Select all that apply" questions require considering each option to decide its merit. Choose the options for the postoperative rehab period. Recall that positioning is very important until the hip structure heals. Review care of clients following hip replacement surgery if you had difficulty answering this question.

Client needs category: Physiological integrity

Client needs subcategory: Reduction of risk potential

Cognitive level: Applying

---

8. A client is suspected of having carpal tunnel syndrome. The nurse assesses for Tinel's sign. Identify the area where the nurse should percuss in an attempt to elicit Tinel's sign.

Answer:

Rationale: Carpal tunnel syndrome is compression of the median nerve in the wrist that supplies feeling and movement to parts of the hand. Tinel's sign may be used to help identify carpal tunnel syndrome. It is elicited by percussing lightly over the median nerve, located on the inner aspect of the wrist. If the client reports tingling, numbness, and pain, the test is considered positive.

Test-taking strategy: Analyze to determine what information the question asks for, which is site of percussion to elicit Tinel's sign. Recall that the cause of carpal tunnel syndrome is compression of the median nerve, thus percussing over the nerve produces definitive symptoms. Review the anatomical basis for carpal tunnel syndrome, and diagnostic clinical findings if you had difficulty answering this question.

Client needs category: Physiological integrity

Client needs subcategory: Reduction of risk potential

Cognitive level: Understanding

9. A client is admitted with a possible diagnosis of osteomyelitis. Based on the documentation below, which laboratory result is the priority for the nurse to report to the physician?

Progress Notes

01/11/10 0900	Pt admitted with elevated temperature, complaining of bone pain and muscle spasms. Laboratory called with the following results: rheumatoid factor negative; blood culture positive for Staphylococcus aureus; alkaline phosphatase 60 International Units/liter; erythrocyte sedimentation rate 10 mm/hr.————————Susan Wright, LPN

- ☐ **1.** Rheumatoid factor
- ☐ **2.** Blood culture
- ☐ **3.** Alkaline phosphatase
- ☐ **4.** ESR

Answer: 2

Rationale: Osteomyelitis is a bacterial infection of the bone and soft tissue that occurs by extension of soft tissue infection, direct bone contamination following surgery, or spreading from other infection sites in the body. A positive blood culture should be reported immediately to the physician so that specific antibiotic therapy can begin or be adjusted based on the positive culture. A negative rheumatoid factor would be expected in a possible diagnosis of osteomyelitis. An alkaline phosphatase level of 60 IU/L is within the normal range, and an ESR of 10 mm/hour is also within the normal range.

Test-taking strategies: Analyze to determine what information the question asks for, which is determining priority laboratory data to be communicated to the physician. Determine laboratory data which are abnormal and then decide the clinical implications. Always contact the physician with important laboratory data. Review the pathophysiology and clinical manifestations of osteomyelitis if you had difficulty answering this question.

Client needs category: Safe and effective care environment

Client needs subcategory: Coordinated care

Cognitive level: Analyzing

10. A client has been prescribed indomethacin (Indocin) for the treatment of gouty arthritis. The orders state 25 mg t.i.d. for first 5 days, then increase by 25 mg per dose at weekly intervals until the daily dose reaches a maximum of 250 mg. The client is on week 3 of treatment and has tolerated the medication without any incident thus far. By week 3, what would the daily dose of medication be? Record your answer as a whole number.

_____ mg

Answer: 225

Rationale: First, determine the first week's daily dosage: 25 mg × 3 = 75 mg. This dosage is increased by 25 mg per dose to equal the second week's daily dosage:

25 mg + 25 mg = 50 mg × 3 = 150 mg. The dosage is then increased by an additional 25 mg to equal the third week's daily dosage: 25 mg + 25 mg + 25 mg = 75 mg × 3 = 225 mg.

Test-taking strategy: Analyze to determine what information the question asks for, which is week 3's Indocin dosage. Read carefully the physician order and carefully increase each dose of medication weekly. Continue with the formula until the maximum dose is reached. Proofread your math calculation. Review the amount of medication per dosage, the number of daily doses, and the amount to increase the dosage weekly if you had difficulty answering this question.

Client needs category: Physiological integrity

Client needs subcategory: Pharmacological therapies

Cognitive level: Applying

---

11. A client is scheduled for an open reduction internal fixation of the right hip. Place the following nursing interventions in chronological order to show the sequence in which the nurse should perform them. Use all of the options.

1. Develop a home care teaching plan.
2. Complete a preoperative checklist.
3. Make sure the client has signed an informed consent form.
4. Encourage coughing, turning, and deep breathing.
5. Monitor vital signs every 15 minutes × 4, every 30 minutes × 2, and every hour × 2.
6. Complete a history and physical examination.

Answer: 6, 3, 2, 5, 4, 1

Rationale: Initially, the nurse will complete the history and physical as part of the admission process. As part of the preoperative interventions, the nurse will witness the signing of the informed consent and complete a preoperative checklist. Postoperatively, the nurse will monitor vital signs frequently and, once the client is awake, alert, and oriented, will encourage the client to turn, cough, and deep-breathe. Finally, a home care teaching plan must be developed before discharge.

Test-taking strategy: Analyze to determine what information the question asks for, which is nursing action for a open reduction internal fixation of the hip. Consider what actions are preoperative and those that are postoperative. Use knowledge of surgical process to chronologically order nursing actions. Review the surgical procedure and related nursing interventions, and recall that client safety is paramount if you had difficulty answering this question.

Client needs category: Health promotion and maintenance

Client needs subcategory: None

Cognitive level: Analyzing

1. A nurse is preparing a client with systemic lupus erythematosus (SLE) for discharge. Which instructions should the nurse include in the teaching plan? Select all that apply.

☐ **1.** Stay out of direct sunlight.
☐ **2.** Do not limit activity between flare-ups.
☐ **3.** Monitor body temperature.
☐ **4.** Taper the corticosteroid dosage as prescribed when symptoms are under control.
☐ **5.** Apply cold packs to relieve joint pain and stiffness.

Answer: 1, 3, 4

Rationale: SLE is a chronic autoimmune disease that can damage any part of the body (skin, joints, and bodily organs). A client with SLE should stay out of direct sunlight and avoid other sources of ultraviolet light because they may trigger severe skin reactions and exacerbate the symptoms. The client's body temperature should be monitored and fevers reported to the primary health care provider. The corticosteroid dosage must be tapered gradually once symptoms are relieved because stopping these drugs abruptly can cause adrenal insufficiency, a potentially life-threatening condition. Fatigue can cause an SLE flare-up, so the client should pace activities and plan for rest periods. The client should apply heat, not cold, to relieve joint pain. Cold packs may aggravate Raynaud's phenomenon, which commonly occurs in clients with SLE.

Test-taking strategy: Analyze to determine what information the question asks for, which is nursing instructions for the teaching plan for a client with SLE. "Select all that apply" questions require considering each option to decide its merit. Review nursing interventions and clinical manifestations for SLE if you had difficulty answering this question.

Client needs category: Physiological integrity

Client needs subcategory: Reduction of risk potential

Cognitive level: Applying

2. A nurse is planning care for a client with human immunodeficiency virus (HIV). The licensed practical nurse (LPN) is delegating responsibilities to a nursing assistant. Which statements by the nursing assistant indicates understanding of HIV transmission? Select all that apply.

☐ **1.** "I will wear a gown, mask, and gloves for all client contact."

☐ **2.** "I do not need to wear any personal protective equipment because nurses have a low risk of occupational exposure."

☐ **3.** "I will wear a mask if the client has a cough caused by an upper respiratory infection."

☐ **4.** "I will wear a mask, gown, and gloves when splashing of body fluids is likely."

☐ **5.** "I will wash my hands after client care."

Answer: 4, 5

Rationale: When the LPN delegates to the nursing assistant, it is important to insure an understanding of client condition and task delegation. In caring for a client with HIV, standard precautions include wearing gloves for any known or anticipated contact with blood, body fluids, tissue, mucous membranes, or nonintact skin. If the task may result in splashing or splattering of blood or body fluids, a mask and goggles or a face shield and a fluid-resistant gown or apron should be worn. Hands should be washed before and after client care and after removing gloves.

Test-taking strategy: Analyze to determine what information the question asks for, which is proper care and understanding of HIV transmission. "Select all that apply" questions require considering each option to decide its merit. Recall that the Centers for Disease Control stresses standard precautions in caring for all clients in all situations where there is blood and body fluid contact. Review standard precautions at the Centers for Disease Control and Prevention isolation guidelines if you had difficulty answering this question.

Client needs category: Safe and effective care environment

Client needs subcategory: Safety and infection control

Cognitive level: Analyzing

---

3. A nurse is caring for a client with moderate rheumatoid arthritis (RA). Which nonpharmacological interventions should a nurse include in the care plan? Select all that apply.

☐ **1.** Massaging inflamed joints

☐ **2.** Avoiding ROM exercises

☐ **3.** Applying splints to inflamed joints

☐ **4.** Using assistive devices at all times

☐ **5.** Selecting clothing that has Velcro fasteners

☐ **6.** Applying moist heat to joints

Answer: 3, 5, 6

Rationale: RA affects more than 2 million Americans, mostly women. RA is a chronic, systematic inflammatory disorder affecting many tissues, organs, and joints. Supportive, nonpharmacological measures for the client with RA include applying splints to rest inflamed joints, using Velcro fasteners on clothing to aid in dressing, and applying moist heat to joints to relax muscles and relieve pain. Inflamed joints should never be massaged because doing so can aggravate inflammation. A physical therapy program, including ROM exercises and carefully individualized therapeutic exercises, prevents loss of joint function. Assistive devices should only be used when marked loss of ROM occurs.

Test-taking strategy: Analyze to determine what information the question asks for, which is nonpharmacological interventions for a client with moderate RA. "Select all that apply" questions require considering each option to decide its merit. Consider the main symptoms of the disease process and link with a helpful nonpharmacological intervention. Review nursing interventions and nonpharmacological pain management therapies if you had difficulty answering this question.

Client needs category: Physiological integrity

Client needs subcategory: Basic care and comfort

Cognitive level: Applying

---

4. A nurse is assessing a young adult with a temperature of 103°, a sore throat, and swollen lymph glands. No adventitious breath sounds or cardiac disorders are noted. To complete an assessment for a potential Epstein-Barr viral infection, place an X on the quadrant of the abdomen which the nurse would be particularly careful to palpate?

Answer:

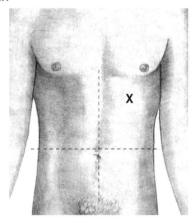

Rationale: An Epstein-Barr infection is a common viral infection. Symptoms include a fever, sore throat, and swollen lymph glands. Additionally, a swollen liver or spleen may develop. Assessment of the liver and spleen is essential. The spleen is located in the left upper quadrant of the abdomen. It is posterior and slightly inferior to the stomach. The nurse should stop palpating immediately if the nurse feels the spleen because compression can cause rupture.

Test-taking strategy: Analyze to determine what information the question asks for, which is area of the abdomen for palpation. The key word is area to pay "particular" attention, providing a clue that one quadrant is more important than the others. Recall the content of the abdomen in the quadrants and relate to the disease process. Review Epstein-Barr assessment techniques if you had difficulty answering this question.

Client needs category: Physiological integrity

Client needs subcategory: Physiological adaptation

Cognitive level: Applying

5. A client presents to the community clinic with a viral infection and swollen lymph nodes. Place an X to identify the area of the submandibular lymph nodes.

Answer:

Rationale: The submandibular lymph nodes are found halfway between the angle and tip of the mandible. The submandibular lymph nodes account for approximately 70% of the salivary volume produced.

Test-taking strategy: Analyze to determine what information the question asks for, which is the location of the submandibular lymph nodes. Use your knowledge of medical terminology to locate the lymph nodes. Break the word into sections such as sub–under and mandibular–mandible and thus make a selection of the lymph node under the mandible on the illustration. Review the anatomy of the lymphatic system and the face if you had difficulty answering this question.

Client needs category: Physiological integrity

Client needs subcategory: Physiological adaptation

Cognitive level: Understanding

---

6. The nurse is caring for a client who is scheduled to undergo a bone marrow aspiration to assess the progression of a hematologic disorder. Which interventions should the nurse include as part of the preprocedural teaching plan? Select all that apply.

☐ **1.** Explain the procedure to the client.

☐ **2.** Maintain a pressure dressing over the aspiration site.

☐ **3.** Encourage the client to ask questions before obtaining the signed informed consent.

☐ **4.** Explain that the client will receive an analgesic prior to the procedure.

☐ **5.** Administer an anxiety-relieving medication prior to the procedure.

☐ **6.** Instruct the client to save all voided urine for 24 hours after the procedure.

Answer: 1, 3, 4

Rationale: The client should understand the procedure and the reason why it is necessary before signing an informed consent form. The client also should be advised of the local analgesia to be administered before the procedure begins. Although the client may receive an anxiety-relieving medication before the procedure, administering the drug is not part of the teaching plan. Likewise, maintaining pressure over the insertion site is a nursing intervention performed after the procedure; it is not a part of the preoperative teaching. Instructing the client to save voided urine would be part of the postprocedural discharge plan.

Test-taking strategies: Analyze to determine what information the question asks for, which is the preprocedure client teaching. "Select all that apply" questions require considering each option to decide its merit. The key word is "preprocedural," indicating that which is done prior to the procedure. Analyze each option with the specific time period in mind. Review preprocedure client teaching, including guidelines on obtaining informed consent and preparation for bone marrow aspiration if you had difficulty answering this question.

Client needs category: Physiological integrity

Client needs subcategory: Basic care and comfort

Cognitive level: Applying

---

7. The nurse is assessing a client who is suspected of having Hodgkin's disease. The client has been admitted with swollen left-sided inguinal lymph nodes. Identify the area where the nurse would be best able to palpate the size of these lymph nodes.

Answer:

Rationale: Hodgkin's disease is a type of neoplasm involving cells of lymphoid origin. It usually begins as a painless enlargement of one or more lymph nodes. Most commonly, the lymph node enlargement involves the nodes in the neck area but it can also involve the inguinal nodes as well. The inguinal nodes are located in the groin area.

Test-taking strategy: Analyze to determine what information the question asks for, which is a location of the left-sided inguinal lymph nodes. The key word is "inguinal" leading to the inguinal or groin region. Also, use anatomical position to distinguish between right and left sides of the body. Review the anatomy of the lymphatic system and abdomen, and pathophysiology of Hodgkin's disease if you had difficulty answering this question.

Client needs category: Physiological integrity

Client needs subcategory: Physiological adaptation

Cognitive level: Applying

8. A multidisciplinary oncology team of physicians, nurses, and the social worker notes that a client who has been undergoing chemotherapy is now experiencing pancytopenia. When reviewing the laboratory data, which values support this diagnosis? Select all that apply.

☐ **1.** Decreased white blood cells
☐ **2.** Increased white blood cells
☐ **3.** Decreased platelets
☐ **4.** Increased platelets
☐ **5.** Decreased RBCs
☐ **6.** Increased RBCs

Answer: 1, 3, 5

Rationale: Pancytopenia is a deficiency of all blood cells which includes a state of simultaneous leukopenia (decreased white blood cells), thrombocytopenia (decreased platelets), and anemia (decreased RBCs). Pancytopenia has widespread effects on the body by leading to oxygen shortage and immune function.

Test-taking strategy: Analyze to determine what information the question asks for, which is laboratory data which supports a diagnosis of pancytopenia. "Select all that apply" questions require considering each option to decide its merit. Notice that there are increased and decreased options of white blood cells, platelets, and red blood cells meaning that there should be three correct answers. Relate each option to chemotherapy side effects. Review laboratory values for the disorder, and review pertinent medical terminology (such as pan, meaning universal, and penia, meaning decreased) if you had difficulty answering this question.

Client needs category: Physiological integrity
Client needs subcategory: Physiological adaptation
Cognitive level: Analyzing

---

9. A nurse is caring for a client scheduled for a Schilling's test to determine the cause of a vitamin B_{12} deficiency. Place the following interventions in the order in which the nurse would perform them. Use all the options.

1. Withhold all food and fluids after midnight before the test.
2. Instruct the client to save all voided urine for 24 hours.
3. Keep the client's urine at room temperature.
4. Answer any questions regarding the procedure for the client.
5. Place the signed informed consent form in the client's chart.
6. Assist with obtaining the client's informed consent.

Answer: 4, 1, 6, 5, 2, 3

Rationale: The nurse assists the physician in explaining and preparing the client. The preprocedure steps consist of answering any further questions regarding the procedure for the client, withholding food and fluids after midnight, obtaining the client's informed consent, and placing the signed forms in the client's chart. Postprocedural nursing interventions include instructing the client to save all voided urine for 24 hours and then keeping the urine at room temperature.

Test-taking strategy: Analyze to determine what information the question asks for, which is the nursing interventions when caring for a client having a Schilling's test. Review routine preprocedural and postprocedural nursing care, and review the procedure for Schilling's test if you had difficulty answering this question.

Client needs category: Physiological integrity
Client needs subcategory: Reduction of risk potential
Cognitive level: Analyzing

10. The nurse is caring for a client who has been newly diagnosed with systemic lupus erythematosus (SLE). Which information should be included in a teaching plan that focuses on home care? Select all that apply.

☐ **1.** Avoid exposure to sunlight.
☐ **2.** Keep exercise to a minimal level.
☐ **3.** Report development of a butterfly rash on the face.
☐ **4.** Avoid over-the-counter (OTC) medications unless approved by the physician.
☐ **5.** Take rest periods as needed.

Answer: 1, 2, 4, 5

Rationale: The client who suffers from SLE has a tendency toward photosensitivity; therefore, the client should avoid exposure to sunlight. The client should also be advised to keep exercise to a minimum, to avoid OTC medications unless directed by the physician, and to rest as needed. Because the butterfly rash associated with lupus is an initial sign, the client would already have the rash and would not be reporting its development after discharge.

Test-taking strategy: Analyze to determine what information the question asks for, which is home care nursing instructions. "Select all that apply" questions require considering each option to decide its merit. The key words are "home care"; thus, instruction is specific in this situation. Review the pathophysiology of SLE, clinical manifestations, and nursing interventions if you had difficulty answering this question.

Client needs category: Physiological integrity

Client needs subcategory: Basic care and comfort

Cognitive level: Applying

Endocrine and Metabolic Disorders

1. A nurse is caring for a client who is being discharged after a thyroidectomy. Which discharge instructions would be appropriate for this client? Select all that apply.

☐ **1.** Report signs and symptoms of hypoglycemia.
☐ **2.** Take thyroid replacement medication as ordered.
☐ **3.** Watch for changes in body functioning, such as lethargy, restlessness, sensitivity to cold, and dry skin, and report these changes to the physician.
☐ **4.** Avoid all OTC medications.
☐ **5.** Carry injectable dexamethasone at all times.

Answer: 2, 3

Rationale: A thyroidectomy is the surgical removal of all or part of the thyroid. After removal of the thyroid gland, the client needs to take thyroid replacement medication. The client also needs to report such changes as lethargy, restlessness, cold sensitivity, and dry skin, which may indicate the need for a higher dosage of medication. The thyroid gland does not regulate blood glucose level; therefore, signs and symptoms of hypoglycemia are not relevant for this client. Injectable dexamethasone is not needed for this client. Some OTC medications (such as non-aspirin products) are allowable.

Test-taking strategy: Analyze to determine what information the question asks for, which is discharge instructions after a thyroidectomy. Use your knowledge of medical terminology to determine procedure such as "ectomy"—removal of. Recall that the thyroid gland releases hormones which affect the body's metabolism. Review the physiology of the thyroid gland, and nursing interventions related to promoting rest, managing pain, and monitoring for potential complications if you had difficulty answering this question.

Client needs category: Safe and effective care environment

Client needs subcategory: Coordinated care

Cognitive level: Applying

2. A client is admitted with a diagnosis of diabetic ketoacidosis. An insulin drip is initiated with 50 units of insulin in 100 mL of normal saline solution administered via an infusion pump set at 10 mL/hour. The nurse determines that the client is receiving how many units of insulin each hour? Record your answer using a whole number.

_____ units/hour

Answer: 5

Rationale: To determine the number of insulin units the client is receiving per hour, first determine the number of units in each milliliter of fluid (50 units ÷ 100 mL = 0.5 unit/mL). Next, multiply the units per milliliter by the rate of milliliters per hour (0.5 unit × 10 mL/hour = 5 units).

Test-taking strategy: Analyze to determine what information the question asks for, which is a number of units of insulin infusing per hour. First, calculate the number of units per milliliter of I.V. solution. Once determined, calculate the number of units per hour. Proofread your math calculations. Review solving for X using the ratio-and-proportion method if you had difficulty answering this question.

Client needs category: Physiological integrity

Client needs subcategory: Pharmacological therapies

Cognitive level: Applying

---

3. A client's glucose level is 365 mg/dL. The physician orders 10 units of regular insulin to be administered. The bottle of regular insulin is labeled 100 units/mL. How many milliliters of insulin should the nurse administer? Record your answer using one decimal place.

_____ mL

Answer: 0.1

Rationale: To find the correct administration amount, use the cross-product principle to set up the following equation:

$$\frac{X}{10 \text{ units}} = \frac{1 \text{ mL}}{100 \text{ units}}$$

Next, cross-multiply:

$$100 \times X \text{ units} = 10 \text{ units} \times 1 \text{ mL.}$$

Then divide both sides of the equation by 100 units to solve for X:

$$X = 0.1 \text{ mL.}$$

Test-taking strategy: Analyze to determine what information the question asks for, which is the milliliters of insulin the nurse should administer. Review ratio-and-proportion calculations as noted above. Proofread your math calculations. Review medical math calculations if you had difficulty answering this question.

Client needs category: Physiological integrity

Client needs subcategory: Pharmacological therapies

Cognitive level: Applying

4. A nurse is performing an admission assessment on a client who has been diagnosed with diabetes insipidus. Which findings does the nurse anticipate during the assessment? Select all that apply.

☐ **1.** Extreme polyuria.
☐ **2.** Excessive thirst.
☐ **3.** Elevated systolic blood pressure.
☐ **4.** Low urine specific gravity.
☐ **5.** Bradycardia.
☐ **6.** Elevated serum potassium level.

Answer: 1, 2, 4

Rationale: Diabetes insipidus is a condition where the kidneys are unable to conserve water. Signs and symptoms of diabetes insipidus include an abrupt onset of extreme polyuria, excessive thirst, dry skin and mucous membranes, tachycardia, and hypotension. Diagnostic studies reveal low urine specific gravity and osmolarity and an elevated serum sodium level. The serum potassium level is likely to be decreased, not increased.

Test-taking strategy: Analyze to determine what information the question asks for, which is assessment findings with diabetes insipidus. "Select all that apply" questions require considering each option to decide its merit. Recall that the disease process is influenced by the pituitary gland's dysregulation of antidiuretic hormone (ADH) causing excessive fluid loss and associated symptoms. Review the pathophysiology and clinical manifestations of diabetes insipidus if you had difficulty answering this question.

Client needs category: Physiological integrity

Client needs subcategory: Physiological adaptation

Cognitive level: Applying

5. A nurse is following the progress of a client being treated for hypothyroidism. Which findings indicate that thyroid replacement therapy has been inadequate? Select all that apply.

☐ **1.** Prolonged QT interval on ECG.
☐ **2.** Tachycardia.
☐ **3.** Low body temperature.
☐ **4.** Nervousness.
☐ **5.** Bradycardia.
☐ **6.** Dry mouth.

Answer: 1, 3, 5

Rationale: In hypothyroidism, the body is in a hypometabolic state. Therefore, a prolonged QT interval with bradycardia and subnormal body temperature would indicate that replacement therapy was inadequate. Tachycardia, nervousness, and dry mouth are symptoms of an excessive level of thyroid hormone; these findings would indicate that the client has received an excessive dose of thyroid hormone.

Test-taking strategy: Analyze to determine what information the question asks for, which is findings which would represent that thyroid replacement therapy is inadequate. "Select all that apply" questions require considering each option to decide its merit. The key word is "inadequate" meaning that symptoms of hypothyroidism still persist. Review the physiology of the thyroid gland clinical manifestations of hypothyroidism if you had difficulty answering this question.

Client needs category: Physiological integrity

Client needs subcategory: Reduction of risk potential

Cognitive level: Evaluating

6. A client is brought to the emergency department after wandering on the street. The client is confused, verbalizes double vision, headache, and shakiness. Laboratory data reveal a serum blood glucose of 52 mg/dL. Which questions, asked by the nurse, may reveal more data related to the client's condition? Select all that apply.

☐ **1.** "What have you eaten today?"
☐ **2.** "Do you take insulin or oral antidiabetic medication?"
☐ **3.** "Have you ever felt this way before?"
☐ **4.** "Can you tell me if you are married?"
☐ **5.** "Are you having any chest pain?"
☐ **6.** "Have you been to this hospital before?"

Answer: 1, 2, 3

Rationale: A serum blood glucose of 52 mg/dL indicates hypoglycemia. Questions that provide information on diet, activity, medications, and daily routine can be helpful in understanding the cause of the low blood sugar. Factors that influence hypoglycemia include missed meals and strenuous activity or taking too high of a dosage of insulin/oral antidiabetic medications. Symptoms of hypoglycemia include shakiness, confusion, headache, sweating, and tingling sensations around the mouth. Questions of marital status, previous hospitalizations, and other symptoms are helpful in determining overall client status but do not provide data on hypoglycemia.

Test-taking strategy: Analyze to determine what information the question asks for, which is pertinent questions related to hypoglycemia. "Select all that apply" questions require considering each option to decide its merit. Read each option to determine how it relates to the disease process. Review the clinical manifestations of and nursing interventions for hypoglycemia if you had difficulty answering this question.

Client needs category: Physiological integrity

Client needs subcategory: Physiological adaptation

Cognitive level: Analyzing

---

7. A nurse is caring for a client with a low calcium level. Place the following options in chronological order to indicate the regulatory feedback mechanism of parathyroid hormone (PTH) release in relation to calcium levels. Use all of the options.

| **1.** High serum calcium level inhibits PTH secretion. |
| **2.** Low serum calcium level stimulates parathyroid gland. |
| **3.** Calcium is reabsorbed. |
| **4.** Parathyroid gland releases PTH. |

Answer: 2, 4, 3, 1

Rationale: Simple feedback occurs when the level of one substance regulates the secretion of hormones. A low calcium level stimulates the parathyroid gland to release PTH, which promotes resorption of calcium, resulting in normalized calcium levels. When calcium levels are elevated, PTH secretion is inhibited.

Test-taking strategy: Analyze to determine what information the question asks for, which is the order when the body uses the regulatory feedback method to maintain serum calcium levels. Recall that the feedback mechanism exists when the body detects an abnormality. Once detected, the body attempts to correct the abnormality by its regulatory process. Once homeostasis reoccurs, the body returns to maintenance of body function. Review the physiology of the parathyroid gland and PTH in relation to the regulatory feedback mechanism if you had difficulty answering this question.

Client needs category: Physiological integrity

Client needs subcategory: Physiological adaptation

Cognitive level: Analyzing

8. A client with Addison's disease is scheduled for discharge after being hospitalized for an adrenal crisis. Which statements by the client would indicate that the nurse's teaching has been effective? Select all that apply.

☐ **1.** "I have to take my steroids for 10 days."
☐ **2.** "I need to weigh myself daily to be sure I don't eat too many calories."
☐ **3.** "I need to call my doctor to discuss my steroid needs before I have dental work."
☐ **4.** "I will call the doctor if I suddenly feel very weak or dizzy."
☐ **5.** "If I feel like I have the flu, I'll carry on as usual because this is an expected response."
☐ **6.** "I need to obtain and wear a Medic Alert bracelet."

Answer: 3, 4, 6

Rationale: Addison's disease is a chronic endocrine disorder that occurs when the adrenal glands do not produce enough hormones such as cortisol and aldosterone. These hormones give instruction to virtually every tissue and organ in the body. Dental work can be a cause of physical stress; therefore, the client's physician needs to be informed about the dental work so adjustments in the dosage of steroids can be made, if necessary. Fatigue, weakness, and dizziness are symptoms of inadequate steroid therapy; the physician should be notified if these symptoms occur. A Medic Alert bracelet allows health care providers to access the client's history of Addison's disease if the client is unable to communicate this information. A client with Addison's disease does not produce enough steroids, so routine administration of steroids is a lifetime treatment. Daily weight should be monitored to monitor changes in fluid balance, not calorie intake. Influenza is an added physical stressor that may require an increased dosage of steroids. The client should notify the physician, not "carry on as usual."

Test-taking strategy: Analyze to determine what information the question asks for, which is a correct statement by the client indicating effective teaching. "Select all that apply" questions require considering each option to decide its merit. Read each option carefully and relate to the disease process. Review the clinical manifestations and nursing interventions for Addison's disease if you had difficulty answering this question.

Client needs category: Physiological integrity

Client needs subcategory: Reduction of risk potential

Cognitive level: Analyzing

9. A client comes to the clinic verbalizing a weight loss of 20 lb over the last month, even with a "ravenous" appetite and no change in activity level. The client is diagnosed with Graves' disease. Which other signs and symptoms of Graves' disease should the nurse assess? Select all that apply.

☐ **1.** Rapid, bounding pulse.
☐ **2.** Bradycardia.
☐ **3.** Heat intolerance.
☐ **4.** Mild tremors.
☐ **5.** Nervousness.
☐ **6.** Constipation.

Answer: 1, 3, 4, 5

Rationale: Graves' disease, or hyperthyroidism, is a hypermetabolic state that is associated with a rapid, bounding pulse; heat intolerance; tremors; and nervousness. Bradycardia and constipation are signs and symptoms of hypothyroidism.

Test-taking strategy: Analyze to determine what information the question asks for, which is signs and symptoms related to Graves' disease. "Select all that apply" questions require considering each option to decide its merit. Relate Graves' disease/hyperthyroidism with "speeding up" the metabolism and the related effects. Note that the correct options all relate an increased metabolism. Review the physiology of the thyroid gland and the pathophysiology of hyperthyroidism (Graves' disease) if you had difficulty answering this question.

Client needs category: Physiological integrity

Client needs subcategory: Physiological adaptation

Cognitive level: Analyzing

---

10. A client who suffered a brain injury after falling off a ladder has recently developed syndrome of inappropriate antidiuretic hormone (SIADH). Which findings indicate that the treatment being received for SIADH is effective? Select all that apply.

☐ **1.** Decrease in body weight.
☐ **2.** Rise in blood pressure and drop in heart rate.
☐ **3.** Absence of wheezing.
☐ **4.** Increase in urine output.
☐ **5.** Decrease in urine osmolarity.

Answer: 1, 4, 5

Rationale: SIADH is an abnormality involving an excessive release of ADH. The predominant feature is water retention with oliguria, edema, and weight gain. Successful treatment should result in a reduction in weight, increased urine output, and a decrease in urine osmolarity (concentration). Wheezes are not typically associated with SIADH. The client's blood pressure should remain the same or decrease after treatment.

Test-taking strategy: Analyze to determine what information the question asks for, which is the reduction of symptoms from SIADH indicating effective treatment. "Select all that apply" questions require considering each option to decide its merit. First, consider which symptoms typically occur in SIADH. Next appraise each option for normalizing of those symptoms indicating effective treatment. Review the clinical manifestations and treatment of SIADH if you had difficulty answering this question.

Client needs category: Physiological integrity

Client needs subcategory: Physiological adaptation

Cognitive level: Evaluating

11. A nurse is about to administer a client's morning dose of insulin. The client's order is for 5 units of regular insulin and 10 units of NPH (neutral protamine Hagedorn) insulin given as a basal dose. The client also is to receive an amount prescribed from the medium-dose sliding scale (shown below) based on morning blood glucose levels. The nurse performs a bedside blood glucose measurement and the result is 264 mg/dL. How many total units of insulin should the nurse administer to the client?

Plasma Glucose (mg/dL)	Low Dose (Regular Insulin)	Medium Dose (Regular Insulin)	High Dose (Regular Insulin)	Very High Dose (Regular Insulin)
<70	←	Call physician	→	
71–140	0 units	0 units	0 units	0 units
141–180	1 unit	2 units	4 units	10 units
181–240	2 units	4 units	8 units	15 units
241–300	4 units	6 units	12 units	20 units
301–400	6 units	9 units	16 units	25 units
>400	8 units	12 units	20 units	30 units
	←	and call physician	→	

_____ units

Answer: 21

Rationale: The basal dose for this client is 5 units of regular insulin and 10 units of NPH insulin. The medium-dose sliding scale indicates that, based on the glucose reading of 264 mg/dL, the client should receive an additional 6 units of regular insulin, totaling 21 units (5 units + 10 units + 6 units = 21 units).

Test-taking strategy: Analyze to determine what information the question asks for, which is total units of insulin. Carefully read the basal order and then add the sliding scale coverage. Proofread your math calculation. Review ordered insulin dosages if you had difficulty answering this question.

Client needs category: Physiological integrity

Client needs subcategory: Pharmacological therapies

Cognitive level: Applying

---

12. A client arrives in the clinic with a possible PTH deficiency. Diagnosis of this condition includes the analysis of serum electrolytes. Which electrolytes would the nurse anticipate to be abnormal? Select all that apply.

☐ **1.** Sodium.
☐ **2.** Potassium.
☐ **3.** Calcium.
☐ **4.** Chloride.
☐ **5.** Glucose.
☐ **6.** Phosphorus.

Answer: 3, 6

Rationale: PTH deficiency is a condition of hypoparathyroidism. Primary hypoparathyroidism is a state of inadequate PTH activity. PTH is essential for maintaining the delicate balance of calcium and phosphorus levels in the blood. Sodium, chloride, potassium, and glucose are not affected by a PTH deficiency.

Test-taking strategy: Analyze to determine what information the question asks for, which is the electrolytes that are abnormal in hypoparathyroidism. "Select all that apply" questions require considering each option to decide its merit. Recall that the parathyroid glands regulate calcium and depending on the calcium level, phosphorus levels are in balance. Review the physiology of the parathyroid gland and its effect on serum electrolytes if you had difficulty answering this question.

Client needs category: Health promotion and maintenance

Client needs subcategory: None

Cognitive level: Applying

13. Two weeks after a partial thyroidectomy, a client is being seen for the postoperative follow-up appointment. The nurse is aware that the client is at increased risk for hypothyroidism. Which signs and symptoms would the nurse anticipate in a client with hypothyroidism? Select all that apply.

- ☐ **1.** Heat intolerance.
- ☐ **2.** Hair loss.
- ☐ **3.** Increased energy.
- ☐ **4.** Dry skin.
- ☐ **5.** Cold intolerance.
- ☐ **6.** Fatigue.

Answer: 2, 4, 5, 6

Rationale: Hypothyroidism refers to suboptimal levels of thyroid hormone. A client with this condition typically has hair loss, dry skin, cold intolerance, and fatigue.

Test-taking strategy: Analyze to determine what information the question asks for, which is signs and symptoms of hypothyroidism. "Select all that apply" questions require considering each option to decide its merit. Recall that in hypothyroidism, metabolism is decreased leading to a reduction in body metabolism. Review the physiology of the thyroid gland and pathophysiology of hypothyroidism if you had difficulty answering this question.

Client needs category: Physiological integrity

Client needs subcategory: Physiological adaptation

Cognitive level: Understanding

---

14. The nurse is caring for a client following a thyroidectomy assessing for a possible low calcium level related to inadvertent removal of parathyroid glands. Identify the part of the body the nurse should assess to determine a positive or negative Chvostek's sign.

Answer:

Rationale: When the facial nerve is stimulated in someone with hypocalcemia, the facial muscles contract, causing twitching of the cheek, mouth, and nose (Chvostek's sign). To elicit Chvostek's sign, tap the nerve about 2 cm anterior to the earlobe, just below the zygomatic arch.

Test-taking strategy: Analyze to determine what information the question asks for, which is the location to assess Chvostek's sign. Recall medical terminology for the definition of Chvostek's sign which will focus you on the assessment of calcium and the facial nerve. Review postthyroidectomy care and assessment techniques if you had difficulty answering this question.

Client needs category: Physiological integrity

Client needs subcategory: Physiological adaptation

Cognitive level: Analyzing

15. The nurse is preparing the morning insulin for a diabetic client on the unit. The order is for 20 units of Humulin 70/30. The nurse knows that this dose contains a mixture of intermediate-acting insulin and fast-acting insulin. How many units of intermediate-acting insulin does this dose contain? Record your answer using a whole number.

_____ units

Answer: 14

Rationale: Recall that Humulin 70/30 insulin contains both intermediate-acting insulin and fast-acting insulin. The 70 and 30 represent the percentages of each kind (the first number always pertains to the percentage of intermediate-acting insulin; the second, to the fast-acting insulin). Therefore, to calculate the amount of intermediate-acting insulin, the nurse must multiply the total number of units to be given by 0.7:

0.7×20 units $= 14$ units of intermediate-acting insulin.

Test-taking strategy: Analyze to determine what information the question asks for, which is the calculation of the combination insulin dose. Use the formula as noted above. Proofread the math calculation. Review calculations involving percentages if you had difficulty answering this question.

Client needs category: Physiological integrity

Client needs subcategory: Pharmacological therapies

Cognitive level: Applying

---

16. A nurse is caring for clients with diabetes insipidus and must be aware of the disorder's pathophysiology. Place the following events in chronological sequence to show the pathophysiologic process. Use all of the options.

1. Thirst occurs.
2. Dehydration occurs.
3. Body has insufficient level of ADH.
4. Polyuria occurs.
5. Distal renal tubules are unable to absorb water.

Answer: 3, 5, 4, 2, 1

Rationale: The pathophysiology of diabetes insipidus begins with a decrease in ADH or with the kidneys' inability to respond to ADH. Without ADH, the distal kidney tubules and collecting ducts cannot absorb water and polyuria occurs. This leads to dehydration and then thirst.

Test-taking strategy: Analyze to determine what information the question asks for, which is the order in which diabetes insipidus progresses. Always begin with the cause of the decrease process (decease in ADH). Focusing then on the end (thirst) narrows the middle to only three options to order. Review the pathophysiology of diabetes insipidus and anatomy and physiology of the kidney if you had difficulty answering this question.

Client needs category: Physiological integrity

Client needs subcategory: Physiological adaptation

Cognitive level: Analyzing

17. The nurse is admitting a client with newly diagnosed diabetes mellitus and left-sided heart failure. Assessment reveals low blood pressure, increased respiratory rate and depth, drowsiness, and confusion. The client complains of headache and nausea. Based on the serum laboratory results below, how would the nurse interpret the client's acid–base balance?

Lab Results	
pH	7.34
HCO_3^-	19 mEq/L
$PaCO_2$	35 mm Hg
PaO_2	88 mm Hg
Potassium	5.3 mEq/L
Chloride	102 mEq/L
Calcium	10.4 mg/dL
Anion gap	30 mEq/L

☐ **1.** Metabolic alkalosis.
☐ **2.** Metabolic acidosis.
☐ **3.** Respiratory acidosis.
☐ **4.** Respiratory alkalosis.

Answer: 2

Rationale: This client has metabolic acidosis, which typically manifests with a low pH, low bicarbonate level, normal to low $PaCO_2$, and normal PaO_2. The client's serum electrolyte levels also support metabolic acidosis, which include an elevated potassium level, normal to elevated chloride level, and normal calcium level. The client's anion gap of 30 mEq/L is high, also indicative of metabolic acidosis. This kind of metabolic acidosis occurs with diabetic ketoacidosis and other disorders.

Test-taking strategy: Analyze to determine what information the question asks for, which is the interpretation of laboratory values. First, consider the diagnosis and then look to the abnormal laboratory values. Decide if there is a respiratory basis or metabolic basis to the disorder. Lastly, look to the alkalosis or acidosis findings. Review the laboratory values and physiological changes associated with diabetic keto-acidosis if you had difficulty answering this question.

Client needs category: Physiological integrity
Client needs subcategory: Physiological adaptation
Cognitive level: Analyzing

---

18. When reviewing the urinalysis report of a client with newly diagnosed diabetes mellitus, the nurse would expect which urine characteristics to be abnormal? Select all that apply.

☐ **1.** Amount.
☐ **2.** Odor.
☐ **3.** pH.
☐ **4.** Specific gravity.
☐ **5.** Glucose level.
☐ **6.** Ketone bodies.

Answer: 1, 2, 5, 6

Rationale: Diabetes mellitus is associated with increased amounts of urine, a sweet or fruity odor, and glucose and ketone bodies in the urine. It does not affect the urine's pH or specific gravity.

Test-taking strategy: Analyze to determine what information the question asks for, which is the changes in urine characteristics associated with diabetes mellitus. "Select all that apply" questions require considering each option to decide its merit. Recall that glucose is found in the urine when elevated in the serum. Also, ketones accumulate in the body when the body breaks down fat to use as energy. Ketones also spill into the urine. Review the pathophysiology and clinical manifestations of diabetes mellitus with focus on urine laboratory values if you had difficulty answering this question.

Client needs category: Physiological integrity
Client needs subcategory: Reduction of risk potential
Cognitive level: Applying

1. A client presents at the physician's office with gray-brown burrows with epidermal curved ridges and follicular papules of the skin. The primary care provider diagnoses scabies. Which teaching points should a nurse review with the client? Select all that apply.

☐ **1.** The disease is only actively contagious when the lesions are open.

☐ **2.** Scabies is transmitted by close person-to-person contact or contact with infected linens and clothing.

☐ **3.** The most commonly infected areas are the hands, feet, and neck.

☐ **4.** Severe itching of the affected areas, especially at night, is a common finding.

☐ **5.** Only the infected individual needs to use the prescribed medication.

☐ **6.** All of the client's linens and clothing should be washed immediately in hot water.

Answer: 2, 4, 6

Rationale: Scabies is a contagious disorder caused by a tiny mite that burrows under the skin; it is transmitted by close person-to-person contact or contact with infected linens or clothing. It causes severe itching, especially at night, in addition to the familiar papular rash. All of the client's linens and clothing should be washed promptly in hot water to reduce the risk of reinfestation. Scabies is transmissible from the time of infection to the time the burrows and papules appear, which may occur several weeks afterward. It remains transmissible until eradicated by a prescription cream or an oral medication. Scabies is most commonly seen in the finger webs, flexor surface of the wrists, and the antecubital fossae. When a family member is diagnosed, all members of the family must be treated with medication, and their clothing and linens washed to prevent transmission and reinfestation.

Test-taking strategy: Analyze to determine what information the question asks for, which is essential teaching points of scabies. "Select all that apply" questions require considering each option to decide its merit. Typical teaching points include what scabies look like, how to treat it, and how to prevent transfer. Review the clinical manifestations of scabies and recommended treatment if you had difficulty answering this question.

Client needs category: Health promotion and maintenance

Client needs subcategory: None

Cognitive level: Applying

2. At an outpatient clinic, a medical assistant interviews a client and documents the findings. The staff nurse reads the progress notes below and begins planning client care based on which nursing diagnosis?

Progress Notes

2/9/10	Client very anxious because new black mole
0900	with shades of brown noted on upper outer
	right thigh. Asymmetrical in shape with an
	irregular border.————M. Rosenfeld, MA

- ☐ **1.** Deficient knowledge related to potential diagnosis of basal cell carcinoma.
- ☐ **2.** Fear related to potential diagnosis of malignant melanoma.
- ☐ **3.** Risk for impaired skin integrity related to potential squamous cell carcinoma.
- ☐ **4.** Readiness for enhanced knowledge of skin care precautions related to benign mole.

Answer: 2

Rationale: Documentation reveals that the client is anxious about the symptoms. These symptoms most closely resemble malignant melanoma. Therefore, fear related to potential diagnosis of malignant melanoma is the most appropriate nursing diagnosis. The nursing note does not indicate that the client presently has deficient knowledge. The characteristics of the lesion are not consistent with a basal or squamous cell carcinoma or a benign nevus (mole).

Test-taking strategy: Analyze to determine what information the question asks for, which is nursing diagnosis from the medical assistant's documentation. Look to the notation for the highest priority problem and relate to the client's symptom or statements. Review prioritizing nursing diagnosis if you had difficulty answering this question.

Client needs category: Physiological integrity

Client needs subcategory: Physiological adaptation

Cognitive level: Analyzing

---

3. A nurse is caring for a client who is admitted from home to a long-term care facility. During the admission assessment, the nurse documents a stage II pressure ulcer and places a referral to the enterostomal therapist (ET). When gathering supplies for a stage II ulcer, what characteristics would the ET anticipate? Select all that apply.

- ☐ **1.** The skin is intact.
- ☐ **2.** Full-thickness skin loss is evident.
- ☐ **3.** Undermining is present.
- ☐ **4.** Sinus tracts have developed.
- ☐ **5.** The ulcer is superficial, like a blister.
- ☐ **6.** Partial-thickness skin loss of the epidermis is evident.

Answer: 5, 6

Rationale: A stage II pressure ulcer involves partial-thickness skin loss of the epidermis or dermis. The ulcer is superficial and presents clinically as an abrasion, blister, or shallow crater. Intact skin is characteristic of a stage I pressure ulcer. Full-thickness skin loss, undermining, and sinus tracts are characteristic of a stage III pressure ulcer.

Test-taking strategy: Analyze to determine what information the question asks for, which is characteristics of a stage II ulcer. "Select all that apply" questions require considering each option to decide its merit. Eliminate option 1 as the skin is intact. Discriminate between the other options to select options through a partial thickness. Review the pathophysiology of pressure ulcers and ulcer staging if you had difficulty answering this question.

Client needs category: Physiological integrity

Client needs subcategory: Physiological adaptation

Cognitive level: Analyzing

4. The nurse is examining the back of a client and notes a rash with a discrete lesion configuration. Which graphic shows a discrete lesion configuration?

☐ 1.

☐ 2.

☐ 3.

☐ 4.

Answer: 1

Rationale: In a discrete pattern, individual lesions are separate and distinct. Option 2 shows a grouped pattern where lesions are clustered together. Option 3 is a confluent pattern. In this configuration, lesions merge so that individual lesions are not visible or palpable. Option 4 is a linear pattern in which lesions form a line.

Test-taking strategy: Analyze to determine what information the question asks for, which is identifying a discrete lesion configuration. Use knowledge of the term "discrete" meaning apart or detached from others to narrow the selection. Review skin lesion configurations and descriptions if you had difficulty answering this question.

Client needs category: Physiological integrity

Client needs subcategory: Physiological adaptation

Cognitive level: Analyzing

---

5. A licensed practical nurse is assisting a triage nurse in the emergency department admit a client with second-degree burns on the anterior and posterior portions of both legs. Based on the Rule of Nines, what percentage of the body is burned?

[figure: front and back body diagrams with Rule of Nines percentages — 4.5% (head, front and back), 18% (front trunk), 18% (back trunk), 4.5% (each arm front), 4.5% (each arm back), 1% (groin), 9% (each leg front), 9% (each leg back)]

_____ %

Answer: 36

Rationale: The anterior and posterior portions of one leg amount to 18%. Because both legs are burned, the total is 36%.

Test-taking strategy: Analyze to determine what information the question asks for, which is percentage of body burned when the anterior and posterior portion of both legs are involved. Recall the Rule of Nines being a quick way of assessing the body and calculating treatment needs. Note the two areas per leg (18%) and multiply by 2. Review the areas affected and the percentage of body surface area calculation if you had difficulty answering this question.

Client needs category: Physiological integrity

Client needs subcategory: Physiological adaptation

Cognitive level: Analyzing

6. A client returns from the operating room with a partial-thickness skin graft on the left arm. The donor tissue was taken from the left hip. In planning immediate postoperative care, which interventions should the nurse include? Select all that apply.

☐ **1.** Change the dressing on the graft site every 8 hours.

☐ **2.** Elevate the left arm and provide complete rest of the grafted area.

☐ **3.** Administer pain medication every 4 hours as ordered for pain at the donor site.

☐ **4.** Perform ROM exercises to the left arm every 4 hours.

☐ **5.** Monitor the pulse in the left arm every 4 hours.

☐ **6.** Encourage the client to ambulate as desired on the first postoperative day.

Answer: 2, 3, 5

Rationale: Skin is the largest organ in the body representing 16% of the body weight. Skin may be harvested from one area and placed on another. In the question, the left arm should be elevated to reduce edema. Complete rest of the arm is needed to allow the graft to adhere. The donor site is usually more painful than the graft site, and the client will require pain medication to obtain relief. Because adequate circulation is needed for graft healing, it is important to monitor for the presence of a pulse. Changing the dressing every 8 hours, performing ROM exercises every 4 hours, and ambulating on the first day are inappropriate because postoperative graft sites require immobilization for 3 to 5 days.

Test-taking strategy: Analyze to determine what information the question asks for, which is the immediate postoperative care required following a skin graft. "Select all that apply" questions require considering each option to decide its merit. The key word is "immediate" and the important consideration is circulation or nourishment to the site. Review postoperative wound care and skin grafts if you had difficulty answering this question.

Client needs category: Physiological integrity

Client needs subcategory: Physiological adaptation

Cognitive level: Applying

---

7. During nursing rounds, a nurse checks on a client on bed rest who reports an itchy rash. The nurse assesses the client's skin for erythematous, slightly edematous areas on the client's back, posterior lower legs, and posterior elbows. The physician's diagnosis is an allergic contact dermatitis. Which teaching points about contact dermatitis are correct? Select all that apply.

☐ **1.** The disorder is contagious.

☐ **2.** This is an allergic reaction.

☐ **3.** Based on the location, it is likely that detergents in the bed linens caused the rash.

☐ **4.** The skin is infected wherever the rash has developed.

☐ **5.** Oatmeal (Aveeno) baths are a good treatment for a rash of this type because of the large area involved.

☐ **6.** Washing with antibacterial soap will help the rash.

Answer: 2, 3, 5

Rationale: Contact dermatitis is classified as a reaction to an allergen and can appear when skin, especially if it's moist from perspiring or other reasons, remains in contact with an irritant for an extended time. It is a hypersensitivity reaction but usually requires extended contact. This client has a presentation often seen when clients remain in bed, perspiring on detergent-cleansed bed linens or gowns. This type of sensitivity to detergents may not have produced a reaction with a shorter time contact. The rash is not contagious or infectious, although areas may become exudative and crusted. Treatment varies according to the intensity of the skin reaction and other factors, but oatmeal (Aveeno) baths are frequently prescribed.

Test-taking strategy: Analyze to determine what information the question asks for, which is teaching points of contact dermatitis. "Select all that apply" questions require considering each option to decide its merit. Consider the name "contact" to lead to answering the question correctly. Review the pathophysiology of contact dermatitis if you had difficulty answering the question.

Client needs category: Physiological integrity

Client needs subcategory: Basic care and comfort

Cognitive level: Applying

8. The nurse is providing an education seminar on skin care to clients and home care families. When discussing interventions, which areas have provided effective outcomes in preventing pressure ulcers? Select all that apply.

☐ **1.** Clean the skin with warm water and a mild cleaning agent, then apply a moisturizer.

☐ **2.** When turning the client, slide and avoid lifting.

☐ **3.** Avoid raising the head of the bed more than 90°.

☐ **4.** Turn and reposition the client every 1 to 2 hours unless contraindicated.

☐ **5.** If the client uses a wheelchair, seat on a rubber or plastic doughnut.

☐ **6.** Use pillows to position the client and increase comfort.

Answer: 1, 4, 6

Rationale: Nursing interventions that are effective in preventing pressure ulcers include cleaning the skin with warm water and a mild cleaning agent, and then applying a moisturizer; lifting—rather than sliding—the client when turning to reduce friction and shear; avoiding raising the head of the bed more than 30°, except for brief periods; repositioning and turning the client every 1 to 2 hours unless contraindicated; and using pillows to position the client and increase comfort. If the client uses a wheelchair, the nurse should offer a pressure-relieving cushion as appropriate. The nurse should not seat the client on a rubber or plastic doughnut because these devices can increase localized pressure at vulnerable points.

Test-taking strategy: Analyze to determine what information the question asks for, which is causes of pressure ulcer development and preventative measures. "Select all that apply" questions require considering each option to decide its merit. When thinking of pressure ulcer development, think of "skin integrity" and "pressure." Ask yourself, does this option maintain skin integrity and not create pressure on a bony prominence? Review preventative measures for pressure ulcers if you had difficulty answering this question.

Nursing process step: Implementation

Client needs category: Safe and effective care environment

Client needs subcategory: Safety and infection control

Cognitive level: Applying

---

9. A client presents to the emergency department with a foot lesion. When documenting the foot lesion in the medical record, which medical terms would a nurse use to classify the pictured lesion found below? Select all that apply.

☐ **1.** Linear.
☐ **2.** Flat.
☐ **3.** Fissure.
☐ **4.** Crack.
☐ **5.** Scale.
☐ **6.** Ulcer.

Answer: 1, 3

Rationale: When documenting in the medical record, it is important to use precise, descriptive terminology when documenting lesions to help aid diagnosis and track healing. The lesion depicted here is best described as a fissure, a linear crack in the skin. This type of lesion is commonly seen on clients with athlete's foot, usually between the toes.

Test-taking strategy: Analyze to determine what information the question asks for, which is accurately documenting a foot lesion. Use knowledge of medical terminology to consider each option against the pictured lesion. Review types of skin lesions and focus on descriptors if you had difficulty answering this question.

Client needs category: Physiological integrity

Client needs subcategory: Physiological adaptation

Cognitive level: Applying

10. The nurse is examining the back of a client who was admitted with a stage III pressure ulcer on the sacral area. Which illustration shows a stage III pressure ulcer?

☐ **1.**

☐ **2.**

☐ **3.**

☐ **4.**

Answer: 1

Rationale: In a stage III pressure ulcer, there is full-thickness skin loss along with damage or necrosis of the subcutaneous tissue. It may or may not extend down to (but not through) the fascia. Undermining may be present. Option 2 shows an unstageable pressure ulcer. In an unstageable pressure ulcer, the true stage of the ulcer cannot be determined until the base of the wound is exposed. Option 3 shows suspected deep tissue injury, which presents as a purple or maroon localized area of intact skin or blood-filled blister. Option 4 shows a stage IV pressure ulcer. In a stage IV ulcer, there is full-thickness skin loss with extensive tissue destruction, tissue necrosis, or damage to the muscle, bone, or support structures.

Test-taking strategy: Analyze to determine what information the question asks for, which is identification of a stage III pressure ulcer. Consider that a stage III ulcer is an advanced ulcer but not as advanced as the stage IV ulcer also depicted. Review the six pressure ulcer stages and characteristics if you had difficulty answering this question.

Client needs category: Physiological integrity

Client needs subcategory: Physiological adaptation

Cognitive level: Analyzing

1. A nurse is caring for a terminally ill cancer client who is being transferred to hospice care. Which information regarding hospice care should the nurse include in the teaching plan? Select all that apply.

- ☐ **1.** The focus of care is on controlling symptoms and relieving pain.
- ☐ **2.** A multidisciplinary team provides care.
- ☐ **3.** Services are provided based on the ability to pay.
- ☐ **4.** Hospice care is provided only in hospice centers.
- ☐ **5.** Bereavement care is provided to the family.
- ☐ **6.** Care is provided in the home, independent of physicians.

Answer: 1, 2, 5

Rationale: Hospice care focuses on controlling symptoms and relieving pain at the end of life. A multidisciplinary team—consisting of nurses, physicians, chaplains, aides, and volunteers—provides the care. After the client's death, hospice provides bereavement care to the grieving family. Hospice services are provided based on need, not on the ability to pay. Hospice care may be provided in a variety of settings, such as freestanding hospice centers, the home, a hospital, or a long-term care facility. Care is provided under the direction of a physician, who is a key member of the hospice team.

Test-taking strategy: Analyze to determine what information the question asks for, which is the concepts and principles of hospice care. "Select all that apply" questions require considering each option to decide its merit. Recall the difference between acute or home health care and hospice care which relates to the needs of a terminally ill client and extends bereavement to the family.

Client needs category: Physiological integrity

Client needs subcategory: Basic care and comfort

Cognitive level: Applying

2. A nurse has identified the nursing diagnosis *Situational low self-esteem related to hair loss and severe fatigue* for a client with cancer. Which nursing interventions would be appropriate for this client's care? Select all that apply.

☐ **1.** Ask how the diagnosis and treatment are affecting the client's personal life and roles.

☐ **2.** Review any anticipated side effects of treatment with the client.

☐ **3.** Teach the client how to resolve specific concerns related to the effects of treatment on the personal life.

☐ **4.** As a behavioral guide, describe the experiences of friends and other clients who have had this disease and treatment.

☐ **5.** Offer information on available counseling services and support groups, if desired, explaining that these techniques are helpful to many clients.

☐ **6.** Maintain eye contact with the client and use touch during interactions, if acceptable to the client.

Answer: 1, 2, 5, 6

Rationale: The nursing diagnosis selected is a psychosocial diagnosis. Discussing the client's feelings about the cancer diagnosis and treatment helps identify coping-related problems. Anticipating potential adverse effects can help the client begin to adapt and prepare to cope with these events. Referral to support groups or counseling services helps provide the client with validation and assistance with problem solving. Touch and eye contact can be therapeutic in affirming individuality and acceptance and can help build self-esteem. Instructing the client in how the nurse believes problems should be resolved is not therapeutic. The nurse should help the client explore options for solving the problems in a manner consistent with the client's beliefs and values. Telling stories about others' experiences without their consent breaches confidentiality and may demonstrate a lack of listening and empathic interaction by the nurse. Validating the client's own personal story is beneficial to rebuilding self-esteem.

Test-taking strategy: Analyze to determine what information the question asks for, which is nursing interventions associated with a specific psychosocial diagnosis. "Select all that apply" questions require considering each option to decide its merit. Recall the clinical manifestations and emotional aspects of cancer which would be a priority. Review expected outcomes for clients with cancer.

Client needs category: Psychosocial integrity

Client needs subcategory: None

Cognitive level: Applying

---

3. A client with laryngeal cancer has undergone a laryngectomy and is now receiving radiation therapy to the head and neck. The nurse should monitor the client for which adverse effects of external radiation? Select all that apply.

☐ **1.** Xerostomia.

☐ **2.** Stomatitis.

☐ **3.** Thrombocytopenia.

☐ **4.** Cystitis.

☐ **5.** Dysgeusia.

☐ **6.** Leukopenia.

Answer: 1, 2, 5

Rationale: Radiation of the head and neck often produces dry mouth (xerostomia), irritation of the oral mucous membranes (stomatitis), and diminished sense of taste (dysgeusia). Thrombocytopenia (reduced platelet count) and leukopenia (reduced white blood cell count) may occur with systemic radiation; cystitis may occur with radiation of the genitourinary system.

Test-taking strategy: Analyze to determine what information the question asks for, which is the adverse effects of radiation therapy for laryngeal cancer. "Select all that apply" questions require considering each option to decide its merit. Recall the specific area being irradiated and relate localized adverse effects of radiation. Review the adverse effects of radiation therapy if you had difficulty answering this question.

Client needs category: Physiological integrity

Client needs subcategory: Reduction of risk potential

Cognitive level: Applying

4. A nurse is teaching a community program on breast self-examination (BSE). The nurse demonstrates the proper procedure for palpating each breast. In what sequence should the following actions be performed for proper self-examination? Use all the options.

1.	Place the hand over the breast to be examined (use the right hand for the left breast and vice versa).
2.	Lie down with one arm behind the head.
3.	Palpate the breast in a perpendicular motion, going across the breast from side to side and top to bottom.
4.	Use a circular motion to feel the breast tissue (with light, medium, and firm pressure).
5.	Use the finger pads of the three middle fingers and touch the breast.

Answer: 2, 1, 5, 4, 3

Rationale: Although the American Cancer Society (ACS) states that monthly BSEs are optional, it remains an important way to discover early breast changes. BSE is a standard procedure described by national organizations designed to ensure palpation of all breast tissue. Examination can begin when lying down, in the shower or standing before a mirror. The examination also includes a visual inspection of the breasts while pressing the hands firmly against the hips and examining the underarms of each breast with the arms slightly raised.

Test-taking strategy: Analyze to determine what information the question asks for, which is the proper sequence for breast evaluation. Recall the assessment standards of palpating all areas of the breast using the pads of the fingers in a perpendicular motion. Review the method for performing BSE if you had difficulty answering this question.

Client needs category: Health promotion and maintenance

Client needs subcategory: None

Cognitive level: Applying

5. A client who is receiving chemotherapy for breast cancer develops myelosuppression. Which instructions should the nurse include in the client's discharge teaching plan? Select all that apply.

☐ **1.** Avoid people who have recently received vaccines.
☐ **2.** Avoid activities that may cause bleeding.
☐ **3.** Wash hands frequently.
☐ **4.** Increase intake of fresh fruits and vegetables.
☐ **5.** Avoid crowded places such as shopping malls.
☐ **6.** Treat a sore throat with OTC products.

Answer: 1, 2, 3, 5

Rationale: Chemotherapy can cause myelosuppression, which is a decreased number of RBCs, white blood cells, and platelets. A client receiving chemotherapy needs to avoid people who have been vaccinated recently, especially by a live virus. Because platelet counts are reduced, the client also needs to avoid activities that could cause trauma and bleeding. The client should wash her hands frequently because hand washing is the best way to prevent the spread of infection. A client receiving chemotherapy should avoid crowded places as well as people with colds during flu season because she has a reduced ability to fight infection. Fresh fruits and vegetables should be avoided because they can harbor bacteria that cannot be removed easily by washing. Signs and symptoms of infection, such as a sore throat, fever, and a cough, should be reported immediately to the primary care provider.

Test-taking strategy: Analyze to determine what information the question asks for, which is the discharge teaching plan of a client with myelosuppression. First, use knowledge of medical terminology to identify that myelo = bone or bone marrow suppression. Next, consider the ramifications related to infection which will identify several discharge teaching points. "Select all that apply" questions require considering each option to decide its merit. Review the clinical manifestations of myelosuppression and review leukopenia, thrombocytopenia, and anemia if you had difficulty answering this question.

Client needs category: Physiological integrity

Client needs subcategory: Reduction of risk potential

Cognitive level: Applying

---

6. A client with bladder cancer undergoes surgical removal of the bladder with construction of an ileal conduit. Which assessment findings indicate that the client is developing complications? Select all that apply.

☐ **1.** Urine output greater than 30 mL/hour.
☐ **2.** Dusky appearance of the stoma.
☐ **3.** Stoma protrusion from the skin.
☐ **4.** Mucus shreds in the urine collection bag.
☐ **5.** Edema of the stoma during the first 24 hours after surgery.
☐ **6.** Sharp abdominal pain with rigidity.

Answer: 2, 3, 6

Rationale: A dusky appearance of the stoma indicates decreased blood supply to the stoma; a healthy stoma should appear beefy red. Protrusion indicates prolapse of the stoma, and sharp abdominal pain with rigidity suggests peritonitis. A urine output greater than 30 mL/hour is a sign of adequate renal perfusion and is a normal finding. Because mucous membranes are used to create the conduit, mucus in the urine is expected. Stomal edema is a normal finding during the first 24 hours after surgery.

Test-taking strategy: Analyze to determine what information the question asks for, which is abnormal findings following placement of an ileal conduit.

"Select all that apply" questions require considering each option to decide its merit. Analyze the options for signs of infection or abnormal ileal conduit structure and function. Review the surgical procedure and potential complications if you had difficulty answering this question.

Client needs category: Physiological integrity

Client needs subcategory: Reduction of risk potential

Cognitive level: Analyzing

---

7. A client is ordered a dose of epoetin alfa (Aranesp) to treat anemia related to chemotherapy. The recommended dose is 150 units/kg. The client weighs 60 kg. The vial is labeled 10,000 units/mL. How many milliliters of epoetin alfa should the nurse administer? Record your answer using one decimal place.

_____ mL

Answer: 0.9

Rationale: First, determine the number of units of epoetin alfa the client is to receive:

$$60 \text{ kg} \times 150 \text{ units} = 9{,}000 \text{ units/kg.}$$

Next, determine the number of milliliters required to deliver that dose:

$$10{,}000 \text{ units} : 1 \text{ mL} = 9{,}000 \text{ units} : X$$

$$\frac{10{,}000 \text{ units} \times X}{10{,}000 \text{ units}} = \frac{9{,}000 \text{ units} \times 1 \text{ mL}}{10{,}000 \text{ units}}$$

$$X = 0.9 \text{ mL.}$$

Test-taking strategy: Analyze to determine what information the question asks for, which is correct dosage of Aranesp. Follow the two-step procedure noted above. Proofread your math calculation. Review drug concentration calculations if you had difficulty answering this question.

Client needs category: Physiological integrity

Client needs subcategory: Pharmacological therapies

Cognitive level: Applying

8. A client who is experiencing colon cancer is scheduled to undergo a colostomy. Which interventions would be appropriate to include in a preoperative teaching plan? Select all that apply.

☐ **1.** Demonstrate turning, coughing, deep breathing, splinting, and leg ROM exercises, and provide rationales for each procedure.

☐ **2.** Encourage the client to rate the current level of discomfort on a 0-to-10 scale.

☐ **3.** Arrange for an ET to speak with the client about colostomy care.

☐ **4.** Explain the need for early postoperative ambulation.

☐ **5.** Instruct the client on signs and symptoms of intestinal obstruction.

☐ **6.** Encourage the client to express feelings about changes in body image.

Answer: 1, 3, 4, 6

Rationale: Preoperatively, the client will require instruction regarding the need for turning, coughing, deep breathing, splinting, and leg ROM exercises. The client will also need to learn about colostomy care and the reason for early postoperative ambulation. Addressing feelings about body image changes is also appropriate at this time. Rating pain and discomfort and instructing the client about signs and symptoms of intestinal obstruction are part of the postoperative care.

Test-taking strategy: Analyze to determine what information the question asks for, which is interventions for the preoperative teaching plan. The key word is "preoperative" meaning instruction which can be given but used in the postoperative period. Review preoperative interventions and colostomy surgery if you had difficulty answering this question.

Client needs category: Physiological integrity

Client needs subcategory: Basic care and comfort

Cognitive level: Applying

---

9. A client has been diagnosed with lung cancer and is scheduled to undergo a left pneumonectomy. The client will have a chest tube inserted as part of the surgical procedure. Identify the area where the nurse will expect to see the chest tube inserted.

Answer:

Rationale: A left pneumonectomy is the surgical removal of the left lung. Removal of one lobe of the lung is called a lobectomy. A chest tube is placed within the thoracic cavity at the site of the removed lung. Therefore, a chest tube would be placed on the left side of the chest.

Test-taking strategy: Analyze to determine what information the question asks for, which is site of chest tube insertion for a left pneumonectomy. Recall from medical terminology that (pneumo—lung, ectomy—removal) meaning as removal of the lung. Also, always use anatomical position when determining between right side and left side placement. Review the clinical manifestations of pneumonectomy and anatomical placement of a chest tube if you had difficulty answering this question.

Client needs category: Physiological integrity

Client needs subcategory: Physiological adaptation

Cognitive level: Applying

10. A client has been diagnosed with breast cancer and is scheduled to begin treatment with the antineoplastic drug doxorubicin hydrochloride. Which side effects should the nurse anticipate? Select all that apply.

- ☐ **1.** Hair thinning.
- ☐ **2.** Blue-green discoloration of urine.
- ☐ **3.** Left ventricular failure.
- ☐ **4.** Complete hair loss within 3 to 4 weeks.
- ☐ **5.** Red discoloration of urine.

Answer: 3, 4, 5

Rationale: Doxorubicin is used in combination with other medications to treat many types of cancers. Primary side effects of this drug include cardiac changes (including left ventricular failure and arrhythmias), complete hair loss within 3 to 4 weeks of receiving the drug, and red discoloration of the urine. Methotrexate rarely causes complete hair loss but may cause thinning or no hair loss. Methocarbamol (Robaxin), a muscle relaxant, causes the urine to turn a blue-green color.

Test-taking strategy: Analyze to determine what information the question asks for, which is side effects of doxorubicin. Recall that a complete cardiac assessment is completed prior to the initiation of chemotherapeutic due to the cardiac changes that may occur. Also note other common side effects of chemotherapeutic therapy. Review common side effects of chemotherapeutic agents, and especially doxorubicin hydrochloride if you had difficulty answering the question.

Client needs category: Physiological integrity

Client needs subcategory: Physiological adaptation

Cognitive level: Applying

---

11. While undergoing treatment with a caustic chemotherapeutic agent, a client experiences extravasation. Indicate how the nurse should respond to extravasation by placing the following nursing interventions in chronological order. Use all the options.

1. Notify the physician.
2. Follow facility policy for dealing with extravasation.
3. Discontinue the intravenous infusion.
4. Implement physician's orders.
5. Document all signs and symptoms thoroughly.
6. Monitor the client throughout the shift and give a detailed report to the oncoming shift.

Answer: 3, 2, 1, 4, 5, 6

Rationale: Extravasation is the accidental administration of I.V. fluid into the extracellular space/tissue. Immediately, the intravenous infusion should be discontinued so that the client will not continue to receive more of the medication and damage the tissue. The facility will have a policy on how to deal with extravasation (usually the application of ice) that can be implemented while the physician is being notified. After the physician is notified, the specific orders will need to be implemented. All signs and symptoms that the client is experiencing should be documented thoroughly in preparation for the report to be given to the oncoming shift.

Test-taking strategy: Analyze to determine what information the question asks for, which is nursing interventions when caring for a client with an extravasation. Safety is always a first concern which includes discontinuing the I.V. administration. Note that options with documentation and monitoring are performed after safety and care of the client. Review the clinical manifestations of extravasation and client safety if you had difficulty answering this question.

Client needs category: Physiological integrity

Client needs subcategory: Pharmacological therapies

Cognitive level: Analyzing

12. The nurse is teaching a client about self-breast examination (SBE). Which pattern of palpation would the nurse encourage based on ACS recommendations?

☐ **1.**

☐ **2.**

☐ **3.**

☐ **4.**

Answer: 3

Rationale: The ACS recommends an up-and-down vertical pattern as the most effective pattern for covering the whole breast. Option 1 (circular pattern) and option 2 (wedged pattern) are alternate methods but may not be as effective. Option 4 (horizontal pattern) is not a recognized method used in SBE.

Test-taking strategy: Analyze to determine what information the question asks for, which is pattern of palpation during an SBE. Consider that the up-and-down method is a common method that covers all breast tissue. Review known patterns of palpation for SBE and the current ACS guidelines if you had difficulty answering this question.

Client needs category: Physiological integrity
Client needs subcategory: Reduction of risk potential
Cognitive level: Analyzing

PART FOUR

Maternal–Neonatal Nursing

1. During her first prenatal visit, a client asks a nurse what physiological changes she can expect during pregnancy. The nurse begins the discussion with the presumptive changes of pregnancy. Put the following presumptive changes in ascending chronological order according to when they occur. Use all of the options.

1. Frequent urination.
2. Breast changes.
3. Quickening.
4. Appearance of linea nigra, melasma, and striae gravidarum.
5. Uterine enlargement in which the uterus can be palpated over the symphysis pubis.

Answer: 2, 1, 5, 3, 4

Rationale: Presumptive changes are subjective and can be caused by other medical conditions. Breast changes occur approximately 2 weeks after implantation of the embryo; frequent urination, at 3 weeks; fatigue and uterine enlargement over the symphysis pubis, at 18 weeks; quickening, between 18 and 20 weeks; and the appearance of linea nigra, melasma, and striae gravidarum, at 24 weeks.

Test-taking strategy: Analyze to determine what information the question asks for, which is the progression of the presumptive changes of pregnancy. The key word is "progression" as the question states that all five options are presumptive changes. The earliest signs can lead from hormonal changes, thus breast changes are first. Next, look to the end and critically think what would be last. The appearance of the linea nigra group of changes refers to a stretched abdomen making it the last choice. Discriminate through the remaining three options to fill in the middle. Review the physiologic changes of pregnancy with presumptive signs if you had difficulty answering this question.

Client needs category: Health promotion and maintenance

Client needs subcategory: None

Cognitive level: Applying

---

2. A 30-year-old client comes to the office for a routine prenatal visit. After reading the chart entry below, the nurse should prepare the client for which study?

Progress Notes	
6/8/10 1320	Pt. is 11 weeks pregnant; urine sample shows glycosuria. Pt. has a family history of diabetes. ———— Chrissy Franks, LPN

☐ **1.** Triple screen.
☐ **2.** Indirect Coombs' test.
☐ **3.** 1-Hour glucose tolerance test.
☐ **4.** Amniocentesis.

Answer: 3

Rationale: A 1-hour glucose tolerance test is recommended to screen for gestational diabetes if the client is obese, has glycosuria or a family history of diabetes, or lost a fetus for unexplained reasons or gave birth to a large-for-gestational-age neonate. A triple screen tests for chromosomal abnormalities. The indirect Coombs' test screens maternal blood for red blood cell antibodies. Amniocentesis is used to detect fetal abnormalities.

Test-taking strategy: Analyze to determine what information the question asks for, which is identifying an abnormal finding, requiring further testing, in the documentation provided. Note that all abnormal findings such as "glycosuria" and "diabetes" lead to a test for gestational diabetes. Review laboratory studies during pregnancy, especially related to gestational diabetes, if you had difficulty answering this question.

Client needs category: Physiological integrity

Client needs subcategory: Reduction of risk potential

Cognitive level: Applying

3. A nurse is preparing to teach a client about fetal growth and development during the first 3 months of pregnancy. The nurse is assembling teaching aids by milestones. In ascending order (month 1, month 2, month 3, and months 4 to 9), how would the nurse arrange the aids? Use all of the options.

1. Teeth and bones begin to appear, the kidneys start to function and, at the end of the month, gender is distinguishable.

2. The embryo has a definite form; the head, trunk, and tiny buds for arms and legs develop; and the cardiovascular system begins to function.

3. Internal and external fetal growth continues at a rapid rate, and the fetus stores the fats and minerals it needs to live outside the womb.

4. The eyes, ears, nose, lips, tongue, and tooth buds develop; the umbilical cord has a definite form; and the external genitalia are present.

Answer: 2, 4, 1, 3

Rationale: Significant growth and development take place during the first 3 months. By the first month, the embryo has a definite form; the head, trunk, and tiny buds for arms and legs develop; and the cardiovascular system begins to function. By the second month, the eyes, ears, nose, lips, tongue, and tooth buds develop; the umbilical cord has a definite form; and the external genitalia are present. By the third month, teeth and bones begin to appear, the kidneys start to function and, at the end of the month, gender is distinguishable. By the fourth month, internal and external fetal growth begins accelerating at a more rapid rate; the fetus stores the fats and minerals it needs to live outside the womb, and growth continues until the fetus is full-term.

Test-taking strategy: Analyze to determine what information the question asks for, which is order of prenatal development milestones. Read each grouping carefully to identify the sequence. Recall that large structures appear first such as head and trunk. Also note the last option, fetal stores for outside the womb. Fill in the middle two options but note umbilical cord development as first. Review fetal development by milestones if you had difficulty answering this question.

Client needs category: Health promotion and maintenance

Client needs subcategory: None

Cognitive level: Applying

4. A woman at 15 weeks of gestation comes to the clinic for an amniocentesis. If an abnormal result is found, which characteristics or problems could be identified? Select all that apply.

☐ **1.** Fetal lung maturity.
☐ **2.** Gestational diabetes.
☐ **3.** Chromosomal defects.
☐ **4.** Neural tube defects.
☐ **5.** Polyhydramnios.
☐ **6.** Sex of the fetus.

Answer: 3, 4, 6

Rationale: In early pregnancy, amniocentesis can be used to identify chromosomal and neural tube defects and to determine the sex of the fetus. It can also be used to evaluate fetal lung maturity during the last trimester of pregnancy. A blood test performed between 24 and 28 weeks of gestation is used to screen for gestational diabetes. Ultrasound is used to identify polyhydramnios; amniocentesis can be used to treat polyhydramnios by removing excess fluid.

Test-taking strategy: Analyze to determine what information the question asks for, which is the characteristics/problems that can be identified with an amniocentesis. "Select all that apply" questions require considering each option to decide its merit. Understanding basic facts, such as fetal development at 15 weeks (approximately 4 months) of gestation and the benefits of amniocentesis, is a must. When considering each option, ask if the option would be able to be identified at that gestation and if amniocentesis would identify it. Both must fit to be chosen for the answer. Review gestational development and amniocentesis if you had difficulty answering this question.

Client needs category: Physiological integrity
Client needs subcategory: Reduction of risk potential
Cognitive level: Applying

---

5. A nurse is caring for a post-term client at 41 weeks of gestation who is about to undergo a biophysical profile (BPP) to evaluate her fetus's well-being. The client asks, "What will be able to be determined from this profile?" The nurse is correct to identify which? Select all that apply.

☐ **1.** Fetal tone.
☐ **2.** Fetal breathing.
☐ **3.** Femur length.
☐ **4.** Amniotic fluid volume.
☐ **5.** Biparietal diameter.
☐ **6.** Crown–rump length.

Answer: 1, 2, 4

Rationale: A BPP is an ultrasound assessment of fetal well-being that includes the following components: nonstress test, fetal tone, fetal breathing, fetal motion, and volume of amniotic fluid. It is used to confirm the health of the fetus or identify abnormalities. Crown–rump length is used to assess gestational age during the first trimester. Biparietal diameter and femur length are also used to assess gestational age and are done in the second and third trimesters.

Test-taking strategy: Analyze to determine what information the question asks for, which is components of a BPP. "Select all that apply" questions require considering each option to decide its merit. First, identify the options that provide information about "well-being." Next, add that information to the five parameters of a BPP. Review BPP information if you had difficulty answering this question.

Client needs category: Physiological integrity
Client needs subcategory: Reduction of risk potential
Cognitive level: Applying

6. A nurse is caring for a client who is at 32 weeks of gestation and performs Leopold's maneuvers to determine that the fetus is in the cephalic position. To identify fetal heart tones, place an X where the nurse should place the Doppler transducer.

Rationale: When the fetus is in the cephalic position (head down), fetal heart tones are best auscultated midway between the symphysis pubis and the umbilicus. When the fetus is in the breech position, fetal heart tones are best heard at or above the level of the umbilicus.

Test-taking strategy: Analyze to determine what information the question asks for, which is placement of transducer to hear fetal heart sound when the fetus is in the cephalic position. Use the clues from medical terminology (cephalo-head). Cephalic position means head first in the birth canal. With that knowledge, visualize where the heart sounds would best be heard. Review fetal positions related to the fetal head placement if you had difficulty answering this question.

Client needs category: Health promotion and maintenance

Client needs subcategory: None

Cognitive level: Analyzing

7. A nurse is caring for a primigravida client. At 20 weeks of gestation, identify the location where the nurse anticipates the uterine fundus.

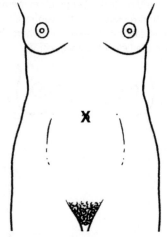

Rationale: At 20 weeks, the uterine fundus should be palpated approximately at the umbilicus. Fundal height should be measured from the symphysis pubis to the top of the uterus (McDonald's method). Serial measurements assess fetal growth over the course of the pregnancy. Between weeks 22 and 34, the number of centimeters measured correlate approximately with the week of gestation. However, if the client is very tall or short, fundal height will differ.

Test-taking strategy: Analyze to determine what information the question asks for, which is the location of the uterine fundus at a specific time (20 weeks of gestation). Recall that the uterine fundus is the top portion of the uterus, opposite the cervix. At 20 weeks, the fundal height is at the level of the umbilicus and increases 1 cm per week thereafter; thus, as pregnancy progresses, the fundal height increases. Review changes in fundal height throughout pregnancy if you had difficulty answering this question.

Client needs category: Health promotion and maintenance

Client needs subcategory: None

Cognitive level: Applying

8. A nurse is caring for a client who is 32 weeks' pregnant and being monitored in the antepartum unit for pregnancy-induced hypertension. The client suddenly complains of continuous abdominal pain and vaginal bleeding. Which nursing interventions are a priority? Select all that apply.

- ☐ **1.** Evaluate maternal vital signs.
- ☐ **2.** Prepare for vaginal delivery.
- ☐ **3.** Reassure the client that she will be able to continue the pregnancy.
- ☐ **4.** Auscultate fetal heart tones.
- ☐ **5.** Monitor the amount of vaginal bleeding.
- ☐ **6.** Monitor intake and output.

Answer: 1, 4, 5, 6

Rationale: The client's symptoms indicate that she is experiencing abruptio placentae. The nurse must immediately evaluate the mother's vital signs, auscultate fetal heart tones, monitor the amount of blood loss, and evaluate volume status by monitoring intake and output. After the severity of the abruption has been determined and blood and fluid have been replaced, a prompt cesarean (not vaginal) delivery is indicated if the fetus is in distress.

Test-taking strategy: Analyze to determine what information the question asks for, which is priority nursing interventions of a client experiencing abdominal pain and vaginal bleeding. "Select all that apply" questions require considering each option to decide its merit. Recall that vaginal bleeding and abdominal pain can be an ominous sign related to life-threatening disorders for the mother and baby. Consider the assessment data needed to relate important data to the physician. Review disorders of pregnancy related to abdominal pain and vaginal bleeding if you had difficulty answering this question.

Client needs category: Physiological integrity

Client needs subcategory: Physiological adaptation

Cognitive level: Analyzing

9. A nurse is obtaining a pregnancy history at the first antepartal visit. The client states symptoms of a nagging abdominal pain and a pulling sensation. Place an X where the nurse anticipates these normal symptoms in early pregnancy.

Answer:

Rationale: As the uterus grows in early pregnancy, it deviates physically to the right. This shift, or dextrorotation, is due to the presence of the rectosigmoid colon in the left lower quadrant. As a result, many women complain of pain in the right lower quadrant.

Test-taking strategy: Analyze to determine what information the question asks for, which is the abdominal site of discomfort in early pregnancy. Consider the effects of a growing fetus in the abdominal cavity and relate to the impact on other abdominal organs. Review maternal anatomy especially with the enlarging uterus if you had difficulty answering this question.

Client needs category: Health promotion and maintenance

Client needs subcategory: None

Cognitive level: Analyzing

---

10. During a prenatal visit, a physician decides to admit a client to the hospital. Based on the nurse's admission note below, which complication of pregnancy would the physician suspect?

Progress Notes	
2/2/10 1100	30-year-old female admitted with nausea and vomiting. Pt. is 16 weeks pregnant and complains of thirst and vertigo. BP 120/70 mm Hg, RR 20, P 104, Temp 100°F. Pt. has had nothing to eat or drink for 24 hours. ————————————S. Thomas, LPN

☐ **1.** Iron-deficiency anemia.
☐ **2.** Placenta previa.
☐ **3.** Pregnancy-induced hypertension.
☐ **4.** Hyperemesis gravidarum.

Answer: 4

Rationale: Hyperemesis gravidarum is severe nausea and vomiting that persists after the first trimester. If untreated, it can lead to weight loss, starvation, dehydration, fluid and electrolyte imbalances, and acid–base disturbances. The client may report thirst, hiccups, oliguria, vertigo, and headache. A rapid pulse and elevated or subnormal temperature can also occur. Signs and symptoms of iron-deficiency anemia include fatigue, pallor, and exercise intolerance. Placenta previa causes painless, bright red, vaginal bleeding after 20 weeks of pregnancy. Pregnancy-induced hypertension usually develops after 20 weeks of pregnancy; the client reports sudden weight gain and presents with hypertension.

Test-taking strategy: Analyze to determine what information the question asks for, which is a complication as documented in the nurse's admission note. Begin by focusing on abnormal findings in the note (nausea/vomiting, thirst, vertigo, and nothing by mouth for 24 hours). Next, relate those symptoms to the options. If unsure, note that hyperemesis contains the word emesis which is an abnormal symptom in the admission note. Review the assessment findings and relate to complications of pregnancy if you had difficulty answering this question.

Client needs category: Physiological integrity

Client needs subcategory: Physiological adaptation

Cognitive level: Applying

---

11. A client at 32 weeks of gestation has mild preeclampsia. She is discharged home with instructions to remain on bed rest. She should also be instructed to call her physician if she experiences which of the following symptoms? Select all that apply.

☐ **1.** Headache.
☐ **2.** Increased urine output.
☐ **3.** Blurred vision.
☐ **4.** Difficulty sleeping.
☐ **5.** Epigastric pain.
☐ **6.** Severe nausea and vomiting.

Answer: 1, 3, 5, 6

Rationale: The care of a client with mild preeclampsia can be managed at home with proper instructions. Headache, blurred vision, epigastric pain, and severe nausea and vomiting can indicate worsening preeclampsia. Decreased, not increased, urine output is a concern because preeclampsia is associated with decreased renal perfusion, leading to a reduction in the glomerular filtration rate and decreased urine output. Difficulty sleeping, a common complaint during the third trimester, is only a concern if it is caused by any of the other symptoms.

Test-taking strategy: Analyze to determine what information the question asks for, which is discharge instructions for mild preeclampsia. "Select all that apply" questions require considering each option to decide its merit. Even though the client's preeclampsia is mild, it is still considered dangerous. Select the options that relate to decreased perfusion and increased blood pressure. Review the management of client symptoms of preeclampsia in the home if you had difficulty answering this question.

Client needs category: Physiological integrity

Client needs subcategory: Reduction of risk potential

Cognitive level: Applying

12. The nurse is caring for a client approaching a term pregnancy. When assessing fetal presentation using Leopold's maneuvers, the nurse alerts the physician to the need of an external version. Place an X where the nurse assesses the fetal head.

Answer:

Rationale: An external version is a procedure that externally rotates the fetus from a breech presentation to a vertex presentation. If the fetal head is palpated at the top of the uterus, the fetus is in the breech position. That is, the head is not the presenting part and the physician may consider external version to convert the fetus to the head-down position. This is accomplished by applying pressure on the maternal abdomen to turn the infant over, as in a somersault.

Test-taking strategy: Analyze to determine what information the question asks for, which is the location of the fetal head if external version is needed. Recall the correct position for the fetus approaching a term pregnancy is in the pelvis preparing for delivery. The client should note lightening at this time marking the decent of the fetus. External version, if successful, will place the head in the correct position for delivery. Review the gestational age of the fetus and the expected fetal position if you had difficulty answering this question.

Client needs category: Physiological integrity

Client needs subcategory: Reduction of risk potential

Cognitive level: Analyzing

13. A nurse is teaching a course on the anatomy and physiology of reproduction. In which location should the nurse identify as the area where fertilization occurs?

Rationale: After ejaculation, the sperm travel by flagellar movement through the cervical mucus into the fallopian tube to meet the descending ovum in the ampulla. Fertilization occurs in the ampulla (outer third) of the fallopian tube.

Test-taking strategy: Analyze to determine what information the question asks for, which is the location of ovum fertilization. Follow the path of the illustration for sperm movement and note the egg erupting from the follicle. Recall that the location of fertilization is different from the area of implantation. Review female anatomy and physiology as related to fertilization if you had difficulty answering this question.

Client needs category: Health promotion and maintenance

Client needs subcategory: None

Cognitive level: Understanding

14. The nurse is providing prenatal instructions to a 32-year-old primagravida. Which nutritional instructions should the nurse review? Select all that apply.

☐ **1.** Caloric intake should be increased by 300 cal/day.
☐ **2.** Protein intake should be increased to more than 30 g/day.
☐ **3.** Vitamin intake should not increase from prepregnancy requirements.
☐ **4.** Folic acid intake should be increased to 800 mg/day.
☐ **5.** Intake of all minerals, especially iron, should be increased.
☐ **6.** Water intake should be doubled.

Answer: 1, 2, 4, 5

Rationale: A pregnant woman should increase her caloric intake by 300 cal/day. The protein requirements (76 g/day) of a pregnant woman exceed those of a non-pregnant woman by 30 g/day. All mineral requirements, especially iron, are increased in a pregnant woman. The woman should also increase her intake of all vitamins; a prenatal vitamin is usually recommended. Folic acid intake is particularly important to help prevent fetal anomalies such as neural tube defect. Intake should be increased from 400 to 800 mg/day. Nonpregnant females are encouraged to drink six 8 oz glasses of water daily. Pregnant females increase that amount to eight.

Test-taking strategy: Analyze to determine what information the question asks for, which is nutritional requirements in pregnancy. "Select all that apply" questions require considering each option to decide its merit. Consider increases needed as the maternal body uses its resources to develop a fetus. Most nutritional building blocks will be increased for this reason. Review nutritional requirements of pregnancy, including calorie, protein, vitamin, and mineral needs if you had difficulty answering this question.

Client needs category: Health promotion and maintenance

Client needs subcategory: None

Cognitive level: Analyzing

15. A nurse is palpating the fundal height of a pregnant woman at 40 weeks of gestation. Identify the area on the abdomen where the nurse would expect to feel the uterine fundus.

Answer:

Rationale: Uterine height is measured from the top of the maternal symphysis pubis to the top of the uterine fundus. By the 36th week, the uterine fundus should touch the xiphoid process. About 2 weeks before term (the 38th week), the fetal head settles into the pelvis to prepare for birth and the uterus returns to the height it was at 36 weeks.

Test-taking strategy: Analyze to determine what information the question asks for, which is fundal height at 40 weeks of gestation, prior to delivery. Recall that the uterus has expanded to largest position and now will decrease due to lightening. Review the fundal height as related to the gestational age and fetal position if you had difficulty answering this question.

Client needs category: Health promotion and maintenance

Client needs subcategory: None

Cognitive level: Applying

---

16. A 35-year-old client who is 28 weeks pregnant is admitted for testing. After reading the nursing notes below, which rationale best explains why a pregnant client should lie on her left side when resting or sleeping in the later stages of pregnancy?

Progress Notes	
5/12/10 1430	Pt. admitted to short-term procedure unit for testing. States "I'm feeling a little faint." Skin slightly diaphoretic to touch. Pt. assisted to left side. VS stable. States "I'm feeling better now." —————— S. Brown, LPN

☐ **1.** To facilitate digestion.
☐ **2.** To facilitate bladder emptying.
☐ **3.** To prevent compression of the vena cava.
☐ **4.** To prevent development of fetal anomalies.

Answer: 3

Rationale: The weight of the pregnant uterus is sufficiently heavy to compress the vena cava, which could impair blood flow to the uterus, possibly decreasing oxygen to the fetus. The client may experience supine hypotension syndrome (faintness, diaphoresis, and hypotension) from the pressure on the inferior vena cava. The side-lying position puts the weight of the fetus on the bed, not on the woman. The side-lying position has not been shown to prevent fetal anomalies, nor does it facilitate bladder emptying or digestion.

Test-taking strategy: Analyze to determine what information the question asks for, which is rationale for left side lying in later stages of pregnancy. Note the documented client symptoms. Analyze the options to relate position change to improvement of condition. Review fetal positioning as related to maternal anatomy, particularly with respect to supine and side-lying positions if you had difficulty answering this question.

Client needs category: Physiological integrity

Client needs subcategory: Reduction of risk potential

Cognitive level: Analyzing

17. A client is at risk for seizures due to pregnancy-induced hypertension. The physician orders 4 g magnesium sulfate in 250 mL D$_5$W to be infused at 1 g/hour following a loading dose. What is the flow rate in milliliters per hour? Round your answer to the nearest whole number.

_____ mL/hour

Answer: 63

Rationale: To solve this, first set up a proportion and then solve for X:

$$4 \text{ g}/250 \text{ mL} = 1 \text{ g}/X \text{ mL}$$
$$4 \times X = 250$$
$$X = \frac{250 \text{ mL}}{4}$$
$$X = 62.5 \text{ mL.}$$

Rounded off to a whole number, this is 63 mL/hour.

Test-taking strategy: Analyze to determine what information the question asks for, which is flow rate in milliliters per hour of a magnesium sulfate infusion. Read the question thoroughly eliminating any extraneous information (loading dose). Solve for X using the ratio–proportion method and aligning both sides of the equation consistently using known data. Proofread the math calculation.

Client needs category: Physiological integrity

Client needs subcategory: Pharmacological therapies

Cognitive level: Applying

---

18. When teaching an antepartum client about the passage of the fetus through the birth canal during labor, the nurse describes the cardinal mechanisms of labor. Place these events in the proper sequence in which they occur. Use all of the options.

1. Flexion.
2. External rotation.
3. Descent.
4. Expulsion.
5. Internal rotation.
6. Extension.

Answer: 3, 1, 5, 6, 2, 4

Rationale: As the fetus moves through the bony and narrow birth canal, it goes through position changes to ensure that the smallest diameter of fetal head presents to the smallest diameter of the birth canal. Termed the cardinal mechanisms of labor, these position changes occur in the following sequence: descent, flexion, internal rotation, extension, external rotation, and expulsion.

Test-taking strategy: Analyze to determine what information the question asks for, which is position changes during the birth process. If unsure, identify the first (descent) and last (expulsion) to narrow the options. Also, consider the birth canal and fetal adjustment to fit through the canal. Review the relationship of the fetal head diameter, diameter of the birth canal, and cardinal movements to aid in birth if you had difficulty answering this question.

Client needs category: Health promotion and maintenance

Client needs subcategory: None

Cognitive level: Applying

19. A nurse is caring for a client who is anxious to know her baby's due date. The nurse instructs the client on how to determine the baby's due date according to Nagele's rule. The client is correct to state which of the following when discussing the use of the rule. Select all that apply.

1. "I need to know the date of intercourse."
2. "I will calculate 9 months from my last menstrual period."
3. "Nagele's rule provides a good approximation of the due date."
4. "I will add seven days to the first day of my last menstrual period and count back 3 months."
5. "Nagele's rule may be used in conjunction with other assessment findings."

Answer: 3, 4, 5

Rationale: Nagele's rule is one method of determining the estimated date of delivery. When using Nagele's rule, add 7 days to the first day of the last menstrual period, and count back 3 months. Nagele's rule may be used with other assessment findings, especially in situations when the last menstrual period is in question. Nagele's rule does not use dates of intercourse nor adding 9 months to the last menstrual period to determine the due date.

Test-taking strategy: Analyze to determine what information the question asks for, which is correct responses indicating an understanding of Nagele's rule. Recall that Nagele's rule uses a calculation based upon the last menstrual period. Consider that it is used frequently along with other assessment data to determine the gestation age of a fetus. Review Nagele's rule if you had difficulty answering this question.

Client needs category: Health promotion and maintenance

Client needs subcategory: None

Cognitive level: Applying

Intrapartum Period

1. A nurse is evaluating a client who is 34 weeks pregnant for preterm rupture of the membranes (PROM). Which findings indicate that PROM has occurred? Select all that apply.

☐ 1. Fernlike pattern when vaginal fluid is placed on a glass slide and allowed to dry.
☐ 2. Acidic pH of fluid when tested with nitrazine paper.
☐ 3. Presence of amniotic fluid in the vagina.
☐ 4. Cervical dilation of 6 cm.
☐ 5. Alkaline pH of fluid when tested with nitrazine paper.
☐ 6. Contractions occurring every 5 minutes.

Answer: 1, 3, 5

Rationale: The fernlike pattern that occurs when vaginal fluid is placed on a glass slide and allowed to dry, the presence of amniotic fluid in the vagina, and an alkaline pH of fluid are all signs of ruptured membranes. The fernlike pattern is a result of the high sodium and protein content of the amniotic fluid. The presence of amniotic fluid in the vagina results from the expulsion of the fluid from the amniotic sac. Amniotic fluid tests as an alkaline, not acidic, fluid. Cervical dilation and regular contractions are signs of progressing labor, but they do not indicate PROM.

Test-taking strategy: Analyze to determine what information the question asks for, which is definitive data of a premature rupture of membranes. "Select all that apply" questions require considering each option to decide its merit. Consider the definitive presence of amniotic fluid as being the pattern displayed on the slide, actual presence of amniotic fluid, and alkaline pH on nitrazine paper. Review the clinical manifestations of PROM if you had difficulty answering this question.

Client needs category: Physiological integrity

Client needs subcategory: Physiological adaptation

Cognitive level: Analyzing

2. A client in the first stage of labor is being monitored using an external fetal monitor. After the nurse reviews the monitoring strip from the client's chart (shown below), into which of the following positions should the nurse assist the client?

☐ **1.** Left lateral.
☐ **2.** Right lateral.
☐ **3.** Supine.
☐ **4.** Prone.

Answer: 1

Rationale: The fetal heart rate monitoring strip shows late decelerations, which indicate uteroplacental circulatory insufficiency and can lead to fetal hypoxia and acidosis if the underlying cause is not corrected. The client should be turned onto her left side to increase placental perfusion and decrease contraction frequency. In addition, the I.V. fluid rate may be increased and oxygen administered. The right lateral, supine, and prone positions do not increase placental perfusion.

Test-taking strategy: Analyze to determine what information the question asks for, which is client position following monitor strip analysis. Interpret the data from the monitor strip by aligning the fetal heart rate (top line) with contraction sequence (bottom line). Compare reaction of fetal heart rate against contractions and conclude late decelerations. Recall that throughout pregnancy having the client lay on the left side aids in placental perfusion. Review fetal heart rate patterns and uterine contractions if you had difficulty answering this question.

Client needs category: Physiological integrity

Client needs subcategory: Reduction of risk potential

Cognitive level: Analyzing

---

3. The nurse is caring for a client in active labor. As the nurse is evaluating the waveform below, identify the area of concern that suggests umbilical cord compression.

Answer:

Rationale: The X is placed at the site where the fetal heart rate decreases. Variable decelerations are decreases in fetal heart rate that are not related to the timing of contractions. They are characteristic of umbilical cord compression, which reduces blood flow between the placenta and fetus. These decelerations generally occur as drops of 10 to 60 beats/minute below the baseline.

Test-taking strategy: Analyze to determine what information the question asks for, which is waveform location suggesting umbilical cord compression. The key term is "compression," indicating an interruption in circulation and heart rate leading to the placement of the X. Review fetal oxygen depletion causing a decrease in fetal heart rate if you had difficulty answering this question.

Client needs category: Physiological integrity

Client needs subcategory: Reduction of risk potential

Cognitive level: Analyzing

4. A client who is 29 weeks' pregnant comes to the labor and delivery unit. She states that she is having contractions every 8 minutes. The client is also 3 cm dilated. Which of the following can the nurse expect to administer? Select all that apply.

- [ ] **1.** Folic acid.
- [ ] **2.** Terbutaline.
- [ ] **3.** Betamethasone.
- [ ] **4.** Rh$_o$(D) immune globulin (RhoGam).
- [ ] **5.** I.V. fluids.
- [ ] **6.** Nalbuphine.

Answer: 2, 3, 5

Rationale: The nurse can expect that terbutaline, a β-2 agonist that relaxes smooth muscle, will be administered to halt contractions; and betamethasone, a corticosteroid, will be administered to decrease the risk of respiratory distress to the neonate if preterm delivery occurs; and that I.V. fluids will be given to expand the intravascular volume and decrease contractions if dehydration is the cause. Folic acid is a mineral recommended throughout pregnancy (especially in the first trimester) to decrease the risk of neural tube defects. RhoGam is given to Rh-negative clients who have been, or may have been, exposed to Rh-positive fetal blood. Nalbuphine is an opioid analgesic used during labor and delivery.

Test-taking strategy: Analyze to determine what information the question asks for, which is medications given to a client who is 29 weeks' pregnant and in labor. "Select all that apply" questions require considering each option to decide its merit. First, determine that the client is in preterm labor (29 weeks). Next, consider the options that would help stop the progression of labor or be beneficial to the fetus. Review interventions to suppress preterm labor and medications used if you had difficulty answering this question.

Client needs category: Physiological integrity

Client needs subcategory: Pharmacological therapies

Cognitive level: Analyzing

---

5. The licensed practical nurse (LPN) is co-assigned with the registered nurse to provide care for a client receiving oxytocin (Pitocin) to induce labor. When discussing adverse side effects of Pitocin, which conditions should the LPN notify the registered nurse of immediately? Select all that apply.

- [ ] **1.** A blood pressure of 170/92 mm Hg.
- [ ] **2.** Jaundice in the sclera.
- [ ] **3.** Lab work suggesting dehydration.
- [ ] **4.** Fluid overload with crackles in the lung fields.
- [ ] **5.** Palpable uterine tetany.
- [ ] **6.** A heart rate of 60 beats/minute.

Answer: 1, 4, 5

Rationale: Adverse effects of oxytocin in the mother include hypertension, fluid overload, uterine tetany, and tachycardia, not bradycardia. The antidiuretic effect of oxytocin increases renal reabsorption of water, leading to fluid overload, not dehydration. Jaundice and bradycardia are adverse reactions that may occur in the neonate.

Test-taking strategy: Analyze to determine what information the question asks for, which is maternal adverse effects of Pitocin. "Select all that apply" questions require considering each option to decide its merit. Recall that the therapeutic action of oxytocin is to induce contractions. When considering adverse reactions, consider effects that suggest an exaggerated effect of the medication. Review the therapeutic action and adverse effects of oxytocin if you had difficulty answering this question.

Client needs category: Physiological integrity

Client needs subcategory: Pharmacological therapies

Cognitive level: Analyzing

6. A nurse is evaluating the external fetal monitoring strip (shown below) of a client who is in labor. Which nursing interventions should the nurse implement?

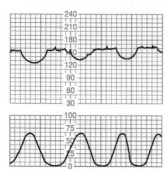

☐ **1.** Increase the I.V. fluid rate to boost intravascular volume.
☐ **2.** Reassure the client and continue to monitor the fetal heart rate.
☐ **3.** Elevate the client's legs.
☐ **4.** Administer supplemental oxygen.
☐ **5.** Require the client to lie on her left side.

Answer: 2

Rationale: The monitoring strip from this client's chart shows early decelerations. These can result from head compression during normal labor and do not indicate fetal distress. The nurse should reassure the client and continue to monitor the fetal heart rate. The other nursing interventions are not appropriate.

Test-taking strategy: Analyze to determine what information the question asks for, which is nursing intervention determined following monitor strip analysis. First, analyze the monitor strip noting timing and sequence of heart rate and contractions. Consider that the heart rate decreases with contraction onset-peak and then returns to baseline. Recall that this occurs in the normal labor process. Review the relationship between fetal heart rate patterns and uterine contraction patterns if you had difficulty answering this question.

Client needs category: Health promotion and maintenance

Client needs subcategory: None

Cognitive level: Analyzing

---

7. A client in labor is 8 cm dilated. The fetus, which is in vertex presentation, is 75% effaced and at 0 station. In the illustration below, identify the level of the fetus's head.

Answer:

Rationale: Station refers to the level of the presenting part in relation to the pelvic inlet and the ischial spines. A 0 station indicates that the presenting part lies at the level of the ischial spines. Other stations are defined by their distance in centimeters above or below the ischial spines.

Test-taking strategy: Analyze to determine what information the question asks for, which is level of the infant's head in the specific circumstance. The key words are "0 station" and the only information needed to answer the question when in the vertex position. Recall that the 0 station is the level of the ischial spines which present inward in the pelvis. Review maternal anatomy as it relates to fetal presentation and position if you had difficulty answering this question.

Client needs category: Health promotion and maintenance

Client needs subcategory: None

Cognitive level: Applying

8. A nurse is evaluating a fetal monitoring strip to time the contractions of a client in labor. Identify the beginning of the contraction in the illustration below.

Answer:

Rationale: An X is placed at the beginning of a contraction, identified by a rise in pressure in the uterus, and indicated on the monitoring strip by movement of the waveform away from the baseline.

Test-taking strategy: Analyze to determine what information the question asks for, which is beginning of a contraction of the monitoring strip. First, identify the baseline on the illustration. Next, recall that any change in the baseline, such as contraction, moves the waveform from baseline. Review uterine contraction waveforms if you had difficulty answering this question.

Client needs category: Health promotion and maintenance

Client needs subcategory: None

Cognitive level: Applying

---

9. A nurse is caring for a client who is in the third stage of labor. Which characteristic behaviors does the nurse anticipate at this stage. Select all that apply.

- ☐ **1.** The client is excited about the process.
- ☐ **2.** The client is focused on the neonate's condition.
- ☐ **3.** The client is exhausted from the labor process.
- ☐ **4.** The client states she has discomfort from uterine contractions.
- ☐ **5.** The client is apprehensive about the process.
- ☐ **6.** The client is feeling embarrassed as she has an urge to defecate.

Answer: 2, 4

Rationale: In the third stage of labor, the client focuses on the neonate's condition. Before the placenta is expelled, she may also state that she is experiencing discomfort from uterine contractions. Excitement and apprehension are characteristic of the first stage of labor. Exhaustion is common in the second stage of labor. The urge to defecate is noted prior to birth at the end of the second stage of labor when the fetus is pushing on the rectum.

Test-taking strategy: Analyze to determine what information the question asks for, which is the behavior of the mother in the third stage of labor. "Select all that apply" questions require considering each option to decide its merit. Recall that during this stage of labor, the focus is on the delivery of the placenta. Consider the process physiologically within the mother and emotionally as the neonate is born. Review maternal behaviors in the stages of labor if you had difficulty answering this question.

Client needs category: Psychosocial integrity

Client needs subcategory: None

Cognitive level: Applying

10. The nurse is caring for a client in labor. Which assessment findings would prompt the nurse to notify the physician? Select all that apply.

☐ **1.** The client is moaning in pain during contractions.

☐ **2.** The fetal heart rate baseline is between 140 and 150 beats/minute

☐ **3.** The client is anxious and requests that someone help her.

☐ **4.** The client's membranes rupture and the amniotic fluid is green.

☐ **5.** Late decelerations are noted on the external fetal monitor strip.

☐ **6.** Blood-tinged mucous is noted upon internal examination.

Answer: 4, 5

Rationale: The presence of green amniotic fluid indicates that the fetus has passed a meconium stool in utero and is an indication of fetal distress. Late decelerations are caused by uteroplacental insufficiency resulting from decreased blood flow and oxygen transfer to the fetus through the intervillous spaces during uterine contractions. Both assessment findings should be related to the physician. Experiencing pain and maternal anxiety are common, especially during the transition period of labor. A fetal heart rate between 140 and 150 beats/minute is normal. Blood-tinged mucous indicates the progression of labor.

Test-taking strategy: Analyze to determine what information the question asks for, which is assessment data prompting physician notification. "Select all that apply" questions require considering each option to decide its merit. Consider any option indicating fetal complications. Recall that amniotic fluid is colorless; thus, green fluid is abnormal and late decelerations also indicate fetal compromise. Review signs and symptoms of fetal distress if you had difficulty answering this question.

Client needs category: Physiological integrity

Client needs subcategory: Pharmacological therapies

Cognitive level: Analyzing

---

11. A client is being admitted to the labor and delivery unit. Her GTPAL classification is 5-2-1-1-2. When providing shift report, which information would the nurse state? Select all that apply.

☐ **1.** The client has had four previous pregnancies.

☐ **2.** The client has had five previous pregnancies.

☐ **3.** The client has had one full-term child, one abortion, and one premature child.

☐ **4.** The client has had two full-term children, one premature child, and one abortion.

☐ **5.** The client has three living children and is pregnant again.

☐ **6.** The client has two living children and is pregnant again.

Answer: 1, 4, 6

Rationale: Detailed information about a client's obstetric history is described using the GTPAL classification system. G represents gravida, or the number of times the client has been pregnant, including the current pregnancy. T is the number of full-term infants born (after 37 weeks); P is the number of preterm infants born (before 37 weeks); A is the number of induced or spontaneous abortions; and L is the number of living children.

Test-taking strategy: Analyze to determine what information the question asks for, which is correct obstetric history as identified by the GTPAL. "Select all that apply" questions require considering each option to decide its merit. Recall what each letter of the GTPAL pregnancy status classification system represents and relate to each option. Realize that each correct option would be included in shift report. Review the GTPAL classification system if you had difficulty answering this question.

Client needs category: Health promotion and maintenance

Client needs subcategory: None

Cognitive level: Applying

12. A nurse is assisting in the delivery room. The physician prepares to perform a midline episiotomy. On the illustration below, identify the area where the physician will place the incision and the nurse will assess healing status.

Answer:

Rationale: An X is placed in the center of the perineum for a midline episiotomy. An episiotomy is surgical enlargement of the vaginal opening that allows easier delivery of the fetus and prevents tearing of the perineum. The incision is made in the perineum and can be midline or right or left mediolateral.

Test-taking strategy: Analyze to determine what information the question asks for, which is location for a midline episiotomy. Use the anatomical terms to determine the location (midline = in the middle) of the perineal incision. Review maternal anatomy and the purpose of an episiotomy if you had difficulty answering this question.

Client needs category: Physiological integrity

Client needs subcategory: Reduction of risk potential

Cognitive level: Applying

13. The nurse is performing Leopold's maneuvers to determine fetal presentation and position. Which illustration shows the third maneuver?

□ **1.**

□ **2.**

□ **3.**

□ **4.**

Answer: 2

Rationale: To perform the third maneuver, the nurse gently grasps the lower portion of the abdomen just above the symphysis pubis between the thumb and index finger and presses them together to determine any movement and whether the part is firm or soft. This maneuver determines the part of the fetus at the inlet and its mobility. Option 1 shows the fourth maneuver of locating the fetal brow; option 3 shows the first maneuver of palpating the upper abdomen to determine the size, shape, and mobility of the fetus; and option 4 shows the second maneuver of determining the location of the fetal back.

Test-taking strategy: Analyze to determine what information the question asks for, which is identifying the third maneuver within Leopold's maneuvers. Visualize the sequence of observing and palpating the client's abdomen to determine fetal presentation and position. Recall that the maneuvers begin with general information with the first and second maneuvers being the fundal grip and then umbilical grip. The third and fourth maneuvers provide data on engagement for the birthing process. Review Leopold's maneuvers if you had difficulty answering this question.

Client needs category: Physiological integrity

Client needs subcategory: Reduction of risk potential

Cognitive level: Applying

14. The nurse is assisting with the delivery of a fetus in a frank breech presentation. Which graphic illustrates that position?

☐ **1.**

☐ **2.**

☐ **3.**

☐ **4.**

Answer: 3

Rationale: In a frank breech presentation, the buttocks are the presenting part, with the hips flexed and the knees remaining straight. In a complete breech (option 1), the knees and hips are flexed. In a footling breech (option 2), neither the hips nor lower legs are flexed, and one or both feet may present. In an incomplete breech (option 4), one or both hips remain extended, and one or both feet or knees lie below the breech.

Test-taking strategy: Analyze to determine what information the question asks for, which is identifying the characteristics of a frank breech presentation. Recall that breech = buttocks. The defining characteristic of the frank breech is the straight legs with feet by head. Review the various breech presentations if you had difficulty answering this question.

Client needs category: Physiological integrity

Client needs subcategory: Reduction of risk potential

Cognitive level: Understanding

15. Assessment of a client progressing through labor reveals the following findings. Place in the order in which they would have occurred. Use all of the options.

1. Uncontrollable urge to push.

2. Cervical dilation of 7 cm.

3. 100% cervical effacement.

4. Strong Braxton Hicks contractions.

5. Mild contractions lasting 20 to 40 seconds.

Answer: 4, 5, 2, 3, 1

Rationale: Strong Braxton Hicks contractions typically occur prior to the onset of true labor and are considered a preliminary sign. During the latent phase of the first stage of labor, contractions are mild, lasting about 20 to 40 seconds. As the client progresses through labor, contractions increase in intensity and duration, and cervical dilation occurs. Cervical dilation of 7 cm indicates that the client has entered the active phase of the first stage of labor. Cervical effacement also occurs, and effacement of 100% characterizes the transition phase of the first stage of labor. Progression into the second stage of labor is noted by the client's uncontrollable urge to push.

Test-taking strategy: Analyze to determine what information the question asks for, which is characteristics of the stages of labor. Sequence the progression through the stages of labor beginning with Braxton Hicks contractions and ending with the uncontrollable urge to push the neonate out. Arrange the middle sections from mild contractions through dilation and effacement. Review the stages of labor if you had difficulty answering this question.

Client needs category: Health promotion and maintenance

Client needs subcategory: None

Cognitive level: Applying

16. A nurse is monitoring the contractions of a client in the first stage of labor. Order the phases of a uterine contraction from the beginning of contraction to its conclusion. Use all of the options.

1. Acme.

2. Relaxation.

3. Decrement.

4. Strong Braxton Hicks contractions.

Answer: 4, 1, 3, 2

Rationale: Braxton Hicks contractions are contractions which occur before actual labor in preparation for the real labor. A contraction consists of three phases: the increment (when the intensity of the contraction increases), the acme (when the contraction is at its strongest), and the decrement (when the intensity decreases). Between contractions, the uterus relaxes. As labor progresses, the relaxation intervals decrease from 10 minutes early in labor to only 2 to 3 minutes later. The duration of contractions also changes, increasing from 20 to 30 seconds to a range of 60 to 90 seconds.

Test-taking strategy: Analyze to determine what information the question asks for, which is order of the phases of the contractions. If unsure, focus on the definition of terms to help determine the sequence. Review the phases as a contraction progresses if you had difficulty answering this question.

Client needs category: Health promotion and maintenance

Client needs subcategory: None

Cognitive level: Applying

1. A nurse is caring for a client with a warm, reddened, painful area in the breast as well as cracked and fissured nipples. The client expresses the desire to continue breast-feeding. Which instructions should the nurse include to prevent a recurrence of this condition? Select all that apply.

- [ ] **1.** Wash the nipples with soap and water.
- [ ] **2.** Change the breast pads frequently.
- [ ] **3.** Expose the nipples to air for part of each day.
- [ ] **4.** Wash hands before handling the breast and breast-feeding.
- [ ] **5.** Make sure that the baby grasps the nipple only.
- [ ] **6.** Release the baby's grasp on the nipple before removing the baby from the breast.

Answer: 2, 3, 4, 6

Rationale: Mastitis is an infection of the breast tissue usually caused by *Staphylococcus aureus*. This infection typically occurs in the second or third postpartum week and is more frequent in primigravidas. To help prevent mastitis, the nurse should suggest measures to prevent cracked and fissured nipples. Changing breast pads frequently and exposing the nipples to air for part of the day help keep the nipples dry and prevent irritation. Washing hands before handling the breast reduces the chance of accidentally introducing organisms into the breast. Releasing the baby's grasp on the nipple before removing the baby from the breast also reduces the chance of irritation. Nipples should be washed with water only; soap tends to remove the natural oils and increases the chance of cracking. The baby should grasp both the nipple and areola.

Test-taking strategy: Analyze to determine what information the question asks for, which is instruction to prevent a reoccurrence of symptoms related to mastitis. "Select all that apply" questions require considering each option to decide its merit. Note that correct options, including hand hygiene, reduce the chances of reopening the fissures and causing infection. Review the principles of infection control and methods to prevent the reoccurrence of mastitis if you had difficulty answering this question.

Client needs category: Health promotion and maintenance

Client needs subcategory: None

Cognitive level: Applying

2. A nurse is caring for a 1-day postpartum client. The progress note below informs the nurse that the client is in which phase of the postpartum period?

Progress Notes	
5/24/10	Mother verbalizing labor and delivery
1715	experience. Doesn't appear confident about
	holding baby or changing diapers. Asking
	appropriate questions.——— J. Conners, LPN

☐ **1.** Letting go.
☐ **2.** Taking in.
☐ **3.** Holding out.
☐ **4.** Taking hold.

Answer: 2

Rationale: The taking-in phase is normally the first postpartum phase. During this phase, the mother feels overwhelmed by the responsibilities of newborn care and is still fatigued from delivery. Taking hold is the next phase, when the client has rested and can learn mothering skills with confidence. Letting go is the final stage, when the client adapts to parenthood, her new role as a caregiver, and her new baby as a separate entity. Holding out is not a valid phase.

Test-taking strategy: Analyze to determine what information the question asks for, which is the phase of the postpartum period as documented in a nursing note. Analyze the nurse's note for clues such as verbalizing labor and delivery, not confident and asking questions. Relate to early stages in the postpartum period. Review the mother's behavior and postpartum phases if you had difficulty answering this question.

Client needs category: Psychosocial integrity

Client needs subcategory: None

Cognitive level: Analyzing

---

3. A nurse observes several interactions between a client and her neonate son. Which behaviors by the mother would the nurse identify as evidence of mother–infant attachment? Select all that apply.

☐ **1.** Talks to and coos at her son.
☐ **2.** Cuddles her son close to her.
☐ **3.** Does not make eye contact with her son.
☐ **4.** Requests that the nurse take the baby to the nursery for feedings.
☐ **5.** Encourages the father to hold the baby.
☐ **6.** Takes a nap when the baby is sleeping.

Answer: 1, 2

Rationale: Talking to, cooing at, and cuddling with her son are positive signs that the client is adapting to her new role as a mother. Eye contact, touching, and speaking help establish attachment with a neonate. Avoiding eye contact is a nonbonding behavior. Feeding a neonate is an important role of a new mother and facilitates attachment. Encouraging the father to hold the neonate will facilitate attachment between the neonate and the father. Resting while the neonate is sleeping will conserve needed energy and allow the mother to be alert and awake when her infant is awake; however, it is not evidence of bonding.

Test-taking strategy: Analyze to determine what information the question asks for, which is evidence of mother–infant attachment. "Select all that apply" questions require considering each option to decide its merit. Consider that evidence means factual actions related to demonstrating bonding. Review behaviors that relate to maternal–infant bonding if you had difficulty answering this question.

Client needs category: Psychosocial integrity

Client needs subcategory: None

Cognitive level: Analyzing

4. A nurse is caring for a postpartum client suspected of developing postpartum psychosis. Which statements accurately characterize this disorder? Select all that apply.

☐ **1.** Symptoms appear at the 6-month screening.
☐ **2.** The disorder is common in postpartum women.
☐ **3.** Symptoms include delusions and hallucinations.
☐ **4.** Suicide and infanticide are uncommon in this disorder.
☐ **5.** The disorder rarely occurs without a psychiatric history.

Answer: 3, 5

Rationale: A postpartum client should be suspected of psychosis if she exhibits delusions or hallucinations, generally starting within 4 weeks of postpartum. Typically, the woman has a past history of a psychiatric disorder and treatment. A history of bipolar disorder is an important risk factor. The disorder occurs in less than 1% of postpartum mothers. It is considered a medical emergency. Suicide and infanticide are common.

Test-taking strategy: Analyze to determine what information the question asks for, which is correct characterization of postpartum psychosis. "Select all that apply" questions require considering each option to decide its merit. The key word is "psychosis." Use your knowledge of medical terminology to identify options related to delusions. Review the onset, symptoms, and etiology of postpartum psychosis and the differences with postpartal blues and depression if you had difficulty answering this question.

Client needs category: Psychosocial integrity

Client needs subcategory: None

Cognitive level: Analyzing

---

5. A mother with a history of varicose veins has just delivered her first baby. The nurse suspects that the mother has developed a pulmonary embolus. Which data below would lead to this nursing judgment? Select all that apply.

☐ **1.** Sudden dyspnea.
☐ **2.** Chills, fever.
☐ **3.** Diaphoresis.
☐ **4.** Cough.
☐ **5.** Confusion.
☐ **6.** Chest pain.

Answer: 1, 3, 4, 5, 6

Rationale: Sudden dyspnea with diaphoresis, chest pain, and confusion are classic signs and symptoms of a pulmonary embolus. The client could also have a cough with blood-tinged sputum. In this disorder, a thrombus (stationary blood clot) dislodges from a varicose vein and becomes lodged in the pulmonary circulation. Chills and fever would indicate an infection.

Test-taking strategy: Analyze to determine what information the question asks for, which is data supporting the possibility of a pulmonary embolism. "Select all that apply" questions require considering each option to decide its merit. Use knowledge of medical terminology to determine pulmonary = lung and embolism = clot. Consider symptoms that would occur with an interruption of blood flow. Review the pathophysiology and clinical manifestations of a pulmonary embolism if you had difficulty answering this question.

Client needs category: Physiological integrity

Client needs subcategory: Physiological adaptation

Cognitive level: Analyzing

6. A nurse is palpating the uterine fundus of a client who delivered her neonate 8 hours ago. Identify the area where the nurse would expect to feel the fundus.

Answer:

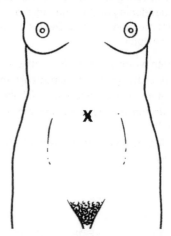

Rationale: Note the X at the level of the umbilicus. The uterus should be felt at the level of the umbilicus from about 1 to 24 hours after birth.

Test-taking strategy: Analyze to determine what information the question asks for, which is fundal height at 8 hours postpartum. Consider the timeframe of 8 hours as key data. Recall the involution process and that fundal height decreases one fingerbreadth (1 cm) per day. Review the involution process if you had difficulty answering this question.

Client needs category: Physiological integrity

Client needs subcategory: Reduction of risk potential

Cognitive level: Applying

---

7. A nurse is caring for a client in the fourth stage of labor. Based on the nurse's note below, which postpartum complication has the client developed?

Progress Notes	
6/7/10 1745	Pt.'s 24-hour blood loss is 600 mL. Uterus is soft and relaxed on palpation and pt. has a full bladder. Assisted pt. in empty-ing bladder and notified Dr. G. McMann of findings. Vital signs stable at present. See graphic sheet for ongoing assessments and perineal pad weights.——— S. Jones, LPN

☐ **1.** Postpartum hemorrhage.
☐ **2.** Puerperal infection.
☐ **3.** Deep vein thrombosis (DVT).
☐ **4.** Mastitis.
☐ **5.** Uterine rupture.

Answer: 1

Rationale: Blood loss from the uterus that exceeds 500 mL in a 24-hour period is considered postpartum hemorrhage. If uterine atony is the cause, the uterus feels soft and relaxed. A full bladder can prevent the uterus from contracting completely, increasing the risk of hemorrhage. Puerperal infection is an infection of the uterus and structures above; its characteristic sign is fever. Two major types of DVT occur in the postpartum period: pelvic and femoral. Each has different signs and symptoms, but both occur later in the postpartum period (femoral, after 10 days postpartum; pelvic, after 14 days). Mastitis is an inflammation of the mammary glands that disrupts normal lactation and usually develops 1 to 4 weeks of postpartum. Uterine rupture is a potentially catastrophic event during childbirth where the wall of the uterus ruptures. A uterine rupture is a life-threatening event for the mother and fetus.

Test-taking strategy: Analyze to determine what information the question asks for, which is a complication during the fourth stage of labor as identified in the nurse's note. Analyze the nurse's note to determine clues (blood loss of 600 mL, uterus soft and relaxed) and relate to the options. Review complications during the fourth stage of labor if you had difficulty answering this question.

Client needs category: Physiological integrity

Client needs subcategory: Reduction of risk potential

Cognitive level: Analyzing

8. A nurse assesses a client's vaginal discharge on the first postpartum day and describes it in the progress note (shown below). Which terms best identifies the discharge?

Progress Notes	
3/30/10 1645	Perineal pad changed two times this shift for moderate amount of red discharge.————————J. Jones, LPN

☐ **1.** Lochia alba.
☐ **2.** Lochia.
☐ **3.** Lochia serosa.
☐ **4.** Lochia rubra.

Answer: 4

Rationale: For the first 3 days after birth, the discharge is called lochia rubra. It consists almost entirely of blood, with only small particles of decidua and mucus. Lochia alba is a creamy white or colorless discharge that occurs 10 to 14 days postpartum. Lochia serosa is a pink or brownish discharge that occurs 4 to 14 days postpartum. The term *lochia* alone is not a correct description of the discharge.

Test-taking strategy: Analyze to determine what information the question asks for, which is the best description of postpartum vaginal discharge. First note that option 2 has no descriptor, eliminating that choice. Recall knowledge of medical terminology that rubra = red. Review vaginal discharge from delivery to 14 days postpartum if you had difficulty answering this question.

Client needs category: Physiological integrity

Client needs subcategory: Physiological adaptation

Cognitive level: Applying

9. A home care lactation nurse has asked a client to keep a record of her intake, including calories, and output for 1 day. After reviewing the flow sheet that the client used to document the results (shown below), the nurse should make which assessments?

Intake and Output			
Time period	Fluids (mL)	Calories	Output (mL)
7 a.m. to 11 a.m.	Milk 240 Orange juice 60	Breakfast 510	60
11 a.m. to 3 p.m.	Coffee 240 Orange juice 120 Water 240	Lunch 350 Snack 80	250 200 200
3 p.m. to 11 p.m.	Water 240 Water 240 Water 240	Dinner 500 Snack 350	100 230 200
11 p.m. to 7 a.m.	Water 240		300

- ☐ **1.** The client consumed an adequate amount of calories and fluids for breast-feeding.
- ☐ **2.** The client consumed an adequate amount of calories but not enough fluids for breast-feeding.
- ☐ **3.** The client consumed an adequate amount of fluids but not enough calories for breast-feeding.
- ☐ **4.** The client consumed an inadequate amount of fluids and calories for breast-feeding.

Answer: 4

Rationale: In general, new mothers who are breast-feeding should consume 2 to 3 L of fluids and 2,300 to 2,700 calories daily. Consuming less than 1,500 to 1,800 calories per day may put the mother's milk supply at risk.

Test-taking strategy: Analyze to determine what information the question asks for, which is analysis of 24-hour intake and output for a lactating mother. First, calculate intake, calories, and output and compare with standard needs. Recall that an increased fluid intake is important to maintain milk production. Also, an increase in calories and nutrients is needed to meet the nutritional requirements of the mother and baby. Calculate the total calories and fluid intake and relate them to the nutritional needs of the lactating client if you had difficulty answering this question.

Client needs category: Health promotion and maintenance

Client needs subcategory: None

Cognitive level: Analyzing

10. During physical assessment of a client who gave birth 3 hours ago, a nurse finds that the client has completely saturated a perineal pad within 15 minutes. Which nursing actions would be appropriate? Select all that apply.

☐ **1.** Begin an I.V. infusion of lactated Ringer's solution.
☐ **2.** Assess the client's vital signs.
☐ **3.** Palpate the client's fundus.
☐ **4.** Place the client in high Fowler's position.
☐ **5.** Administer a pain medication.

Answer: 2, 3

Rationale: Saturating a perineal pad within 15 minutes indicated excessive bleeding. Checking vital signs provides information about the client's circulatory status and identifies significant changes that may need to be reported to the physician. By palpating the client's fundus, the nurse also gains valuable data. A boggy uterus may lead to excessive bleeding. Starting an I.V. infusion requires a physician's order. Placing the client in high Fowler's position may lower the blood pressure and be harmful to the client. Administration of a pain medication does not address the current problem.

Test-taking strategy: Analyze to determine what information the question asks for, which is nursing actions when assessment findings reveal a saturated perineal pad indicating excessive bleeding. "Select all that apply" questions require considering each option to decide its merit. Choose the options that directly relate to interventions for bleeding. Review nursing actions related to excessive bleeding if you had difficulty answering this question.

Client needs category: Physiological integrity

Client needs subcategory: Reduction of risk potential

Cognitive level: Applying

11. The nurse is caring for a postpartum client with symptoms of swelling and tenderness in the left leg. The nurse suspects a developing DVT. When assessing for a DVT, identify the area on the body below, where the nurse would perform a focused assessment.

Answer:

Rationale: Note that an X is placed on the calf. To assess for the presence of a DVT, the nurse performs a Homans' sign. To elicit Homans' sign, the client dorsiflexes her ankle and then the nurse assesses for pain in the calf during that motion. If a positive Homans' sign is noted, the physician may order an ultrasound or venography for a definitive diagnosis.

Test-taking strategy: Analyze to determine what information the question asks for, which is site of a focused assessment when a DVT is suspected. Recall the area where thrombosis usually develops and consider how to assess if a thrombosis blocking blood flow is present. Review Homans' sign for assessing a DVT if you had difficulty answering this question.

Client needs category: Physiological integrity

Client needs subcategory: Physiological adaptation

Cognitive level: Applying

12. The nurse is assessing a client who is 4 hours postpartum. Based on the findings documented by the nurse below, which action is most appropriate at this time?

Progress Notes	
06/11/10	Pt.'s vital signs stable at present. Perineal
1830	pad changed for moderate amount of red
	drainage. Uterus palpated at the level of
	the umbilicus and to the left side of the
	abdomen.————————N. Green, LPN

☐ **1.** Ask the client to empty her bladder.
☐ **2.** Raise the head of the bed.
☐ **3.** Straight-catheterize the client immediately.
☐ **4.** Call the client's primary health-care provider for direction.
☐ **5.** Straight-catheterize the client for half of her urine volume.
☐ **6.** Notify the charge nurse of the assessment findings.

Answer: 1

Rationale: A full bladder may displace the uterine fundus to the left or right of the abdomen. A straight catheterization is unnecessarily invasive if the client can urinate on her own. Nursing interventions should be completed before notifying the primary health-care provider or charge nurse in a nonemergency situation. Raising the head of the bed is not helpful to change the position of the uterus.

Test-taking strategy: Analyze to determine what information the question asks for, which is nursing action needed following focused assessment and documentation. Analyze the nurse's note to determine any abnormal data. Note the position of the uterus and consider causes. Recall that a filled bladder sits adjacent to the uterus and can dislocate the uterus. Review assessment findings as they relate to the postpartal uterus if you had difficulty answering this question.

Client needs category: Physiological integrity

Client needs subcategory: Physiological adaptation

Cognitive level: Applying

---

13. A postpartum client has been ordered 500 mg of ampicillin oral suspension. The label reads *ampicillin 125 mg/5 mL.* How many milliliters should the client receive? Record your answer using a whole number.

_____ mL

Answer: 20

Rationale: To solve this problem, set up proportions as follows:

$$5 \text{ mL}/125 \text{ mg} = X \text{ mL}/500 \text{ mg}$$

$$X \times 125 \text{ mg} = 5 \text{ mL} \times 500 \text{ mg}.$$

Solve for X by dividing both sides of the equation by 125 mg:

$$\frac{X \times 125 \text{ mg}}{125 \text{ mg}} = \frac{5 \text{ mL} \times 500 \text{ mg}}{125 \text{ mg}}$$

$$X = \frac{2{,}500 \text{ mL}}{125}$$

$$X = 20 \text{ mL}.$$

Test-taking strategy: Analyze to determine what information the question asks for, which is dosage of ampicillin oral suspension. Use the proportion method aligning both sides of the equation consistently using known data. Proofread the math calculation. Review calculations using proportions and solving for *X* if you had difficulty answering this question.

Client needs category: Physiological integrity

Client needs subcategory: Pharmacological therapies

Cognitive level: Applying

14. A postpartum client is experiencing thoughts and behaviors common to the taking-hold phase. Which items are characteristic of this phase? Select all that apply.

☐ **1.** Prefers having the nurse care for her.
☐ **2.** Holds new child and breastfeeds without prompting.
☐ **3.** Rests to regain physical strength and calm her swirling thoughts.
☐ **4.** Expresses a strong interest in taking care of her child.
☐ **5.** Gives up fanaticized image of her child and accepts the real one.

Answer: 2, 4

Rationale: The taking-in phase occurs in the first 24 hours after birth. The mother is concerned with her own needs and requires support from staff and relatives. She holds her new child with a sense of wonder and rests to gain her physical strength and calm her thoughts. The taking-hold phase occurs when the mother is ready to take responsibility for her care, as well as her neonate's care. The letting-go phase begins when the mother accepts her real child and incorporates the neonate into the family unit.

Test-taking strategy: Analyze to determine what information the question asks for, which is characteristics of the taking-hold phase. "Select all that apply" questions require considering each option to decide its merit. Consider the term "taking hold" meaning to take control of the care of herself and her neonate. Consider each option or data that the mother is actively participating in care. Review transitional maternal roles during the postpartum period if you had difficulty answering this question.

Client needs category: Health promotion and maintenance

Client needs subcategory: None

Cognitive level: Analyzing

---

15. The nurse is preparing to perform a fundal massage on a client who is 2 hours postpartum. Order the sequence of events for performing this procedure. Use all of the options.

1. Rotate the upper hand to massage the uterus until firm.
2. Place the client in supine position.
3. Gently press the fundus between the hands using slight downward pressure.
4. Place one hand around the top of the fundus.
5. Ask the client to void.
6. Place one hand on the abdomen just above the symphysis pubis.

Answer: 5, 2, 6, 4, 1, 3

Rationale: Fundal massage is performed to promote uterine tone and consistency and to minimize the risk of hemorrhage. First, have the client void to prevent displacement of the bladder and allow an accurate assessment of uterine tone. Then, place the client in proper supine positioning to allow for good visualization. To anchor the lower part of the uterus, place one hand on the abdomen just above the symphysis pubis and then place the other hand around the top of the fundus. Next, rotate the upper hand to massage the uterus until it is firm. Finally, when the uterus is firm, push gently on the fundus, using slight downward pressure against the lower hand.

Test-taking strategy: Analyze to determine what information the question asks for, which is the procedure to perform a fundal massage. Visualize the fundal massage procedure including placement of the hands on the abdomen. Review the fundal massage sequence and the reason for performing maneuvers if you had difficulty answering this question.

Client needs category: Physiological integrity

Client needs subcategory: Reduction of risk potential

Cognitive level: Applying

The Neonate

1. A nurse is performing a neurologic assessment on a 1-day-old neonate in the nursery. Which findings would indicate possible asphyxia in utero? Select all that apply.

☐ **1.** The neonate grasps the nurse's finger when put in the palm of the neonate's hand.

☐ **2.** The neonate does stepping movements when held upright with the sole of the foot touching a surface.

☐ **3.** The neonate's toes do not curl downward when the soles of the feet are touched.

☐ **4.** The neonate does not respond when the nurse claps hands.

☐ **5.** The neonate turns toward the nurse's finger when touching the cheek.

☐ **6.** The neonate displays weak, ineffective sucking.

Answer: 3, 4, 6

Rationale: Perinatal asphyxia is an insult to the fetus or newborn due to the lack of oxygen. If the neonate's toes do not curl downward when the soles of the feet are touched and the neonate does not respond to a loud sound, neurologic damage from asphyxia may have occurred. A normal neurologic response would be the downward curling of the toes when touched and extension of the arms and legs in response to a loud noise. Weak, ineffective sucking is another sign of neurologic damage. A neonate should grasp a person's finger when it is placed in the palm of the neonate's hand, do stepping movements when held upright with the sole of the foot touching a surface, and turn toward the nurse's finger when touching the cheek.

Test-taking strategy: Analyze to determine what information the question asks for, which is assessment findings that indicate asphyxia. Recall that the brain is especially susceptible to hypoxia as it has one of the highest oxygen requirement; thus, neurological deficits are common. "Select all that apply" questions require considering each option to decide its merit. When assessing each option, note that all options are neonatal reflexes. Select the options that indicate abnormal findings. Review normal neurologic assessment findings if you had difficulty answering this question.

Client needs category: Health promotion and maintenance

Client needs subcategory: None

Cognitive level: Applying

2. What information would the nurse include when teaching postcircumcision care to the parents of a neonate prior to discharge from the hospital? Select all that apply.

☐ **1.** The infant must void before being discharged home.

☐ **2.** Petroleum jelly or antibiotic ointment should be applied to the glans of the penis with each diaper change.

☐ **3.** The infant can have tub baths while the circumcision heals.

☐ **4.** Any amount of blood noted on the front of the diaper should be reported.

☐ **5.** The circumcision will require care for 2 to 4 days after discharge.

Answer: 1, 2, 5

Rationale: Circumcision is a common surgical procedure when the foreskin of the penis is removed. The infant must void prior to discharge to ensure that the urethra is not obstructed. A lubricating or antibiotic ointment should be applied with each diaper change. Typically, the penis heals within 2 to 4 days, and circumcision care is needed for that period only. To prevent infection, the infant should not have tub baths until the circumcision is healed; sponge baths are appropriate. A small amount of bleeding is expected following a circumcision; parents should report only a large amount of bleeding.

Test-taking strategy: Analyze to determine what information the question asks for, which is post circumcision care. "Select all that apply" questions require considering each option to decide its merit. Recall that parents need to understand abnormal findings and appropriate care for healing. Also, consider standards of clean technique and infection control. Review teaching guidelines and actions related to circumcision care if you had difficulty answering this question.

Client needs category: Safe and effective care environment

Client needs subcategory: Coordinated care

Cognitive level: Applying

---

3. A nurse is caring for a 14-day-old neonate admitted for aspiration pneumonia. The physician ordered a barium swallow to confirm a diagnosis of gastroesophageal reflux with resulting aspiration pneumonia. When instructing the parents, in which area of the stomach would the nurse stress as the area of concern?

Answer:

Rationale: Gastroesophageal reflux is a neuromotor disturbance in which the cardiac sphincter located between the stomach and the esophagus is weak. This allows easy regurgitation of gastric contents into the esophagus, causing possible aspiration into the lungs.

Test-taking strategy: Analyze to determine what information the question asks for, which is site of gastroesophageal reflux. Use knowledge of medical terminology to lead to the correct answer. (gastro = stomach and esophageal = esophagus). Review the anatomy of the gastrointestinal system and pathophysiology of gastroesophageal reflux if you had difficulty answering this question.

Client needs category: Physiological integrity

Client needs subcategory: Physiological adaptation

Cognitive level: Applying

4. A nurse is evaluating the return demonstration of cord care by the mother of a neonate. Which actions would the nurse encourage the mother to perform? Select all that apply.

☐ **1.** Placing the diaper below the cord.
☐ **2.** Tugging gently on the cord as it begins to dry.
☐ **3.** Applying antibiotic ointment to the cord twice daily.
☐ **4.** Sponge-bathing the infant until the cord falls off.
☐ **5.** Cleaning the length of the cord with alcohol several times daily.
☐ **6.** Washing the cord with mild soap and water.

Answer: 1, 4, 5

Rationale: The diaper should be positioned below the cord to allow it to air-dry and to prevent urine from getting on the cord. The nurse should instruct the parents to sponge-bathe the infant until the cord falls off. Soap and water should not be used as a part of cord care. The entire cord should be cleaned with alcohol, using a cotton swab or another appropriate method, several times a day. Parents should also be instructed to never pull on the cord, but to allow it to fall off naturally. Antibiotic ointments are contraindicated unless there are signs of infection.

Test-taking strategy: Analyze to determine what information the question asks for, which is proper cord care. "Select all that apply" questions require considering each option to decide its merit. Consider that the umbilicus is similar to a scab and must be kept clean and dry so that it is allowed to dry and fall off naturally. Select any option that decreases the risk of infection and promotes healing. Review teaching guidelines and care unique to cord care if you had difficulty answering this question.

Client needs category: Safe and effective care environment

Client needs subcategory: Coordinated care

Cognitive level: Applying

5. At 5 minutes of age, a neonate is pink with acrocyanosis; has flexed knees, clenched fists, a whimpering cry, and a heart rate of 128 beats/minute; and withdraws the foot when slapped on the sole. What 5-minute Apgar score would the nurse record for this neonate?

Sign	Apgar Score		
	0	1	2
Heart rate	Absent	Less than 100 beats/minute (slow)	More than 100 beats/minute
Respiratory effort	Absent	Slow, irregular	Good cry
Muscle tone	Flaccid	Some flexion and resistance to extension of extremities	Active motion
Reflex irritability	No response	Grimace or weak cry	Vigorous cry
Color	Pallor, cyanosis	Pink body, blue extremities	Completely pink

☐ **1.** 5.
☐ **2.** 7.
☐ **3.** 8.
☐ **4.** 10.

Answer: 3

Rationale: The Apgar score provides an assessment of a neonate's health immediately after birth and at 5 minutes of age. Criteria assessed include heart rate, respiratory effort, muscle tone, reflex irritability, and color, each receiving a score from 0 (poor) to 2 (normal). This neonate has a heart rate above 100 beats/minute (score of 2); a weak cry (score of 1); good flexion (score of 2); a good response to a slap on the sole (score of 2); and pink color with acrocyanosis (score of 1). Thus, the total Apgar score is 8.

Test-taking strategy: Analyze to determine what information the question asks for, which is Apgar score using the neonatal data. Match the data provided with scored table data to determine numerical classification. Add the totals from each column to determine the final score. Review the Apgar scale and focus on the data given in the question if you had difficulty answering this question.

Client needs category: Physiological integrity

Client needs subcategory: Physiological adaptation

Cognitive level: Analyzing

6. A nurse is administering vitamin K to a neonate following delivery. The medication comes in a concentration of 2 mg/mL, and the ordered dose is 0.5 mg to be given subcutaneously. How many milliliters should the nurse administer? Record your answer using two decimal places.

_____ mL

Answer: 0.25

Rationale: Use the following formula to calculate drug dosages:

Dose on hand/quantity on hand = dose desired/X

2 mg/mL = 0.5 mg/X

X = 0.25 mL.

Test-taking strategy: Analyze to determine what information the question asks for, which is calculating the dosage of vitamin K in milliliters using two decimal places. Recall dosage calculations using ratio and proportion and solving for X. Use known data to insert into the calculation. Proofread the math calculation. Be careful to follow decimal instructions. Review dosage calculation if you had difficulty answering this question.

Client needs category: Physiological integrity

Client needs subcategory: Pharmacological therapies

Cognitive level: Analyzing

---

7. A nurse is eliciting reflexes in a neonate during a physical examination. Identify the area that the nurse would touch to elicit a plantar grasp reflex.

Answer:

Rationale: To elicit a plantar grasp reflex, the nurse should touch the sole of the foot near the base of the digits, causing flexion or grasping. This reflex disappears at around age 9 months.

Test-taking strategy: Analyze to determine what information the question asks for, which is assessment of the plantar grasp reflex. Use knowledge of medical terminology to lead to the answer (plantar = sole of the feet). Review neonatal reflexes if you had difficulty answering this question.

Client needs category: Health promotion and maintenance

Client needs subcategory: None

Cognitive level: Applying

8. A nurse is providing care to a neonate. Place the following steps in the order that the nurse should implement them to properly perform ophthalmia neonatorum prophylaxis. Use all of the options.

1. Close and manipulate the eyelids to spread the medication over the eye.

2. Shield the neonate's eyes from direct light, and tilt the head slightly to the side that will receive the treatment.

3. Repeat the procedure for the other eye.

4. Wash hands and put on gloves.

5. Instill the ointment in the lower conjunctival sac.

6. Gently raise the neonate's upper eyelid with the index finger and pull the lower eyelid down with the thumb.

Answer: 4, 2, 6, 5, 1, 3

Rationale: Ophthalmia neonatorum prophylaxis involves the instillation of 0.5% erythromycin or 1% tetracycline ointment into a neonate's eyes. This procedure is performed to prevent gonorrheal and chlamydial conjunctivitis. All 50 states mandate that this treatment be given within 1 hour after delivery to decrease the risk of permanent eye damage and blindness.

Test-taking strategy: Analyze to determine what information the question asks for, which is the procedure to perform ophthalmia neonatorum prophylaxis. When ordering responses, begin with determining the first and last actions to narrow the middle options. Notice that washing hands is a standard first option. The last option would be to conclude the actions of the first eye and move to the next eye. Visualize the procedure to fill in the middle options. Review instilling eye ointment associated with the ophthalmia neonatorum prophylaxis procedure if you had difficulty answering this question.

Client needs category: Physiological integrity

Client needs subcategory: Physiological adaptation

Cognitive level: Applying

---

9. A nurse is completing a physical assessment of a neonate following birth. When completing the musculoskeletal assessment, which findings would indicate developmental dysplasia of the hip (DDH)? Select all that apply.

☐ **1.** Negative Ortolani test.
☐ **2.** Positive Barlow test.
☐ **3.** Asymmetrical leg skin folds.
☐ **4.** Limitation in adduction of the affected leg.
☐ **5.** Lengthening of the affected leg.

Answer: 2, 3

Rationale: Developmental dysplasia (dislocation) of the hip is an abnormal formation of the hip joint in which the ball on the top of the femur is not held firmly in the socket. A neonate with DDH will have a positive Ortolani test, a positive Barlow test, and asymmetrical skin folds in the thigh. The affected leg has limited abduction and appears shorter than the unaffected leg in a neonate with DDH.

Test-taking strategy: Analyze to determine what information the question asks for, which is physical assessment findings that indicate a DDH. "Select all that apply" questions require considering each option to decide its merit. Consider the pathophysiology of the hip (dislocated) and look to the options. Review the characteristics of developmental hip dysplasia if you had difficulty answering this question.

Client needs category: Physiological integrity

Client needs subcategory: Physiological adaptation

Cognitive level: Applying

10. Following the admission assessment of a neonate born at 42 weeks of gestation, the nurse documents which findings as normal? Select all that apply.

- [ ] **1.** A three-vessel umbilical cord.
- [ ] **2.** Peeling skin on the feet.
- [ ] **3.** Absence of sole creases.
- [ ] **4.** Absence of vernix caseosa.
- [ ] **5.** Cyanosis of the hands and feet.
- [ ] **6.** Large amounts of frothy oral secretions.

Answer: 1, 2, 3, 4, 5

Rationale: All of the answers are expected findings in a healthy infant at 42 weeks of gestation except for large amounts of frothy oral secretions. This is indicative of tracheoesophageal fistula; it is an abnormal finding in any neonate, regardless of gestational age at the time of birth.

Test-taking strategy: Analyze to determine what information the question asks for, which is normal findings of a post-term neonate. "Select all that apply" questions require considering each option to decide its merit. Consider the effects of remaining in the uterus, within amniotic fluid, past normal gestation. While anatomically the neonates are normal, some post-term neonates have a distinctive appearance as noted above. Review normal assessment findings for full-term neonates and post-term neonates if you had difficulty answering this question.

Client needs category: Health promotion and maintenance

Client needs subcategory: None

Cognitive level: Applying

---

11. A neonate has been placed on cardiac and apnea monitoring in the neonatal nursery. The nurse notes that apnea alarm repeatedly triggers. Place the following actions in the order in which they should be completed by the nurse. Use all of the options.

1. Silence the alarm to decrease environmental stimuli.

2. Perform a focused assessment on the neonate.

3. Count the respiratory rate for 60 seconds.

4. Document the assessment findings, interventions, and neonate's response.

5. Check all connects on apnea monitor.

Answer: 2, 3, 1, 5, 4

Rationale: The priority action is to perform a focused assessment on the neonate. Afterward, the nurse should evaluate the respiratory rate by counting respirations for 60 seconds. Afterward, the nurse should silence the alarm, check all connection on the apnea monitor, and, finally, document the information. Remember to "nurse the client," not the equipment.

Test-taking strategy: Analyze to determine what information the question asks for, which is nursing actions when the apnea monitor repeatedly triggers. Standards of care dictate that the neonate is to be assessed immediately following alarm. Completing a focused assessment including respiratory count ensures neonatal safety. Once it is determined that the neonate is safe, the nurse addresses the apnea monitor and documentation. Recall the ABCs (airway, breathing, and circulation) of care when prioritizing actions if you had difficulty answering this question.

Client needs category: Physiological integrity

Client needs subcategory: Physiological adaptation

Cognitive level: Applying

12. A 2-week-old neonate is admitted to the hospital with a diagnosis of possible sepsis. The neonate weighs 3.2 kg. The physician writes the following orders for the neonate and signs the order sheet. Which order should the nurse question?

Progress Notes	
05/12/10	Acetaminophen (Tylenol) 10 mg/kg per
1000	rectum, Q4-6 hours prn pain Ampicillin
	200 mg/kg I.V. Q6 hrs, D₅½ Normal saline
	IV @ 125 mL/hr. Mom may breastfeed ad
	lib. Draw blood cultures x 3 in a.m. Send
	Urine C & S in a.m.
	———————— R. Richard, M.D.

☐ **1.** Acetaminophen (Tylenol) 10 mg/kg per rectum, q4–6h prn pain.

☐ **2.** Ampicillin 200 mg/kg I.V. q6h.

☐ **3.** Mom may breastfeed ad lib.

☐ **4.** Draw blood cultures × 3 in a.m.

Answer: 4

Rationale: After the administration of ampicillin, the neonate's blood cultures will be invalid; the cultures should be obtained prior to the administration of the antibiotics. It is the nurse's responsibility to notify the physician and seek further clarification before carrying out this order. All of the other physician orders are appropriate as written.

Test-taking strategy: Analyze to determine what information the question asks for, which is identification of questionable physician order. Questioning a physician order indicates that one of the orders documented is incorrect. Analyze each option for validity. Recall normal protocol for the timing of blood cultures and administration of antibiotics. Note that all other orders are typical for an infant diagnosed with possible sepsis.

Client needs category: Physiological integrity

Client needs subcategory: Pharmacologic therapies

Cognitive level: Analyzing

13. The nurse is caring for a neonate who has a suspected neonatal sepsis. The physician's order is for ampicillin 100 mg/kg/day to be given in four divided doses. The client weighs 7 lb, 8 oz. How many milligrams should the nurse give with each dose? Record your answer using a whole number.

_____ mg/dose

Answer: 85

Rationale: First, convert the weight to kilograms:

$$7 \text{ lb}, 8 \text{ oz} = 7.5 \text{ lb}$$
$$1 \text{ lb} = 2.2 \text{ kg}$$
$$7.5 \text{ lb} \div 2.2 \text{ kg} = 3.4 \text{ kg}.$$

Then, multiply the kilograms of body weight by 100 mg (dose given):

$$3.4 \text{ kg} \times 100 \text{ mg} = 340 \text{ mg/kg}.$$

Next, divide 340 mg/kg by four doses per day:

$$340 \div 4 = 85 \text{ mg per dose}.$$

Test-taking strategy: Analyze to determine what information the question asks for, which is medication dose per dose. Consider that there are three steps to this calculation. As usual, weight must be converted to kilograms. Next, the daily (24-hour) dose is calculated. Lastly, calculate to mg/dose as required in the question. Be sure to carefully read how the dosage is to be reported. Proofread the math calculation. Review conversions and dosage calculations based on body weight if you had difficulty answering this question.

Client needs category: Physiological integrity

Client needs subcategory: Pharmacological therapies

Cognitive level: Applying

14. The nurse is caring for a newborn with a heart defect that involves mixing blood from the pulmonary and systemic circulation. Which illustration shows a congenital heart disorder with mixed blood flow?

☐ **1.**

☐ **2.**

☐ **3.**

☐ **4.**

Answer: 2

Rationale: In transposition of the great arteries (option 2), the aorta arises from the right ventricle instead of the left and the pulmonary artery arises from the left ventricle instead of the right. In most instances, atrial and ventricular defects also occur, making the entire heart have one mixed circulatory system. Option 1 shows patent ductus arteriosus, an increased pulmonary blood flow disorder. Option 3 depicts coarctation of the aorta, an obstruction to blood flow disorder. Option 4 shows tetralogy of Fallot, a decreased pulmonary blood flow disorder.

Test-taking strategy: Analyze to determine what information the question asks for, which is which illustration identifies a congenital heart disorder with mixed blood flow. Mixed blood flow indicates that oxygenated blood is in contact with deoxygenated blood. Consider that this mixing of the blood occurs with blood prior to oxygenation in the lungs. Review the hemodynamic and blood flow patterns of congenital heart disorders if you had difficulty answering this question.

Client needs category: Physiological integrity

Client needs subcategory: Physiological adaptation

Cognitive level: Analyzing

PART FIVE

Pediatric Nursing

The Infant

1. A physician orders an I.V. infusion of dextrose 5% in quarter-normal saline solution to be infused at 7 mL/kg/hour for a 10-month-old infant. The infant weighs 22 lb. How many milliliters of the ordered solution should the nurse infuse each hour? Record your answer using a whole number.

_____ mL/hour

Answer: 70

Rationale: To perform this calculation, the nurse should first convert the infant's weight to kilograms:

$$2.2 \text{ lb/kg} = 22 \text{ lb/}X \text{ kg}$$
$$X = 22/2.2$$
$$X = 10 \text{ kg.}$$

Next, the nurse should multiply the infant's weight by the ordered rate:

$$10 \text{ kg} \times 7 \text{ mL/kg/hour} = 70 \text{ mL/hour.}$$

Test-taking strategy: Analyze to determine what information the question asks for, which is the dose in milliliter per hour. Use knowledge of drug calculations and the calculation method of solving for X (see above). Proofread your math calculation for accuracy. Review basic drug calculations and basic conversions if you had difficulty answering this question.

Client needs category: Physiological integrity

Client needs subcategory: Pharmacological therapies

Cognitive level: Applying

---

2. A nurse is teaching the parents of a 6-month-old infant about normal growth and development. Which statements regarding infant development are true? Select all that apply.

☐ **1.** A 6-month-old infant has difficulty holding objects.

☐ **2.** A 6-month-old infant can usually roll from prone to supine and supine to prone positions.

☐ **3.** A teething ring is appropriate for a 6-month-old infant.

☐ **4.** Stranger anxiety usually peaks at age 12 to 18 months.

☐ **5.** Head lag is commonly noted in infants at age 6 months.

☐ **6.** Lack of visual coordination usually resolves by age 6 months.

Answer: 2, 3, 6

Rationale: Gross motor skills of the 6-month-old infant include rolling from front to back and back to front. Teething usually begins around age 6 months and, therefore, a teething ring is appropriate. Visual coordination is usually resolved by age 6 months. At age 6 months, fine motor skills include purposeful grasping and releasing of objects and transferring objects from one hand to another. Stranger anxiety normally peaks at 8 months. The 6-month-old infant also should have good head control and no longer display head lag when pulled up to a sitting position.

Test-taking strategy: Analyze to determine what information the question asks for, which is normal growth and development for a 6-month-old infant. "Select all that apply" questions require considering each option to decide its merit. Memorization of growth and development milestones is a must when answering many pediatric questions. Grouping development into ages may be helpful in recalling milestones on a continuum. Review infant growth and development if you had difficulty answering this question.

Client needs category: Health promotion and maintenance

Client needs subcategory: None

Cognitive level: Applying

3. A nurse is caring for an infant who weighs 8 kg and is ordered to receive ampicillin (Omnipen) 25 mg/kg I.V. every 6 hours. How many milligrams should a nurse administer per dose? Record the answer as a whole number.

_____ mg/dose

Answer: 200

Rationale: The nurse should calculate the correct dose by multiplying the infant's weight by the ordered rate:

$$8 \text{ kg} \times 25 \text{ mg/kg} = 200 \text{ mg.}$$

Critical thinking strategy: Analyze to determine what information the question asks for, which is the number of milligrams in each dose. Use knowledge of drug calculations to multiply the weight (kg) per milligrams. Proofread your math calculation for accuracy and remember the opportunity to use the drop-down calculator during your NCLEX. Review basic drug calculations if you had difficulty answering this question.

Client needs category: Physiological integrity

Client needs subcategory: Pharmacological therapies

Cognitive level: Applying

---

4. A nurse is conducting a physical examination on a 2-month-old infant at the well-child examination. When measuring chest circumference, identify the standard anatomical landmark used?

Answer:

Rationale: Chest circumference is most accurately measured by placing the measuring tape around the infant's nipples. Measuring above or below the nipples will yield a false measurement. The measurement should be taken after exhalation.

Test-taking strategy: Analyze to determine what information the question asks for, which is the anatomical site used when measuring chest circumference. When assessing the chest, the nipple line is the most notable landmark on the chest area. This provides a standard reference point for comparison. Review assessment of chest circumference if you had difficulty answering this question.

Client needs category: Health promotion and maintenance

Client needs subcategory: None

Cognitive level: Applying

5. A healthy 2-month-old infant is being seen in the local clinic for a well-child checkup and initial immunizations. When analyzing the pediatric record, which immunizations should the nurse anticipate administering at this appointment? Select all that apply.

☐ **1.** DTaP (diphtheria, tetanus, and acellular pertussis).
☐ **2.** MMR (measles, mumps, and rubella).
☐ **3.** Hep B (hepatitis B vaccine).
☐ **4.** Varicella (chickenpox) vaccine.
☐ **5.** Hib (*Haemophilus influenzae* vaccine).
☐ **6.** PCV (pneumococcal vaccine).

Answer: 1, 3, 5, 6

Rationale: At age 2 months, the American Academy of Pediatrics recommends the administration of DTaP, IPV (inactivated polio vaccine), Hep B, Hib, Rotavirus vaccine, and PCV. The MMR and varicella immunizations should be administered at 12 to 15 months.

Test-taking strategy: Analyze to determine what information the question asks for, which is immunizations to be administered at a 2-month well-child check. "Select all that apply" questions require considering each option to decide its merit. Memorization or a working knowledge of the immunization schedule is a necessity in determining the correct immunizations. Consider grouping immunization by months or on a timeline to assist in remembering the schedule. Review the immunization schedule if you had difficulty answering this question.

Client needs category: Health promotion and maintenance

Client needs subcategory: None

Cognitive level: Applying

---

6. The nurse is caring for an emergency room infant who has symptoms of irritability and a high fever. When assessing for increased intracranial pressure using the anterior fontanel, identify the area where a nurse should palpate.

Answer:

Rationale: The anterior fontanel is formed by the junction of the sagittal, frontal, and coronal sutures. It is shaped like a diamond and normally measures 4 to 5 cm at its widest point. The posterior fontanel closes during the first several months of life and the anterior fontanel closes around 2 years of age. A widened, bulging fontanel is a sign of increased intracranial pressure.

Test-taking strategy: Analyze to determine what information the question asks for, which is location of the anterior fontanel for assessment of increased intracranial pressure. The key words are "anterior," meaning before, and "fontanel," meaning opening covered by a membrane. Look to the illustration to select the opening on the top of the head. Review anterior and posterior fontanel placement and characteristics if you had difficulty answering this question.

Client needs category: Health promotion and maintenance

Client needs subcategory: None

Cognitive level: Applying

7. A parent is planning to enroll a 9-month-old infant in a day-care facility. The parent asks a nurse what to look for as indicators that the facility is adhering to good infection control measures. The nurse identifies which as an indication of meeting proper infection control standards? Select all that apply.

- ☐ **1.** The facility keeps boxes of gloves in the director's office.
- ☐ **2.** Soiled diapers are discarded in covered receptacles.
- ☐ **3.** Toys are kept on the floor for the children to share.
- ☐ **4.** Disposable papers are used on the diaper-changing surfaces.
- ☐ **5.** Facilities for hand hygiene are located in every classroom.
- ☐ **6.** Soiled clothing and cloth diapers are sent home in labeled paper bags.

Answer: 2, 4, 5

Rationale: A parent can assess infection control practices by appraising steps taken by the facility to prevent the spread of disease. Placing soiled diapers in covered receptacles, covering the diaper-changing surfaces with disposable papers, and ensuring that hand sanitizers and sinks are available for personnel to wash their hands after activities are all indicators that infection control measures are being followed. Gloves should be readily available to personnel and, therefore, should be kept in every room—not in an office. Toys typically are shared by numerous children; however, this contributes to the spread of germs and infections. All soiled clothing and cloth diapers should be placed in a sealed plastic bag before being sent home.

Test-taking strategy: Analyze to determine what information the question asks for, which is standard precautions for infection control. "Select all that apply" questions require considering each option to decide its merit. Discriminate between each option to identify how that option meets the criteria for ensuring proper infection control practices. Review infection control practices if you had difficulty answering this question.

Client needs category: Safe and effective care environment

Client needs subcategory: Safety and infection control

Cognitive level: Analyzing

---

8. A neonatal intensive care nurse is performing cardiopulmonary resuscitation (CPR) on an infant. Between cycles of breathing and compressions, place an X where the nurse should assess for a pulse.

Answer:

Rationale: The X is placed over the brachial pulse best assessed just above the antecubital of the arm. The brachial pulse is the pulse to assess when performing infant CPR. The carotid pulse, which is used in children and adults, is extremely difficult to locate in an infant because of the infant short neck.

Test-taking strategy: Analyze to determine what information the question asks for, which is site for pulse assessment during infant CPR. Recall that pulse assessment sites vary according to age of the child. Review infant CPR if you had difficulty answering this question.

Client needs category: Physiological adaptation

Client needs subcategory: Physiological integrity

Cognitive level: Understanding

9. A nurse is assessing a 10-month-old infant during a checkup. Which developmental milestones would the nurse expect the infant to display? Select all that apply.

- ☐ **1.** Holding the head erect.
- ☐ **2.** Self-feeding.
- ☐ **3.** Demonstrating good bowel and bladder control.
- ☐ **4.** Sitting on a firm surface without support.
- ☐ **5.** Bearing the majority of weight on legs.
- ☐ **6.** Walking alone.

Answer: 1, 4, 5

Rationale: By age 4 months, an infant should be able to hold the head erect. By age 9 months, the infant should be able to sit on a firm surface without support and bear the majority of weight on the legs (for example, walking while holding onto furniture). Self-feeding and bowel and bladder control are developmental milestones of toddlers. By age 12 months, the infant should be able to stand alone and may take the first steps.

Test-taking strategy: Analyze to determine what information the question asks for, which is developmental milestones of a 10-month-old. "Select all that apply" questions require considering each option to decide its merit. Memorization of growth and development milestones is a must when answering many pediatric questions. Grouping development into ages may be helpful in recalling milestones on a continuum. Another helpful point may be to visualize the actions of a child at this age. Review growth and development of infants and toddlers if you had difficulty answering this question.

Client needs category: Health promotion and maintenance

Client needs subcategory: None

Cognitive level: Applying

---

10. A nurse is conducting an infant nutrition class for parents. Which foods should the nurse tell parents that they may introduce during the first year of life? Select all that apply.

- ☐ **1.** Sliced beef.
- ☐ **2.** Pureed fruits.
- ☐ **3.** Whole milk.
- ☐ **4.** Rice cereal.
- ☐ **5.** Strained vegetables.
- ☐ **6.** Fruit drink.

Answer: 2, 4, 5

Rationale: The first food provided to a neonate is breast milk or formula. Between ages 4 and 6 months, rice cereal can be introduced, followed by pureed or strained fruits and vegetables, then strained or ground meat. Meats must be chopped or ground before they are fed to an infant to prevent choking. Infants should not be given whole milk until they are at least 1 year old. Fruit drinks, many times with added sweeteners, provide no nutritional benefit and should not be encouraged.

Test-taking strategy: Analyze to determine what information the question asks for, which is foods to be introduced during the first year of life. "Select all that apply" questions require considering each option to decide its merit. The key words are "during the first year of life." Review each option for introduction into the child's system during the select timeframe. If unsure, recall the progression of oral intake. Review infant feeding schedules, including timing and type of solid foods introduced in the first year of life if you had difficulty answering this question.

Client needs category: Health promotion and maintenance

Client needs subcategory: None

Cognitive level: Applying

11. A nurse is teaching parents about the developmental milestones of an infant. Place the following developmental activities for an infant in order of occurrence by age from earliest to latest. Use all the options.

1.	Crawling on hands and knees.

2.	Sitting alone.

3.	Turning self from supine to prone.

4.	Turning self from prone to supine.

5.	Effectively using pincer grasp.

Answer: 4, 3, 2, 1, 5

Rationale: Infants turn first from prone to supine, and then supine to prone by age 3 to 4 months. Sitting alone usually occurs at about age 6 months. Crawling occurs at around age 7 to 8 months. The use of pincer grasp usually occurs at around 9 to 10 months.

Test-taking strategy: Analyze to determine what information the question asks for, which is identifying the proper progression of developmental milestones. Consider the progression of motor skills from gross to refined. Review infant developmental milestones if you had difficulty answering this question.

Client needs category: Health promotion and maintenance

Client needs subcategory: None

Cognitive level: Applying

---

12. The nurse is assessing the primitive reflexes of a 1-month-old infant. Which of the reflexes shown in photos below should not be present after the age of 2 months?

☐ **1.**

☐ **2.**

☐ **3.**

☐ **4.**

Answer: 4

Rationale: Option 4 shows the tonic neck reflex. Persistence of this reflex beyond 2 months suggests asymmetric central nervous system development. Option 1 shows the palmer grasp reflex. This reflex disappears around age 3 to 4 months. Option 2 shows the plantar grasp reflex. This reflex disappears at age 6 to 8 months. Option 3 shows the Moro reflex. This reflex disappears around age 4 months.

Test-taking strategy: Analyze to determine what information the question asks for, which is identification of reflexes that should not be present after 2 months of age. Analyze each illustration to identify the reflex being demonstrated and relate to the time period in which the reflex should disappear. Review when each primitive reflex is present and how it is assessed if you had difficulty answering this question.

Client needs category: Physiological integrity

Client needs subcategory: Reduction of risk potential

Cognitive level: Analyzing

13. A child is brought to the emergency depart-ment severely dehydrated after having gastroenteritis for 4 days. The physician orders an I.V. to maintain fluid replacement for this child. If the child weights 18 kg, what is the hourly flow rate in milliliters. Use the stan-dard, 100 mL/kg/day for the first 10 kg of body weight, 50 mL/kg/day for the next 10 kg of body weight, 20 mL/kg/day for each kilogram above 20 kg of body weight for daily maintenance.

_____ mL

Answer: 58

To find the answer, use the given formula as a guide. The client is 18 kg meaning that this is a two-step problem.

$$\text{Step 1: }100\text{ mL}/10\text{ kg} = 1,000\text{ mL.}$$
$$\text{Step 2: }50\text{ mL} \times 8\text{ kg} = 400\text{ mL.}$$

Total: 1,400 mL of daily maintenance fluids

Next, to find the hourly flow rate, divide by 24:

1,400 mL divided by 24 = 58.3 mL.

Test-taking strategy: Analyze to determine what information the question asks for, which is calculation of hourly fluid maintenance. Look for key informa-tion in the problem to place in the standard equation and calculate. Make sure that the answer provided answers the intended question, as in this question it was not daily amount but hourly. Proofread the math calculation. Review fluid maintenance calculations if you had difficulty answering this question.

Client needs category: Physiological integrity

Client needs subcategory: Pharmacological therapies

Cognitive level: Applying

The Toddler

1. A nurse is preparing a dose of amoxicillin for a 3-year-old with acute otitis media. The child weighs 33 lb. The dosage prescribed is 50 mg/kg/day in divided doses for every 8 hours. The concentration of the drug is 250 mg/5 mL. How many milliliters should the nurse administer? Record your answer using a whole number.

_____ mL

Answer: 5

Rationale: To calculate the child's weight in kilograms, the nurse should use the following formula:

$$2.2\text{ lb}/1\text{ kg} = 33\text{ lb}/X\text{ kg}$$
$$X = 33 \div 2.2$$
$$X = 15\text{ kg.}$$

Next, the nurse should calculate the daily dosage for the child:

$$50\text{ mg/kg/day} \times 15\text{ kg} = 750\text{ mg/day.}$$

To determine divided daily dosage, the nurse should know that "every 8 hours" means three times per day. So, the nurse should perform the calculation in this way:

Total daily dosage ÷ 3 times per day = divided daily dosage

$$750\text{ mg/day} \div 3 = 250\text{ mg.}$$

The drug's concentration is 250 mg/5 mL, so the nurse should administer 5 mL.

Test-taking strategy: Analyze to determine what information the question asks for, which is milliliters of medication to be administered per dose. Follow the steps above thinking through the process of determin-ing kilograms, then calculating daily dose, and then each dose. Lastly, use the known concentration to determine the milliliters to be administered. Proofread the math calculations. Review multistep dosage calculations if you had difficulty answering this question.

Client needs category: Physiological integrity

Client needs subcategory: Pharmacological therapies

Cognitive level: Applying

---

2. A 3-year-old is to receive 500 mL of dextrose 5% in normal saline solution over 8 hours. At what rate (in milliliters per hour) should a nurse set the infusion pump? Round your answer to a whole number.

_____ mL/hour

Answer: 63

Rationale: To calculate the rate per hour for the infusion, the nurse should divide 500 mL by 8 hours:

500 mL ÷ 8 hours = 62.5 mL/hour (63 mL/hour).

Test-taking strategy: Analyze to determine what information the question asks for, which is infusion rate in milliliters per hour. Recall that there are two types of infusion calculations: (1) looking at quantity in milliliter per hour and (2) drip factor rates in gtts per minute. Quantity of fluid (mL/hour) calculations divides the amount of fluid by the number of hours to be infused. Proofread all mathematical calculations. Review dosage calculations for hourly flow rates if you had difficulty answering this question.

Client needs category: Physiological integrity

Client needs subcategory: Pharmacological therapies

Cognitive level: Applying

---

3. A 2-year-old is being treated for pneumonia. After reviewing the respiratory section of the client care flow sheet (shown below), the nurse concludes that which position is most beneficial to maximize oxygenation?

Flow Sheet			
Date: 4/2/10	2300–0700	0700–1500	1500–2300
Breath sounds	Diminished BS LLL	Diminished BS LLL	Crackles LLL
Treatment/ results	------	CPT and postural drainage	CPT and postural drainage
Cough/results	Nonproductive	Nonproductive	Yellow sputum
Oxygen therapy	Humidifier	Humidifier	Humidifier

☐ **1.** Left-side lying.
☐ **2.** Right-side lying.
☐ **3.** Supine.
☐ **4.** Supine with the head of the bed elevated 30°.

Answer: 2

Rationale: The client should be positioned on the right side. Gravity will help mobilize secretions from the affected (left) lung, thereby allowing for improved blood flow and oxygenation.

Test-taking strategy: Analyze to determine what information the question asks for, which is the analysis of the nurse's note to determine the status of the client and progression of symptoms. Identify that breath sounds, cough results, and treatment results provide data that secretion status is a priority. Determine which position would eliminate secretions from the lung fields. Review respiratory data and postural drainage treatment if you had difficulty answering this question.

Client needs category: Physiological integrity

Client needs subcategory: Physiological adaptation

Cognitive level: Analyzing

4. A 15-month-old has just received routine immunizations, including DTaP, IPV, and MMR. What information should the nurse give to the parents before they leave the office? Select all that apply.

☐ **1.** Minor symptoms can be treated with acetaminophen (Tylenol).

☐ **2.** Minor symptoms can be treated with aspirin.

☐ **3.** Call the office if the toddler develops a fever above 103°F (39.4°C), seizures, or difficulty breathing.

☐ **4.** Soreness at the immunization site and mild fever are common.

☐ **5.** The immunizations prevent the toddler from contracting their associated diseases.

☐ **6.** The parents should restrict toddler activity for the remainder of the day.

Answer: 1, 3, 4

Rationale: Minor symptoms, such as soreness at the immunization site and mild fever, can be treated with acetaminophen or ibuprofen. Aspirin should be avoided in children because of its association with Reye's syndrome. The parents should notify the clinic if serious complications (such as a fever above 103°F, seizures, or difficulty breathing) occur. Minor discomforts, such as soreness and mild fever, are common after immunizations. Immunizing the child decreases the health risks associated with contracting certain diseases; it does not prevent the toddler from acquiring them. Although the child may prefer to rest after immunizations, it is not necessary to restrict activity.

Test-taking strategy: Analyze to determine what information the question asks for, which is parent teaching following immunizations. "Select all that apply" questions require considering each option to decide its merit. Note routine standards that can be eliminated for inaccurate information such as providing aspirin to a child and immunizations preventing diseases. Recall the rationale for immunizations and side effects which can occur if you had difficulty answering this question.

Client needs category: Health promotion and maintenance

Client needs subcategory: None

Cognitive level: Applying

---

5. A nurse is assessing the apical impulse of a 28-month-old child. Identify the area where the nurse should locate the apical impulse.

Answer:

Rationale: The heart's apex for a toddler is located at the fourth intercostal space, immediately to the left of the midclavicular line. It is one or two intercostal spaces above what is considered normal for an adult because the heart's position in a child of this age is more horizontal and larger in diameter than that of an adult.

Test-taking strategy: Analyze to determine what information the question asks for, which is anatomical location for the apical pulse. First, identify the point of maximal impulse, then count the number of ribs to identify the intercostal spaces. Review procedure for obtaining an apical pulse if you had difficulty answering this question.

Client needs category: Health promotion and maintenance

Client needs subcategory: None

Cognitive level: Applying

---

6. A nurse is caring for a 3-year-old diagnosed with viral meningitis. Which signs and symptoms would the nurse expect to find during the admission assessment? Select all that apply.

- ☐ **1.** Bulging anterior fontanel.
- ☐ **2.** Fever.
- ☐ **3.** Nuchal rigidity.
- ☐ **4.** Petechiae.
- ☐ **5.** Irritability.
- ☐ **6.** Photophobia.

Answer: 2, 3, 5, 6

Rationale: Common signs and symptoms of viral meningitis include fever, nuchal rigidity, irritability, and photophobia. A bulging anterior fontanel is a sign of hydrocephalus, which is not likely to occur in a toddler because the anterior fontanel typically closes by age 24 months. A petechial, purpuric rash may be seen with bacterial meningitis.

Test-taking strategy: Analyze to determine what information the question asks for, which is signs and symptoms associated with viral meningitis. "Select all that apply" questions require considering each option to decide its merit. When determining pediatric assessment questions, always note the child's age to ensure that the symptoms compare with the age. Also, if unsure, use knowledge of terminology to break the word apart (meninges = layer of the brain; itis = infection). Review the clinical findings of viral meningitis if you had difficulty answering this question.

Client needs category: Physiological integrity

Client needs subcategory: Physiological adaptation

Cognitive level: Applying

7. The nurse is caring for a 3-year-old client being treated for severe status asthmaticus. After comparing clinical manifestations with laboratory results (reported below), a nurse determines evidence that this client has progressed to which condition?

Progress Notes	
4/5/10	Pt. was acutely restless, diaphoretic, and
0600	with SOB at 0530. Dr. T. Smith notified
	and ordered ABG analysis. ABG drawn from
	R radial artery. Stat results as follows: pH
	7.28, Paco₂ 55 mm Hg, HCO₃ 26 mEg/L.
	Dr. Smith with pt. now. ———— J. Collins,
	LPN.

☐ **1.** Metabolic acidosis.
☐ **2.** Respiratory alkalosis.
☐ **3.** Respiratory acidosis.
☐ **4.** Metabolic alkalosis.

Answer: 3

Rationale: A pH less than 7.35 and a partial pressure of arterial carbon dioxide ($PaCO_2$) greater than 45 mm Hg indicate respiratory acidosis. Status asthmaticus is a medical emergency characterized by respiratory distress. At first, the client hyperventilates; then respiratory alkalosis occurs, followed by metabolic acidosis. If treatment is ineffective or has not begun, symptoms can progress to hypoventilation and respiratory acidosis, both of which are life-threatening. A client with respiratory alkalosis would have a pH greater than 7.45 and a $PaCO_2$ less than 35 mm Hg. Metabolic acidosis is characterized by a pH less than 7.35 and a bicarbonate (HCO_3^-) level less than 22 mEq/L. Metabolic alkalosis is characterized by a pH greater than 7.45 and HCO_3^- above 26 mEq/L.

Test-taking strategy: Analyze to determine what information the question asks for, which is the selection of correct metabolic state coordinating with reported data. Use the data provided and reference ranges to analyze blood gases. If unsure, recall the normal range for blood gas values to determine either acidosis or alkalosis and that the admission disease process is respiratory in nature. Review analysis techniques of ABG (arterial blood gas) values if you had difficulty answering this question.

Client needs subcategory: Physiological integrity

Client needs subcategory: Physiological adaptation

Cognitive level: Analyzing

8. A 30-month-old toddler is being evaluated for a ventricular septal defect (VSD). When teaching the parents about the condition, identify the area where a VSD occurs.

Answer:

Rationale: A VSD is a small hole between the right and left ventricles that allows blood to shunt between them, causing right ventricular hypertrophy and, if left untreated, biventricular heart failure. It is a common congenital heart defect and accounts for 20% to 30% of all heart lesions.

Test-taking strategy: Analyze to determine what information the question asks for, which is anatomical location where a VSD occurs. *Use knowledge of medical terminology to guide to the location (ventricular = ventricles; septal = septum or wall defect or between the two ventricles).* Review congenital heart defects and how blood flow is altered by each defect if you had difficulty answering this question.

Client needs category: Physiological integrity

Client needs subcategory: Physiological adaptation

Cognitive level: Applying

9. A child weighing 44 lb is to receive 45 mg/kg/day of penicillin V potassium oral suspension in four divided doses for every 6 hours. The suspension that is available is penicillin V potassium 125 mg/5 mL. How many milliliters should the nurse administer for each dose? Record your answer using a whole number.

_____ mL

Answer: 9

Rationale: First, convert the child's weight to kilograms:

$$44 \text{ lb} \div 2.2 \text{ kg/lb} = 20 \text{ kg.}$$

Next, determine the daily dose:

$$45 \text{ mg} : 1 \text{ kg} = X \text{ mg} : 20 \text{ kg}$$
$$45 \times 20 = 1 \times X$$
$$900 = X.$$

Then, determine the dose to administer every 6 hours (four doses):

$$900 \text{ mg} \div 4 = 225 \text{ mg.}$$

Finally, determine the volume to be given at each dose:

$$225 \text{ mg} : X = 125 \text{ mg} : 5 \text{ mL}$$
$$1{,}125 \text{ mg/mL} = 125 \text{ mg/}X$$
$$9 \text{ mL} = X.$$

Test-taking strategy: Analyze to determine what information the question asks for, which is milliliters to be administered per dose. First, recall the conversion of pounds to kilograms. Next, follow the steps above to determine daily dose and then single dose. Use caution to ensure that the question is answered in the proper measuring units such as milliliter per dose administered. Proofread math calculations. Review drug dose calculations if you had difficulty answering this question.

Client needs category: Physiological integrity

Client needs subcategory: Pharmacological therapies

Cognitive level: Applying

---

10. A nurse is caring for a 34-month-old who is hospitalized for a lengthy illness. Which behaviors would the nurse identify as examples of expected developmental regression for the child's age group? Select all that apply.

☐ **1.** Enuresis.
☐ **2.** Encopresis.
☐ **3.** Immature speech patterns.
☐ **4.** Altered gait.
☐ **5.** Loss of fine motor skills.

Answer: 1, 2, 3

Rationale: Enuresis (uncontrolled voiding) and encopresis (uncontrolled stooling) are often seen in toddlers who were previously toilet trained and return to diapers during hospitalization. Language regression ("baby talk") is often observed during hospitalization. Altered gait and loss of fine motor skills are not typical regressive behaviors; when seen in a child, they may indicate musculoskeletal or neurological problems.

Test-taking strategy: Analyze to determine what information the question asks for, which is behaviors that are characteristic of developmental regression. "Select all that apply" questions require considering each option to decide its merit. Consider each option listed against current age of the child to decide if that milestone has been previously reached. Review the developmental milestones of toddlers, which may regress if hospitalized, if you had difficulty answering this question.

Client needs category: Health promotion and maintenance

Client needs subcategory: None

Cognitive level: Applying

11. A nurse is caring for a group of toddlers in a large urban hospital. When considering providing care, which clients require contact precautions? Select all that apply.

☐ **1.** A toddler with scabies.
☐ **2.** A toddler with mumps.
☐ **3.** A toddler with streptococcal pharyngitis.
☐ **4.** A toddler with pulmonary tuberculosis.
☐ **5.** A toddler with a multidrug-resistant organism.

Answer: 1, 5

Rationale: According to the Centers for Disease Control, in addition to standard precautions, contact isolation precautions are used for clients with known or suspected infections. Scabies is a skin infection and requires contact precautions. Multidrug-resistant infection also requires contact precautions because of potential contamination. A toddler with mumps or streptococcal pharyngitis requires droplet precautions. Pulmonary tuberculosis requires airborne precautions.

Test-taking strategy: Analyze to determine what information the question asks for, which is determining conditions which need to be placed in contact isolation. "Select all that apply" questions require considering each option to decide its merit. Recall that contact isolation means that the client is preferred to be in a private room with disposable equipment if possible, and gowns and gloves are required and removed prior to leaving the room. Review the pathophysiology of the listed diseases and transmission-based precautions if you had difficulty answering this question.

Client needs category: Safe and effective care environment

Client needs subcategory: Safety and infection control

Cognitive level: Applying

---

12. A nurse, on the pediatric unit, received shift report on a 15-month-old with the following needs. Using Maslow's hierarchy framework, prioritize the following nursing care activities for the toddler. Use all of the options.

1. Progressing the diet after surgery.
2. Clearing the airway of secretions.
3. Changing a soiled diaper.
4. Administering antipyretics for an axillary temperature of 104°F.
5. Notifying the practitioner about suspected compartment syndrome.

Answer: 2, 5, 3, 4, 1

Rationale: According to Maslow's hierarchy framework, the five categories, or hierarchy of needs in order of priority, are as follows: physiologic needs, safety, love, esteem, and self-actualization. Within the physiologic needs category are the essentials for existence: air, nutrition, water, elimination, sleep and rest, thermoregulation, and sex. Therefore, maintaining a patent airway is the first priority, followed by notifying the practitioner of suspected compartment syndrome because of the risk of loss of limb. Changing a soiled diaper would be next because this is necessary to prevent skin breakdown. Administering antipyretics for fever primarily provides comfort to the child. The lowest priority, although important, is progressing the child's diet following surgery.

Test-taking strategy: Analyze to determine what information the question asks for, which is prioritizing the care of a toddler. Recall Maslow's hierarchy of needs and the levels that guide decision making about care. Consider that clearing an airway is typically a top priority, followed by potential safety concerns. Review Maslow's hierarchy of needs associated with a variety of client scenarios if you had difficulty answering this question.

Client needs category: Safe and effective care environment

Client needs subcategory: Coordinated care

Cognitive level: Applying

13. The nurse is preparing to insert an intravenous catheter into an anxious toddler. Place the following steps in the order the nurse should follow. Use all of the options.

| 1. Wash hands and gather supplies. |
| 2. Prepare the equipment. |
| 3. Inform the toddler of the procedure. |
| 4. Inform the parents of the procedure. |
| 5. Select and prep the appropriate site. |
| 6. Insert the I.V. catheter and secure it appropriately. |

Answer: 4, 1, 2, 3, 5, 6

Rationale: It is important to inform the parents and gain their support for the procedure first, especially if the child is anxious. A toddler does not understand the concept of time, so the nurse should not inform the toddler until very shortly before the I.V. insertion. Next, the nurse should wash hands and prepare the supplies and equipment, keeping them out of the child's sight to decrease anxiety. Finally, the nurse should inform the toddler of what is about to happen, then perform the procedure by selecting and prepping the site, inserting the I.V. catheter, and securing it.

Test-taking strategy: Analyze to determine what information the question asks for, which is considerations when performing a procedure on an anxious toddler. Use knowledge of growth and development and psychosocial skills to plan care realizing that skill and efficiency are important. For any invasive procedure, informed consent, which would be provided by the parents, is completed first. Next, the efficient nurse prepares and gathers all supplies. Lastly, the child is told and procedure completed. Review prioritizing nursing actions for an anxious toddler if you had difficulty answering this question.

Client needs category: Physiological integrity

Client needs subcategory: Basic care and comfort

Cognitive level: Applying

The Preschooler

1. A 4½-year-old is ordered to receive 25 mL/hour of I.V. solution. The nurse is using a pediatric microdrip chamber to administer the medication. For how many drops per minute should the microdrip chamber be set? Record your answer using a whole number.

_____ drops/minute

Answer: 25

Rationale: When using a pediatric microdrip chamber (60 gtts/minute), the number of milliliters per hour equals the number of drops per minute. If 25 mL/hour is ordered, the I.V. solution should infuse at 25 drops/minute.

For example:

$$\frac{\text{Volume} \times \text{drip factor}}{\text{Minutes}} = \text{gtts/minute.}$$

Thus, if the drip factor on a microdrip IV tubing is 60 and the infusion time is 60 minutes, these cancel and the answer is the volume (mL).

Test-taking strategy: Analyze to determine what information the question asks for, which is the number of drops per minute. Use the math calculation above and quick check to provide the answer. Be sure that the I.V. tubing is a microdrip set to be able to use the quick check of canceling the microdrip and time per hour. Review I.V. infusion rates if you had difficulty answering this question.

Client needs category: Physiological integrity

Client needs subcategory: Pharmacological therapies

Cognitive level: Applying

2. While assessing a child experiencing respiratory distress, the nurse notes subcostal retractions. Which graphic highlights the area where subcostal retractions are seen?

☐ **1.**

☐ **2.**

☐ **3.**

☐ **4.**

Answer: 2

Rationale: Subcostal retractions are retractions seen below the lower costal margin of the rib cage. Option 2 highlights the area where subcostal retractions are seen. Option 1 shows the areas where intercostal retractions would be seen. Option 3 shows the area for suprasternal retraction. Option 4 shows the areas for clavicular retractions.

Test-taking strategy: Analyze to determine what information the question asks for, which is location of subcostal retractions. Use knowledge of medical terminology to guide to the location. (Sub = below; costal = ribs.) Review the definition of retractions and the anatomical landmarks associated if you had difficulty answering this question.

Client needs category: Physiological integrity

Client needs subcategory: Physiological adaptation

Cognitive level: Applying

3. A nurse is performing a Denver Developmental Screening Test II on a 4½-year-old child. What behaviors should the nurse expect the child to demonstrate? Select all that apply.

- ☐ **1.** The child balances on each foot for at least 6 seconds.
- ☐ **2.** The child copies a circle that is closed or very nearly closed.
- ☐ **3.** The child speaks clearly.
- ☐ **4.** The child draws a person with at least three body parts.

Answer: 2, 3, 4

Rationale: By age 4½, a child should be able to copy a circle, speak clearly, and draw a person with at least three body parts. The majority of children do not achieve balancing on each foot for 6 seconds until about age 5½.

Test-taking strategy: Analyze to determine what information the question asks for, which is anticipated behaviors of a 4½-year-old on the Denver Developmental Screening II. "Select all that apply" questions require considering each option to decide its merit. Recall that cognitive growth is substantial during these years, and each year during this period marks a major step forward in gross motor, fine motor, and language development. If unsure, consider that preschoolers draw circles and stick figures and are able to communicate through speaking but are uncoordinated at this age. Review the Denver Developmental Screening II assessment tool if you had difficulty answering this question.

Client needs category: Health promotion and maintenance

Client needs subcategory: None

Cognitive level: Analyzing

---

4. The nurse is caring for a 4-year-old recently diagnosed with acute lymphocytic leukemia (ALL). Which statement, made by the parents, indicates the need for clarification of teaching. Select all that apply.

- ☐ **1.** "I read that ALL is a rare form of childhood leukemia."
- ☐ **2.** "I understand that ALL affects all blood-forming organs and systems throughout the body."
- ☐ **3.** "Because of the increased risk of bleeding, I will eliminate evening teeth brushing."
- ☐ **4.** "I realize that the adverse effects of chemotherapy includes sleepiness, alopecia, and stomatitis."
- ☐ **5.** "I am glad that there's a 95% chance of obtaining a first remission with treatment."
- ☐ **6.** "I will not discipline my child during this difficult time."

Answer: 1, 3, 6

Rationale: In ALL, immature white blood cells (WBCs) crowd out healthy WBCs, red blood cells, and platelets in the bone marrow. These abnormal WBCs affect all blood-forming organs and systems. Common adverse effects of chemotherapy and radiation include nausea, vomiting, diarrhea, sleepiness, alopecia, anemia, stomatitis, pain, and increased susceptibility to infection. A first remission occurs in about 95% of cases. Brushing teeth does not result in increased or abnormal bleeding. A child with leukemia still needs appropriate discipline and limits because a lack of consistent parenting may lead to negative behaviors and fear. ALL is the most common cancer in children.

Test-taking strategy: Analyze to determine what information the question asks for, which is inaccurate statements, made by the parent, regarding issues of ALL. "Select all that apply" questions require considering each option to decide its merit. Consider each option for a wrong statement. Review the pathophysiology of ALL and parent teaching guidelines if you had difficulty answering this question.

Client needs category: Physiological integrity

Client needs subcategory: Reduction of risk potential

Cognitive level: Applying

5. A school nurse is gathering registration data for a child entering first grade. Which immunizations should the school nurse verify that the child has had? Select all that apply.

- ☐ **1.** Hepatitis B series.
- ☐ **2.** Diphtheria–tetanus–pertussis series.
- ☐ **3.** *Haemophilus influenzae* type b series.
- ☐ **4.** Varicella vaccine.
- ☐ **5.** Pneumonia vaccine.
- ☐ **6.** Oral polio series.

Answer: 1, 2, 3, 4

Rationale: Hepatitis B series, diphtheria–tetanus–pertussis series, *H. influenzae* type b series, varicella, and inactivated (not oral) polio series are the immunizations that the child should receive before entering first grade. The oral polio vaccine was discontinued; the safer IPV is now used. Pneumonia vaccine is not required or routinely given to children.

Test-taking strategy: Analyze to determine what information the question asks for, which is immunizations needed to begin school. "Select all that apply" questions require considering each option to decide its merit. Consider immunization received in childhood as the basis of those needed prior to school. These vaccines are typically those administered from birth, as infants and then preschool years. Review immunization and infection control recommendations provided by the American Academy of Pediatrics and the Centers for Disease Control and Prevention if you had difficulty answering this question.

Client needs category: Physiological integrity

Client needs subcategory: Physiological adaptation

Cognitive level: Analyzing

6. A 4-year-old child is brought to the emergency department in cardiac arrest. During CPR, identify the area where the child's pulse should be assessed.

Answer:

Rationale: The carotid artery should be used to assess for a pulse when performing CPR on children and adults. The brachial pulse should be used when performing CPR on an infant.

Test-taking strategy: Analyze to determine what information the question asks for, which is site for assessment of a pulse during the child's CPR. Consider that children have the same assessment site for a pulse as adults. The rationale for the change in pulse site for infants is due to the shortness of the neck. Review the recommendations for CPR in infants, children, and adults if you had difficulty answering this question.

Client needs category: Physiological integrity

Client needs subcategory: Physiological adaptation

Cognitive level: Understanding

7. A nurse is caring preoperatively for a preschooler scheduled for a Wilms' tumor removal. When explaining the location of the tumor to the parents, identify the area of the urinary system impacted.

Answer:

Rationale: Wilms' tumor, also known as a nephroblastoma, is located on the kidney. The most common intra-abdominal tumor in children, Wilms' tumor, usually affects children ages 6 months to 4 years and favors the left kidney.

Test-taking strategy: Analyze to determine what information the question asks for, which is location of a Wilms' tumor. Since this is a common pediatric tumor, memorization of the location, signs and symptoms, and nursing actions is important. Review the anatomy of the urinary system and the pathophysiology of Wilms' tumor if you had difficulty answering this question.

Client needs category: Physiological integrity

Client needs subcategory: Physiological adaptation

Cognitive level: Applying

8. A nurse is caring for a 5-year-old child who is in the terminal stages of cancer. Which statements about the child's impending death are most likely to be true? Select all that apply.

☐ **1.** The parents may be at different stages of grief in dealing with the child's impending death.

☐ **2.** The child is thinking about the future and knows he/she may not be able to participate.

☐ **3.** The dying child may become clingy and act like a toddler.

☐ **4.** Whispering in the child's room will help the child to cope.

☐ **5.** The death of a child may have long-term disruptive effects on the family.

☐ **6.** The child does not fully understand the concept of death.

Answer: 1, 3, 5, 6

Rationale: When dealing with a dying child, parents may be at different stages of grief at different times. The child may regress in behaviors. The stress of a child's death commonly results in divorce of parents and behavioral problems in siblings. Preschoolers see illness and death as a form of punishment. They fear separation from parents and might worry about who will provide care for them. Preschoolers have only a rudimentary concept of time; thinking about the future is typical of an adolescent facing death, not a preschooler. Whispering in front of the child only increases fear of death.

Test-taking strategy: Analyze to determine what information the question asks for, which is correct statements about a child's impending death. "Select all that apply" questions require considering each option to decide its merit. Recall the stages of the grief process (adults and children) and developmental stage of preschoolers when selecting an option. Review psychosocial concepts associated with childhood death if you had difficulty answering this question.

Client needs category: Psychosocial integrity

Client needs subcategory: None

Cognitive level: Analyzing

---

9. A 3-year-old boy has arrived in the emergency department. The nurse documents the following assessment findings in the client's chart, knowing that they are consistent with which disease process?

Progress Notes	
5/15/10 1100	Pt. admitted to ER with T. 103.6°F, HR 100, RR 24. Respirations are shallow, and breath sounds are decreased, with rales auscultated bilaterally. Pt. has a harsh cough and mother states he has had a discolored productive cough at home.——S. Jones, LPN

☐ **1.** Bronchiolitis.

☐ **2.** Pneumonia.

☐ **3.** Asthma.

☐ **4.** Cystic fibrosis.

Answer: 2

Rationale: The elevated fever, shallow respirations, decreased breath sounds, rales, harsh cough, and productive mucus are findings associated with pneumonia. Typically, there is no fever with asthma and cystic fibrosis, and bronchiolitis presents with a low-grade fever. Wheezing is associated with asthma and bronchiolitis; however, this was not found upon physical examination of this client. Bronchiolitis produces a dry cough, and pneumonia causes a productive, harsh cough. The client with cystic fibrosis typically presents with wheezing, rhonchi, and thick, tenacious mucus.

Test-taking strategy: Analyze to determine what information the question asks for, which is assessment findings associated with a respiratory disease process. Compare and contrast the clinical findings as documented to the findings associated with the illness. Focus on specific details such as temperature and breath sounds that either confirm or disprove a disease process. Review disorders of the respiratory tract if you had difficulty answering this question.

Client needs category: Physiological integrity

Client needs subcategory: Physiological adaptation

Cognitive level: Analyzing

10. A 4-year-old postoperative child is found unresponsive. Place the following actions in the correct sequence to perform CPR after the child has been assessed for responsiveness and help has been called. Use all of the options.

| 1. Open the airway. |
| 2. Feel for the carotid pulse. |
| 3. Check for breathing. |
| 4. Perform 30 compressions. |
| 5. Provide 2 rescue breaths. |

Answer: 2, 4, 1, 3, 5

Rationale: Following the 2010 American Heart Association guidelines for CPR, the rescuer should activate the emergency response system and get an automatic external defibrillator (AED) or appoint another person to do this. The next step is to check the pulse for no more than 10 seconds. If no pulse is detected, the rescuer gives 30 chest compressions. Next, the rescuer opens the airway with the head tilt-chin lift or jaw thrust maneuver and checks for breathing. If breathing is not detected, the rescuer gives 2 rescue breaths and immediately resumes chest compressions at a cycle of 30 compressions to 2 breaths. The rescuer should use the AED as soon as it arrives.

Test-taking strategy: Analyze to determine what information the question asks for, which is the sequence for CPR on a child. Visualize the steps in the process by first determining the need for CPR then circulating blood through manual compressions and lastly providing breaths. Review the CPR steps and checking the ABCs (airway, breathing, and circulation) if you had difficulty answering this question.

Client needs category: Physiological integrity

Client needs subcategory: Physiological adaptation

Cognitive level: Applying

11. A nurse is caring for a 4-year-old child who developed acute renal failure after a traumatic injury and hemorrhaging. Place the following events in the order in which they most likely occurred during progression of the severe renal deterioration. Use all of the options.

| 1. Acidosis. |
| 2. Severe hypocalcemia. |
| 3. Azotemia. |
| 4. Oliguria. |

Answer: 4, 3, 1, 2

Rationale: The first symptom of acute renal failure is oliguria (urine output less than 1 mL/kg of the child's body weight per hour). The inability to produce urine causes azotemia, an accumulation of nitrogen waste in the bloodstream, which leads to rising blood urea nitrogen levels. This leads to acidosis because of the body's inability to excrete H+ ions. The acidotic state results in hyperphosphatemia (high phosphorus levels), which in turn causes hypocalcemia (low calcium levels). When hypocalcemia is severe, muscle twitching and tetany can occur.

Test-taking strategy: Analyze to determine what information the question asks for, which is sequence of events during acute renal failure. Consider the definition of each term and place from simple to complex. Note that as the disease process continues more symptoms become involved. Review the pathophysiology of acute renal failure if you had difficulty answering this question.

Client needs category: Physiological integrity

Client needs subcategory: Physiological adaptation

Cognitive level: Analyzing

1. A 7-year-old child is admitted to the hospital for a course of I.V. antibiotics. What actions should the nurse take before inserting the peripheral I.V. catheter? Select all that apply.

- ☐ **1.** Explain the procedure to the child immediately before the procedure.
- ☐ **2.** Apply a topical anesthetic to the I.V. site before the procedure.
- ☐ **3.** Ask the child which hand he/she uses for drawing.
- ☐ **4.** Explain the procedure to the child using abstract terms.
- ☐ **5.** Do not let the child see the equipment to be used in the procedure.
- ☐ **6.** Tell the child that the procedure will not hurt.

Answer: 2, 3

Rationale: Topical anesthetics reduce the pain of a venipuncture. The cream should be applied about 1 hour before the procedure and requires a physician's order. The I.V. should be inserted into the hand opposite the one the child identifies as his/her drawing hand. The procedure should be explained to the child in simple, concrete words well before it takes place so that he/she has time to ask questions. Unfamiliar terms should be defined. To help ease anxiety, the child should be shown the equipment that will be used for the procedure. The use of dolls for roleplay can also be utilized. Although the topical anesthetic will relieve some pain, there is usually some pain or discomfort involved in venipuncture, so the child should not be told otherwise.

Test-taking strategy: Analyze to determine what information the question asks for, which is nursing actions related to peripheral I.V. insertion. "Select all that apply" questions require considering each option to decide its merit. Visualize the steps in placing an I.V. catheter then consider the age-appropriate adjustments needed for a school-aged pediatric client. Recall that the cognitive development of a school-age child is concrete operational thinking. Review the nursing process for administration of I.V. fluids to a school-aged child if you had difficulty answering this question.

Client needs category: Health promotion and maintenance

Client needs subcategory: None

Cognitive level: Applying

2. A mother brings her child to the pediatrician's office for evaluation of chronic stomach pain. The mother states that the pain seems to go away when she keeps the child home from school. The physician diagnoses school phobia. Which other behaviors or symptoms may the child exhibit? Select all that apply.

- ☐ **1.** Nausea.
- ☐ **2.** Headaches.
- ☐ **3.** Weight loss.
- ☐ **4.** Dizziness.
- ☐ **5.** Fever.

Answer: 1, 2, 4

Rationale: Children with school phobia commonly complain of vague symptoms, such as stomachaches, nausea, headaches, and dizziness, to avoid going to school. These symptoms typically do not occur on weekends. A careful history must be taken to identify a pattern of school avoidance. Weight loss and fever are more likely to have a physiological cause and are uncommon in children with school phobia.

Test-taking strategy: Analyze to determine what information the question asks for, which is symptoms of school phobia. "Select all that apply" questions require considering each option to decide its merit.

Relate school phobia to symptoms of anxiety as the children are anxious about going to school. Recall that anxiety and fears manifest with acute episodes of symptoms (such as gastrointestinal problems). Review symptoms associated with school phobia if you had difficulty answering this question.

Client needs category: Psychosocial integrity

Client needs subcategory: None

Cognitive level: Applying

---

3. A child with sickle cell anemia is being discharged after treatment for a crisis. Which instructions for avoiding future crises should the nurse provide to the child and family? Select all that apply.

- ☐ **1.** Avoid foods high in folic acid.
- ☐ **2.** Drink plenty of fluids.
- ☐ **3.** Use cold packs to relieve joint pain.
- ☐ **4.** Report a sore throat to an adult immediately.
- ☐ **5.** Restrict activity to quiet board games.
- ☐ **6.** Wash hands before meals and after playing.

Answer: 2, 4, 6

Rationale: Sickle cell anemia is a disease passed down through families in which red blood cells form an abnormal sickle or crescent shape. Fluids should be encouraged to prevent stasis in the bloodstream, which can lead to sickling. Sore throats and all other cold symptoms should be reported promptly because they may indicate an infection, which can precipitate a crisis (red blood cells sickle and obstruct blood flow to tissues). Children with sickle cell anemia should learn appropriate measures to prevent infection, such as proper hand-washing techniques and good nutrition. Folic acid intake should be encouraged to help support new cell growth; new cells replace fragile sickled cells. Warm packs should be applied to promote comfort and relieve pain; cold packs cause vasoconstriction. The child should maintain an active, normal life but should avoid excessive exercise, which can precipitate an attack. When the child experiences a crisis, the child will typically limit his/her own activity according to his/her pain level.

Test-taking strategy: Analyze to determine what information the question asks for, which is nursing instructions helpful to avoid a sickle cell crisis. "Select all that apply" questions require considering each option to decide its merit. Recall that infants and children are at an increased risk for a crisis because of exposure to various bacterial infections which could cause dehydration and infection. Daily penicillin therapy may be prescribed. Also encouraging fluids such as water is important as a daily routine, especially during the summer when outside playing. Review the events that may trigger a sickle cell crisis if you had difficulty answering this question.

Client needs category: Physiological integrity

Client needs subcategory: Reduction of risk potential

Cognitive level: Applying

4. A nurse is caring for an 8-year-old postoperative tonsillectomy client. When performing a postoperative assessment, which signs and symptoms of bleeding should be monitored for by the nurse? Select all that apply.

☐ **1.** Frequent clearing of the throat.
☐ **2.** Breathing through the mouth.
☐ **3.** Frequent swallowing.
☐ **4.** Sleeping for long intervals.
☐ **5.** Pulse rate of 98 beats/minute.
☐ **6.** Blood red vomitus.

Answer: 1, 3, 6

Rationale: A classic sign of bleeding after tonsillectomy is frequent swallowing; this occurs because blood drips down the back of the throat, tickling it. Other signs include frequent clearing of the throat and vomiting of bright red blood. Vomiting of dark blood may occur if the child swallowed blood during surgery, but this does not indicate postoperative bleeding. Breathing through the mouth is common because of dried secretions in the nares. Sleeping for long intervals is normal after receiving sedation and anesthesia. A pulse rate of 98 beats/minute is in the normal range for this age group.

Test-taking strategy: Analyze to determine what information the question asks for, which is signs of postoperative tonsillectomy bleeding. "Select all that apply" questions require considering each option to decide its merit. Consider the location of the tonsils and what sign may be present if there was bleeding. Bleeding at the rear of the oral cavity would lead to clearing of the throat, swallowing, and bright red bleeding down the gastrointestinal tract. Review the postoperative management of a child after a tonsillectomy and the signs and symptoms of complications if you had difficulty answering this question.

Client needs category: Physiological integrity

Client needs subcategory: Reduction of risk potential

Cognitive level: Applying

---

5. A 6-year-old child with complaints of fever, malaise, and anorexia is diagnosed with varicella (chickenpox). The nurse explains to the mother how skin lesions will develop. Place the following descriptions in the order that they will occur as the disease progresses. Use all of the options.

1. As initial lesions progress through stages, new lesions form on the trunk and extremities.
2. Papules develop into clear vesicles on an erythematous base.
3. Itchy red macules on the face, scalp, and trunk progress to papules.
4. Vesicles become cloudy and break easily.
5. Scabs form.

Answer: 3, 2, 4, 5, 1

Rationale: Varicella (chickenpox) is a common childhood illness, which is usually mild but can be serious. Fever, malaise, and anorexia occur 24 to 48 hours before a rash develops. The rash begins as itchy red macules on the face, scalp, and trunk. These macules progress to papules, which develop into clear vesicles on an erythematous base. The vesicles become cloudy and break, forming scabs. New lesions continue to form on the trunk and extremities.

Test-taking strategy: Analyze to determine what information the question asks for, which is sequence of chicken pox (shingles). If unsure, identify the first and last option to narrow the middle options. Consider the development of the clear to cloudy vesicles before being scabbed. Review the pathophysiology of varicella, and characteristics of lesions if you had difficulty answering this question.

Client needs category: Physiological integrity

Client needs subcategory: Basic care and comfort

Cognitive level: Analyzing

6. The school nurse is assessing the chest of a first-grade child and notes a pectus excavatum. Which graphic depicts this abnormality?

☐ **1.**

☐ **2.**

☐ **3.**

☐ **4.**

Answer: 3

Rationale: Pectus excavatum is an indentation of the lower portion of the sternum (option 3). Option 1 shows a normal chest contour. Option 2 shows a barrel chest contour. Option 4 shows a thoracic scoliosis chest contour.

Test-taking strategy: Analyze to determine what information the question asks for, which is the graphic which denotes a pectus excavatum. Use knowledge of medical terminology (pectus = chest, excavatum = hollow) to determine the type of abnormality and then compare with illustration. Review disorders of the thoracic region if you had difficulty answering this question.

Client needs category: Physiological integrity

Client needs subcategory: Reduction of risk potential

Cognitive level: Applying

---

7. A 10-year-old child visits the pediatrician's office for an annual sports examination. When a nurse asks how he is doing, he becomes quiet and states that his grandmother died last week. Which statements by the child show that he understands the concept of death? Select all that apply.

☐ **1.** "Death is final."
☐ **2.** "All people must die."
☐ **3.** "My grandmother's death has been hard to understand."
☐ **4.** "My grandmother died because she was sick and nothing could make her better."
☐ **5.** "My grandmother is dead, but she'll come back."
☐ **6.** "My grandmother died because someone in the family did something bad."

Answer: 1, 3, 4

Rationale: By age 10, most children know that death is irreversible and final. However, a child may still have difficulty understanding the death of a specific loved one or understanding that children can die. School-age children should be able to identify cause-and-effect relationships, such as when a terminal illness causes someone to die. Adolescents, not school-age children, understand that death is a universal process. Preschoolers see death as temporary and may think of it as a punishment.

Test-taking strategy: Analyze to determine what information the question asks for, which is a 10-year-old's concept of death. "Select all that apply" questions require considering each option to decide its merit. Recall the cognitive stages of development for a school-age child as having a more realistic understanding of death. They may be curious about the physical process of death and what happens after a person dies. Review children's concept of death at various ages if you had difficulty answering this question.

Client needs category: Psychosocial integrity

Client needs subcategory: None

Cognitive level: Analyzing

8. The pediatric cardiac nurse is assessing the heart sounds of a 3-year-old child with a mitral valve regurgitation. Which graphic shows the area where the nurse would assess the site of the insufficiency?

☐ **1.**

☐ **2.**

☐ **3.**

☐ **4.**

Answer: 1

Rationale: Mitral valve regurgitation or insufficiency is a heart disorder where the mitral valve does not close properly when the heart pumps out blood; thus, causing an abnormal leaking of blood from the left ventricle through the mitral valve and into the left atrium. The mitral valve is heard best at the fourth left intercostal space at the nipple line (option 1). The aortic valve is heard best at the second intercostal space to the right of the sternum (option 2). The pulmonic valve is heard best at the second intercostal space to the left of the sternum (option 3). The tricuspid valve is heard best in the fourth intercostal space to the right of the sternum (option 4).

Test-taking strategy: Analyze to determine what information the question asks for, which is the location of the mitral valve. Recall that the mitral valve is like a one-way gate helping blood flow in one direction through the heart. Recall that the mitral valve is on the left side of the heart and lets blood flow from the upper to the lower chambers. Review where each heart valve is located if you had difficulty answering this question.

Client needs category: Physiological integrity

Client needs subcategory: Reduction of risk potential

Cognitive level: Analyzing

9. An 11-year-old girl comes into the physician's office complaining of dysuria. The nurse suspects a urinary tract infection. Which findings on the laboratory report is consistent with a urinary tract infection?

Laboratory Results	
Test: Urinalysis **Date:** 07/16/10	**Time collected:** 0700
Parameter	*Results*
Color	Pale yellow
Turbidity	Clear
pH	7.8
Specific gravity	1.015
Protein	Negative
Glucose	Positive
Ketones	Positive
Red blood cells	<1 per high-power field
White blood cells	20 per high-power field
Casts	None

☐ **1.** WBCs: 20 per high-power field.
☐ **2.** pH 7.8.
☐ **3.** Ketones: positive.
☐ **4.** Glucose: positive.

Answer: 1

Rationale: Urinary tract infections are more common in school-aged girls than in school-aged boys. A normal urinalysis would show less than 5 WBCs per high-power field. An elevated WBC count of 20 is an indication of bacteria and urinary tract infection. The normal range of urinary pH is 4.6 to 8.0. The presence of glucose or ketones in the urine does not indicate a urinary tract infection, but may indicate diabetes mellitus.

Test-taking strategy: Analyze to determine what information the question asks for, which is laboratory evidence of a urinary tract infection. Discriminate through the lab report for abnormal results, then identify if that result would indicate a urinary tract infection. Review the normal and abnormal findings for a urinalysis if you had difficulty answering this question.

Client needs category: Physiological integrity

Client needs subcategory: Reduction of risk potential

Cognitive level: Analyzing

---

10. A 10-year-old child has been admitted to the hospital with Reye's syndrome. Place the following findings in chronological order to show the clinical stages of Reye's syndrome. Use all of the options.

1. Flaccid paralysis.
2. Coma.
3. Vomiting.
4. Presence of a viral infection.
5. Deepened coma.
6. Disorientation.

Answer: 4, 3, 6, 2, 5, 1

Rationale: Reye's syndrome is an acute multisystem disorder that causes encephalopathy and predominately affects school-age children. Symptoms develop within a few days to weeks after a viral infection, beginning with vomiting, sleepiness, and liver dysfunction. About 24 to 48 hours after onset of symptoms, the child's condition rapidly deteriorates, causing disorientation, hallucinations, and sometimes a coma with decorticate posturing. The coma may progress to a deepened coma with decerebrate posturing and, eventually, flaccid paralysis. The majority of children who survive the acute stage of illness completely recover.

Test-taking strategy: Analyze to determine what information the question asks for, which is progression of Reye's syndrome symptoms. Recall that symptoms begin quickly after a viral infection and quickly deteriorate with significant neurological findings. If unsure, select the most generalized symptom first and end with the most severe symptoms of neurological compromise. Review the clinical findings and deteriorating stages of Reye's syndrome if you had difficulty answering this question.

Client needs category: Physiological integrity

Client needs subcategory: Reduction of risk potential

Cognitive level: Analyzing

1. A nurse is caring for an adolescent who was admitted to the hospital's medical unit after attempting suicide by ingesting acetaminophen (Tylenol). Which interventions should the nurse incorporate into the client's care plan? Select all that apply.

☐ **1.** Limit care until the client initiates a conversation.

☐ **2.** Ask the client's parents if they keep firearms in their home.

☐ **3.** Ask the client if he/she is currently having suicidal thoughts.

☐ **4.** Assist the client with bathing and grooming as needed.

☐ **5.** Inspect the client's mouth after giving oral medications.

☐ **6.** Assure the client that anything said will be held in strict confidence.

Answer: 2, 3, 4, 5

Rationale: Safety is the primary consideration when caring for suicidal clients. Because firearms are the most common method used in suicides, the client's parents should be taught to lock firearms and ammunition in separate locations and not give the client access to the keys. Safety also includes assessing for current suicidal ideation. Many suicidal people are depressed and do not have the energy to care for themselves, so the client may need assistance with bathing and grooming. Because depressed and suicidal clients may hide pills in their cheeks, the nurse should inspect the client's mouth after giving oral medications. Rather than limit care, the nurse should try to establish a trusting relationship through nursing interventions and therapeutic communication. The client cannot be guaranteed confidentiality when self-destructive behavior is an issue.

Test-taking strategy: Analyze to determine what information the question asks for, which is nursing interventions for a client who attempted suicide. "Select all that apply" questions require considering each option to decide its merit. Consider the nursing care of the suicidal adolescent with emphasis that safety is the priority. Review care of the client who attempted suicide if you had difficulty answering this question.

Client needs category: Physiological integrity

Client needs subcategory: Reduction of risk potential

Cognitive level: Applying

2. A nurse is teaching a 16-year-old female client with inflammatory bowel disease about corticosteroid treatment. Which adverse effects are likely to be concerns for this client? Select all that apply.

☐ **1.** Acne.
☐ **2.** Hirsutism.
☐ **3.** Mood swings.
☐ **4.** Osteoporosis.
☐ **5.** Growth spurts.
☐ **6.** Adrenal suppression.

Answer: 1, 2, 3, 4, 6

Rationale: Adverse effects of corticosteroids include acne, hirsutism, mood swings, osteoporosis, and adrenal suppression. Steroid use in children and adolescents may cause delayed growth, not growth spurts.

Test-taking strategy: Analyze to determine what information the question asks for, which is adolescent concerns about corticosteroid use. "Select all that apply" questions require considering each option to decide its merit. Consider side effects of the corticosteroid use which may impact typical growth and development issues in adolescents. Since adolescents place great influence on relationships with peers, appearance and mood swings are of particular concern. Review the pharmacology of corticosteroids and how the adverse effects of corticosteroids relate to adolescents if you had difficulty answering this question.

Client needs category: Physiological integrity

Client needs subcategory: Pharmacological therapies

Cognitive level: Applying

3. A nurse is caring for a 17-year-old female client with cystic fibrosis who has been admitted to the hospital for administration of I.V. antibiotics and respiratory treatment for exacerbation of a lung infection. The client states, "I have a number of questions about my future and the consequences of this disease." Which statements about the course of cystic fibrosis are true? Select all that apply.

☐ **1.** Breast development is commonly delayed.
☐ **2.** The client is at risk for developing diabetes.
☐ **3.** Pregnancy and childbearing are not affected.
☐ **4.** Normal sexual relationships can be expected.
☐ **5.** Only males carry the gene for the disease.
☐ **6.** By age 20, the client is able to decrease the frequency of respiratory treatments.

Answer: 1, 2, 4

Rationale: Cystic fibrosis delays growth and the onset of puberty. Children with cystic fibrosis tend to be smaller than the average size and develop secondary sex characteristics later in life. In addition, they are at risk for developing diabetes mellitus because the pancreatic duct becomes obstructed as pancreatic tissues are destroyed. Clients with cystic fibrosis can expect to have normal sexual relationships, but thick secretions that obstruct the cervix and block sperm entry may impair fertility. Males and females carry the gene for cystic fibrosis. Pulmonary disease commonly progresses as the client ages, requiring additional respiratory treatment, not less.

Test-taking strategy: Analyze to determine what information the question asks for, which is providing accurate information about the disease process as it relates to a young adult. "Select all that apply" questions require considering each option to decide its merit. Consider that cystic fibrosis has metabolic consequences that impact every stage of development due to the metabolic effects on body systems. Review the pathophysiology of cystic fibrosis and its effects on sexual development and reproduction if you had difficulty answering the question.

Client needs category: Physiological integrity
Client needs subcategory: Physiological adaptation
Cognitive level: Analyzing

4. The nurse is caring for a diabetic adolescent who admits to consuming many simple sugars and carbohydrates at a graduation party. The parents brought the client to the emergency room with unusual behavior. The serum glucose level was 375 mg/dL.

The physician provided a coverage schedule:

150 to 200 mg/dL—2 units of Humulin R.

201 to 250 mg/dL—4 units of Humulin R.

251 to 300 mg/dL—6 units of Humulin R.

301 to 350 mg/dL—8 units of Humulin R.

351 to 399 mg/dL—10 units of Humulin R.

Over 400 mg/dL—call the physician.

Indicate with and draw a line on the low-dose insulin syringe, which amount of insulin should be drawn into the syringe.

Answer:

Rationale: The adolescent's blood sugar is 375 mg/dL, thus falling within the 10 unit range (351 to 399 mg/dL). The nurse would drawn up 10 units of Humulin R to administer as per physician's orders.

Test-taking strategy: The key words are "blood sugar of 375." The nurse must obtain the blood sugar and then compare with the sliding schedule to determine the correct amount of coverage. Recall that the low-dose syringe uses 1 unit increments to document amounts. Review types of insulin syringes and the use of insulin sliding scales if you had difficulty answering this question.

Client needs category: Physiological integrity

Client needs subcategory: Pharmacological therapies

Cognitive level: Applying

5. A nurse is caring for a 14-year-old boy who arrives in the physician's office complaining of abdominal pain with nausea and vomiting for the past 24 hours. The mother reports the client experiencing sharp pain when hitting a pothole along the road. The vital signs are: temperature, 101.6°F; pulse, 92 beats/minute; respirations, 24 breaths/minute; blood pressure, 142/82 mm Hg. As the nurse is collecting all data, in which location of the abdomen will the nurse obtain definitive assessment data?

Answer:

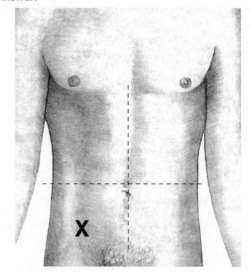

Rationale: The X is placed in the right lower quadrant. All of the data provided (abdominal pain, nausea with vomiting, elevated temperature, and rebound tenderness when hitting a pothole) indicate a potential appendicitis. Appendicitis typically begins with anorexia, nausea, and vomiting for the first 12 to 24 hours. Abdominal pain, a late sign, is usually diffuse at first and gradually localizes to the right lower quadrant. The sharpest pain should be noted at McBurney's point, which is one-third of the way between the anterior and superior iliac crest and the umbilicus.

Test-taking strategy: Analyze to determine what information the question asks for, which is site for abdominal assessment of a potential appendicitis. Use the data listed to focus on an abdominal disease process. Once appendicitis is selected, recall the classic assessment point (McBurney's point) and assessment finding (rebound tenderness) in the right lower quadrant. Review the anatomy of the gastrointestinal system and the organs within each of the abdominal quadrants if you had difficulty answering this question.

Client needs category: Physiological integrity

Client needs subcategory: Reduction of risk potential

Cognitive level: Analysis

6. A 17-year-old client visits the family planning clinic to discuss with a nurse regarding safe sex practices. In instructing the client on how to correctly use a condom, which information should be stressed? Select all that apply.

☐ **1.** The condom only needs to be placed on the penis immediately before ejaculation.

☐ **2.** Condoms should be stored in a cool, dry place to prevent damage.

☐ **3.** A condom should be applied to the penis before it becomes fully erect.

☐ **4.** Leave a ½ inch space at the end of the condom.

☐ **5.** Never reuse a condom.

☐ **6.** The condom should be applied on an erect penis.

Answer: 2, 4, 5, 6

Rationale: At a family planning center, condoms can be a reliable method of birth control offered with proper instruction. Condoms should be stored in a cool, dry place to prevent heat damage. A ½ inch space should be left at the tip of the condom to allow for collection of the ejaculate and to prevent tearing of the condom. A condom is applied after the penis is erect. A condom should not be reused.

Test-taking strategy: Analyze to determine what information the question asks for, which is instruction for proper use of a condom. "Select all that apply" questions require considering each option to decide its merit. Recall that maintaining the integrity of the condom is key in proper use and to prevent pregnancy and sexually transmitted diseases. Review the proper use of condoms if you had difficulty answering this question.

Client needs category: Health promotion and maintenance

Client needs subcategory: None

Cognitive level: Applying

7. The nurse is examining an adolescent boy. The nurse classifies his sexual maturity as Tanner stage 3. Which graphic depicts this stage?

☐ **1.**

☐ **2.**

☐ **3.**

☐ **4.**

Answer: 2

Rationale: Because the onset and progression of puberty is variable, the Tanner stage is a widely acceptable scale to describe progression. In Tanner stage 3, pubic hair extends across the pubis. Testes and scrotum begin to enlarge more, and the penis increases in length. Option 1 shows Tanner stage 2, option 3 shows Tanner stage 4, and option 4 shows Tanner stage 5. Tanner also has a scale for females.

Test-taking strategy: Analyze to determine what information the question asks for, which is proper classification of sexual development using Tanner stages. Recall that Tanner stage 1 begins in the preadolescent period and Tanner stage 5 progresses to the adult. Tanner stage 3 is in the middle, where hair is located across the pubis. Review secondary sex changes in male adolescents (genital and pubic hair development) and the Tanner stages 1 to 5 if you had difficulty answering this question.

Client needs category: Physiological integrity

Client needs subcategory: Reduction of risk potential

Cognitive level: Applying

PART SIX

Psychiatric and Mental Health Nursing

1. A hospitalized client becomes angry and belligerent toward a nurse after speaking on the phone with his mother. The nurse learns that the mother cannot visit as expected. Which interventions might the nurse use to help the client deal with the displaced anger? Select all that apply.

- ☐ **1.** Explore the client's unmet needs.
- ☐ **2.** Avoid the client until he apologizes.
- ☐ **3.** Suggest that the client direct the anger at his mother.
- ☐ **4.** Invite the client to a quiet place to talk.
- ☐ **5.** Assist the client in identifying alternate ways of approaching the problem.

Answer: 1, 4, 5

Rationale: Feelings of displacement or directing his anger toward the nurse need to be identified and understood by the client before the nurse can help guide him to choose appropriate actions. Avoiding the client or having him direct anger at another person is inappropriate. Approaching the client in a calm manner and offering to assist in the problem-solving process allows the client to identify needs that are not being met and explore constructive ways of dealing with his anger.

Test-taking strategy: Analyze to determine what information the question asks for, which is nursing interventions to deal with displaced anger. "Select all that apply" questions require considering each option to decide its merit. Recall therapeutic behaviors to have the client explore his feelings and be able to verbalize thoughts. This strategy is helpful in clarifying thoughts and defusing anger. Focus on the optimal therapeutic approach and effective anger management techniques if you had difficulty answering this question.

Client needs category: Psychosocial integrity

Client needs subcategory: None

Cognitive level: Applying

---

2. The nurse is caring for a client with severe depression. In which conditions would the nurse support the use of electroconvulsive therapy (ECT)? Select all that apply.

- ☐ **1.** The client also has dementia.
- ☐ **2.** The client cannot tolerate tricyclic antidepressants.
- ☐ **3.** The client lives in a long-term care facility.
- ☐ **4.** The client is undergoing a stressful life change.
- ☐ **5.** The client is having acute suicidal thoughts.

Answer: 2, 5

Rationale: ECT is used to treat acute depressive illnesses in an attempt to rapidly reverse a life-threatening situation, such as disturbing delusions, agitation, and attempted suicide. It is also used when the client cannot tolerate tricyclic antidepressants, since other medication regimens for depression can take weeks to become effective. ECT is usually not indicated for situational depression caused by intense stress. Clients with dementia are not given ECT because ECT may further exacerbate cognitive impairment. The decision to use ECT is not based on where the client lives.

Test-taking strategy: Analyze to determine what information the question asks for, which is when to support the use of ECT. "Select all that apply" questions require considering each option to decide its merit. Recall that the use of ECT is supported when the client is experiencing severe mental health problems or tradition therapy is ineffective. Using that rationale leads to the correct answers. Recall the major symptoms of depression and treatment options for depression if you had difficulty answering this question.

Client needs category: Psychosocial integrity

Client needs subcategory: None

Cognitive level: Applying

---

3. A nurse is working in the emergency room when a police officer walks in with a rape victim to be examined. To decrease client anxiety, which interventions would be appropriate? Select all that apply.

☐ **1.** Admit the client to the treatment area right away.

☐ **2.** Encourage the client to undergo an examination immediately in order to get it behind her.

☐ **3.** Assure the client that she is safe in the examination room.

☐ **4.** Touch the client early on so that she knows the nurse is supportive.

☐ **5.** Allow a third party to be present if the client requests it.

☐ **6.** Ask "what" questions to determine the type of assault.

Answer: 1, 3, 5, 6

Rationale: Immediately admitting a rape victim to the treatment area may help her feel cared for and safe. Allowing a third party to remain with her, if requested, also increases her feeling of safety. "What" questions help to clarify events in a nonjudgmental way. At a time of great distress, the nurse should pace the interview and examination according to the client's level of comfort. Touching a client who has recently been assaulted may increase her anxiety. The nurse should wait for the client to initiate contact or ask permission prior to initiating physical contact.

Test-taking strategy: Analyze to determine what information the question asks for, which is interventions to decrease a rape victim's anxiety. "Select all that apply" questions require considering each option to decide its merit. Consider that victims of violent crimes often feel violated and build trust slowly. Offering of oneself in a nonjudgmental way reduces anxiety. Review the client's physical and emotional needs after experiencing rape if you had difficulty answering this question.

Client needs category: Psychosocial integrity

Client needs subcategory: None

Cognitive level: Applying

4. A nurse is engaging in a therapeutic relationship with a client. Which nursing actions are appropriate with this type of relationship? Select all that apply.

☐ **1.** Identify and meet the needs and specific desires of the client.
☐ **2.** Help the client explore different problem-solving techniques.
☐ **3.** Encourage the practice of new coping skills.
☐ **4.** Give advice to the client.
☐ **5.** Exchange personal information with the client.
☐ **6.** Discuss the client's feelings with family members.

Answer: 2, 3

Rationale: The goal of a therapeutic relationship is to enhance the personal growth of the client. This is achieved by helping clients explore problem-solving techniques and develop coping skills. Giving advice, exchanging personal information, and striving to meet the personal needs and special desires of the client are characteristic of social relationships. Discussing the client's feelings with family members is a breach of confidentiality, unless previously approved by the client.

Test-taking strategy: Analyze to determine what information the question asks for, which is actions within a therapeutic relationship. "Select all that apply" questions require considering each option to decide its merit. The key words are "therapeutic relationship," meaning that it benefits the client in some way to meet specific goals. Review how the nurse assists the client to meet basic needs and review therapeutic communication if you had difficulty answering this question.

Client needs category: Psychosocial integrity
Client needs subcategory: None
Cognitive level: Applying

---

5. A nurse is explaining the Bill of Rights for psychiatric patients to a client who has voluntarily sought admission to an inpatient psychiatric facility. Which rights should the nurse include in the discussion? Select all that apply.

☐ **1.** Right to select health care team members.
☐ **2.** Right to refuse treatment.
☐ **3.** Right to a written treatment plan.
☐ **4.** Right to obtain disability benefits.
☐ **5.** Right to confidentiality.
☐ **6.** Right to personal mail.

Answer: 2, 3, 5, 6

Rationale: An inpatient client usually receives a copy of the Bill of Rights for psychiatric patients, which includes the right to refuse treatment, to have a written treatment plan, to have all medical information kept confidential, and to receive mail. A client in an inpatient setting does not have the right to select health care team members. Although the client may apply for disability benefits as a result of a chronic or incapacitating illness, obtaining disability compensation is not a patient right and members of a psychiatric institution do not decide who should receive it.

Test-taking strategy: Analyze to determine what information the question asks for, which is components within the Patient Bill of Rights for psychiatric patients. "Select all that apply" questions require considering each option to decide its merit. Recall that the Bill of Rights provides guarantees of essential rights such as the right to information, autonomy, and fair treatment. Review the rights of clients in hospitalized settings and the responsibilities of health care providers if you had difficulty answering this question.

Client needs category: Psychosocial integrity
Client needs subcategory: None
Cognitive level: Applying

6. In the emergency department, a client reveals to the nurse a lethal plan for committing suicide and agrees to a voluntary admission to the psychiatric unit. Which information should the nurse discuss with the client to answer the question "How long do I have to stay here?" Select all that apply.

☐ **1.** "You may leave the hospital at any time unless you're suicidal or homicidal or unable to meet your basic needs."
☐ **2.** "Let's talk more after the health care team has assessed you."
☐ **3.** "Once you've signed the papers, you have no say."
☐ **4.** "Because you could hurt yourself, you must be safe before being discharged."
☐ **5.** "You need a lawyer to help you make that decision."
☐ **6.** "There must be a court hearing before you can leave the hospital."

Answer: 1, 2, 4

Rationale: A person who is admitted to a psychiatric hospital may voluntarily sign out of the hospital unless the health care team determines that the person is harmful to himself or others. The health care team evaluates the client's condition before discharge. If there is reason to believe that the client may be harmful to himself or others, a hearing can be held to determine if the admission status should be changed from voluntary to involuntary. The client still has rights after committing himself to a psychiatric unit. The client does not need a lawyer to leave the hospital. A court hearing is held only if the client may pose a threat to himself or others and requires further treatment.

Test-taking strategy: Analyze to determine what information the question asks for, which is answering a client's question of "how long do I have to stay here?" "Select all that apply" questions require considering each option to decide its merit. Recall guidelines for voluntary commitment and subsequent release. Consider safety issues, especially in light of suicide concerns. Review factors that determine length of stay and patient rights if you had difficulty answering this question.

Client needs category: Psychosocial integrity
Client needs subcategory: None
Cognitive level: Applying

---

7. A nurse has developed a relationship with a client who has an addiction problem. Which actions would indicate that the therapeutic interaction is in the working phase? Select all that apply.

☐ **1.** The client discusses how the addiction has contributed to family distress.
☐ **2.** The client reluctantly shares the family history of addiction.
☐ **3.** The client verbalizes difficulty identifying personal strengths.
☐ **4.** The client discusses the financial problems related to the addiction.
☐ **5.** The client expresses uncertainty about what topic to discuss.
☐ **6.** The client acknowledges the addiction's effects on his children.

Answer: 1, 3, 4, 6

Rationale: Acknowledging the addiction's effects on the family and discussing its financial impact will help the client to identify personal strengths in dealing with addiction and strengthen the therapeutic relationship in the process. Discussing the family history of addiction and expressing uncertainty about what topics to address with the nurse typically happen during the introductory phase of a nurse–client relationship.

Test-taking strategy: Analyze to determine what information the question asks for, which is analyzing for a therapeutic interaction. "Select all that apply" questions require considering each option to decide its merit. Note the client statements that suggest open communication with the nurse. Also, analyze each option for characteristics that the client is open to working on goals and displaying personal introspection. Review the dynamics occurring in the working phase of a therapeutic relationship if you had difficulty answering this question.

Client needs category: Psychosocial integrity
Client needs subcategory: None
Cognitive level: Evaluating

8. A nurse is caring for a client who has exhibited testing behaviors. When discussing this behavior at a multidisciplinary team conference, which behaviors would the nurse provide as examples of this behavior? Select all that apply.

☐ **1.** Placing the nurse in the role of parent.
☐ **2.** Dressing in a flamboyant or seductive manner.
☐ **3.** Requesting personal information from the nurse.
☐ **4.** Following the contract established between the nurse and client.
☐ **5.** Stating information to try to shock the nurse.
☐ **6.** Violating the nurse's personal space.

Answer: 1, 3, 5, 6

Rationale: A client will test the nurse–client relationship by acting in ways to control the relationship or to elicit an emotional response from the nurse. Examples of the testing behavior include speaking about things that will shock the nurse, violating personal space, requesting personal information, and placing the nurse in the role of parent. Dressing in a flamboyant or seductive manner demonstrates a lack of rules or expected behaviors; this is a violation of boundary setting. A contract is used to develop or negotiate an agreement between the nurse and the client to achieve a mutual goal.

Test-taking strategy: Analyze to determine what information the question asks for, which is examples of client testing behaviors. "Select all that apply" questions require considering each option to decide its merit. Recall that client testing behaviors test a nurse's response/behavior and deal with controlling the situation by catching the nurse off guard or creating an uncomfortable situation. Review what behaviors test the nurse's professional demeanor if you had difficulty answering this question.

Client needs category: Psychosocial integrity
Client needs subcategory: None
Cognitive level: Analyzing

Anxiety Disorders

1. A nurse is caring for a client with agoraphobia. Which signs and symptoms would the nurse anticipate? Select all that apply.

☐ **1.** Hallucinations.
☐ **2.** Panic attacks.
☐ **3.** Inability to leave home.
☐ **4.** Eating disorders.
☐ **5.** Alcohol consumption.
☐ **6.** Tobacco use.

Answer: 2, 3

Rationale: Agoraphobia is characterized by extreme anxiety and a fear of being in open places. Panic attacks and an inability to leave home are symptoms associated with the disorder. No correlation exists between fear of open spaces and hallucinations, eating disorders, alcohol consumption, or tobacco use.

Test-taking strategy: Analyze to determine what information the question asks for, which is signs and symptoms anticipated with the diagnosis of agoraphobia. "Select all that apply" questions require considering each option to decide its merit. Use your knowledge of medical terminology to recall the definition of agoraphobia (agora = gathering place; phobia = fear of). Once understood, analyze the options for related symptoms. Review conditions that commonly occur with phobias or unrealistic fears if you had difficulty answering this question.

Client needs category: Psychosocial integrity
Client needs subcategory: None
Cognitive level: Applying

2. A client is being seen in the clinic after returning from military service abroad. The nurse documents restlessness at night with nightmares leaving the veteran irritable and fatigued during the day. When discussing the possibility of posttraumatic stress disorder (PTSD), which statements about PTSD are accurate? Select all that apply.

☐ **1.** PTSD is a syndrome that affects only those who have experienced traumatic episodes during war.
☐ **2.** PTSD is characterized by nightmares and flashbacks.
☐ **3.** Hypervigilance is characteristic of clients with PTSD.
☐ **4.** Substance abuse is a common coping mechanism used by clients with PTSD.
☐ **5.** Psychotic episodes can occur in clients with PTSD.
☐ **6.** Clients with PTSD may complain of feeling empty inside.

Answer: 2, 3, 4, 5, 6

Rationale: PTSD is a serious condition that develops after a person has witnessed a traumatic or terrifying event in which serious physical harm has occurred or is threatened. Although PTSD is commonly associated with combat, it can manifest itself after any kind of trauma. If symptoms occur within 6 months of the traumatic event, the disorder is considered acute. If symptoms occur more than 6 months after the traumatic event, PTSD is considered delayed or chronic. PTSD is characterized by nightmares or flashbacks. Clients are hypervigilant but typically describe themselves as "empty inside." Sometimes, the events can present as a psychotic episode. Substance abuse is a common "symptom" used for coping.

Test-taking strategy: Analyze to determine what information the question asks for, which is accurate statements of PTSD. "Select all that apply" questions require considering each option to decide its merit. If unsure, consider the full name of PTSD and relate symptoms stemming from a trauma or stress. Review the defining characteristics and clinical manifestations of PTSD if you had difficulty answering this question.

Client needs category: Psychosocial integrity
Client needs subcategory: None
Cognitive level: Analyzing

3. An 8-year-old child, diagnosed with obsessive-compulsive disorder, is admitted by the nurse to a psychiatric facility. During the admission assessment, which behaviors would be characterized as compulsions? Select all that apply.

☐ **1.** Checking and rechecking that the television is turned off before going to school.
☐ **2.** Repeatedly washing the hands.
☐ **3.** Brushing teeth three times per day.
☐ **4.** Routinely climbing up and down a flight of stairs three times before leaving the house.
☐ **5.** Feeding the dog the same meal every day.
☐ **6.** Wanting to play the same video game each night.

Answer: 1, 2, 4

Rationale: Compulsions involve symbolic rituals that relieve anxiety when they are performed. The disorder is caused by anxiety from obsessive thoughts, and acts are seen as irrational. Examples include repeatedly checking the television set, washing hands, or climbing stairs. An activity such as playing the same video game each night may be indicative of normal development for a school-age child. Frequent brushing of the teeth and feeding the dog a consistent meal are not abnormal.

Test-taking strategy: Analyze to determine what information the question asks for, which is behaviors that indicate a compulsion. "Select all that apply" questions require considering each option to decide its merit. Analyze each option for behaviors that are considered irrational in nature and, many times, repetitive. Review the symptoms of compulsive behavior if you had difficulty answering this question.

Client needs category: Psychosocial integrity
Client needs subcategory: None
Cognitive level: Analyzing

4. A nurse selects a priority nursing diagnosis of *fear related to being embarrassed in the presence of others* for a client who exhibits symptoms of social phobia. Which outcomes, if met, would demonstrate improvement in client's symptoms? Select all that apply.

- ☐ **1.** The client manages fear in group situations.
- ☐ **2.** The client develops a plan to avoid situations that may cause stress.
- ☐ **3.** The client verbalizes feelings that occur in stressful situations.
- ☐ **4.** The client develops a plan for responding to stressful situations.
- ☐ **5.** The client denies feelings that may contribute to irrational fears.
- ☐ **6.** The client uses suppression to deal with underlying fears.

Answer: 1, 3, 4

Rationale: When selecting an outcome for a nursing diagnosis, choose a statement that would demonstrate the progressing toward or achievement of the short-term or long-term goal. Improving stress management skills, verbalizing feelings, and anticipating and planning for stressful situations are adaptive responses to stress. Avoidance, denial, and suppression are maladaptive defense mechanisms.

Test-taking strategy: Analyze to determine what information the question asks for, which is outcomes that demonstrate improvement in social phobia symptoms. "Select all that apply" questions require considering each option to decide its merit. Analyze each option for evidence of positive progress in handling and coping with social phobia. Review client outcomes related to acceptable behaviors in social situations if you had difficulty answering this question.

Client needs category: Psychosocial integrity

Client needs subcategory: None

Cognitive level: Evaluating

---

5. A nurse recognizes improvement in a client with the nursing diagnosis of *ineffective role performance related to the need to perform rituals.* Which behaviors indicate improvement? Select all that apply.

- ☐ **1.** The client refrains from performing rituals during stress.
- ☐ **2.** The client verbalizes using "thought stopping" when obsessive thoughts occur.
- ☐ **3.** The client verbalizes the relationship between stress and ritualistic behaviors.
- ☐ **4.** The client avoids stressful situations.
- ☐ **5.** The client rationalizes ritualistic behavior.
- ☐ **6.** The client performs ritualistic behaviors in private.

Answer: 1, 2, 3

Rationale: Refraining from performing rituals demonstrates that the client manages stress appropriately. Using "thought stopping" demonstrates the client's ability to employ appropriate interventions for obsessive thoughts. Verbalizing the relationship between stress and behaviors indicates that the client understands the disease process. Avoiding stressful situations and rationalizing or hiding ritualistic behaviors are maladaptive methods of managing stress and anxiety.

Test-taking strategy: Analyze to determine what information the question asks for, which is behaviors that demonstrate improvement in the nursing diagnosis of ineffective role performance in relation to ritualistic behavior. "Select all that apply" questions require considering each option to decide its merit. Look for data in the option related to or characteristic of less ritualistic behavior. Review options that promote healthy behaviors if you had difficulty answering this question.

Client needs category: Psychosocial integrity

Client needs subcategory: None

Cognitive level: Evaluating

6. A nurse is caring for a client recently diagnosed with cancer and experiencing severe anxiety. Which interventions should the nurse include in the care plan? Select all that apply.

- ☐ **1.** Maintain a calm, nonthreatening environment.
- ☐ **2.** Explain relevant aspects of chemotherapy.
- ☐ **3.** Encourage the client to verbalize concerns regarding the diagnosis.
- ☐ **4.** Encourage the client to use deep-breathing exercises and other relaxation techniques during periods of increased stress.
- ☐ **5.** Provide distractions for the client during periods of stress.
- ☐ **6.** Teach the stages of grieving to the client.

Answer: 1, 3, 4

Rationale: During periods of acute stress, interventions that help the client regain control will help master this new threat. Providing a calm, nonthreatening environment and encouraging verbalization of concerns will help the client face the unknown. Relaxation techniques have a physiologic and psychological effect in calming the client, which in turn allows further exploration of thoughts and feelings as well as problem solving. The ability to learn is limited during extreme stress, so teaching the client about grief and chemotherapy would not be effective at this stage. Providing distractions would be ineffective at this point in the grief process.

Test-taking strategy: Analyze to determine what information the question asks for, which is nursing intervention for a client with extreme stress and anxiety. "Select all that apply" questions require considering each option to decide its merit. Consider anxiety-relieving measures that will assist the client in coping with the diagnosis and regaining control. Review interventions that relieve stress and promote relaxation if you had difficulty answering this question.

Client needs category: Psychosocial integrity

Client needs subcategory: None

Cognitive level: Applying

7. The nurse is teaching a client diagnosed with a generalized anxiety disorder how to effectively cope with severe distress. Which interventions would the nurse use to promote effective coping with anxiety? Select all that apply.

☐ **1.** Discuss previous methods that were effective in handling stress.

☐ **2.** Encourage the client to limit the time spent worrying to only 15 minutes per day.

☐ **3.** Help the client to establish a goal and develop a plan to meet the goal.

☐ **4.** Teach the client how to label feelings and how to express them.

☐ **5.** Examine ways to differentiate between realistic and unrealistic thoughts.

☐ **6.** Assist the client to acknowledge the major consequences of blaming others.

Answer: 1, 2, 3, 4

Rationale: To promote effective skills, the nurse should focus on having the client identify successful coping skills used in the past and on building on the client's knowledge of the disorder. Setting a limit on the amount of time spent worrying gives him boundaries and acknowledges his concerns. Establishing a goal and planning to meet the goal allows the client to engage in solving the problem and exercise control over the stressful situation. Labeling and expressing feelings is a healthy way to acknowledge feelings. Clients with schizophrenia, not generalized anxiety disorder, require help with focusing on reality-based behaviors. Clients who demonstrate oppositional behavior tend to blame others instead of taking responsibility for their inappropriate behavior.

Test-taking strategy: Analyze to determine what information the question asks for, which is interventions on how to cope with anxiety. "Select all that apply" questions require considering each option to decide its merit. Consider each option for anxiety-reducing strategies and coping skills. Review the defining characteristics and clinical manifestations of generalized anxiety disorder and related coping skills if you had difficulty answering this question.

Client needs category: Psychosocial integrity

Client needs subcategory: None

Cognitive level: Applying

Mood, Adjustment, and Dementia Disorders

1. A nurse is conducting a group session for children and adolescents who have been diagnosed with depression. Which behaviors would a nurse anticipate in this group? Select all that apply.

☐ **1.** Delusions.

☐ **2.** Anxiety.

☐ **3.** Sadness.

☐ **4.** Irritability.

☐ **5.** Somatic symptoms, such as headache and stomachache.

☐ **6.** Suicidal thoughts.

Answer: 2, 4, 5, 6

Rationale: Children and adolescents with depression commonly experience anxiety and irritability (rather than sadness) as well as somatic symptoms. Suicide is a serious risk in these age groups. These age groups seldom experience psychotic symptoms. If psychotic symptoms do occur, they are more likely to be auditory hallucinations, not delusions.

Test-taking strategy: Analyze to determine what information the question asks for, which is behaviors of children and adolescents diagnosed with depression. "Select all that apply" questions require considering each option to decide its merit. Consider maturity level, impulsivity, and fluctuating hormones in addition to depressive symptoms. Review the symptoms of children and adolescents with depression if you had difficulty answering this question.

Client needs category: Psychosocial integrity

Client needs subcategory: None

Cognitive level: Applying

2. A nurse is caring for a client diagnosed with dysthymia. Which defining characteristics are associated with this disorder? Select all that apply.

☐ **1.** Insomnia or hypersomnia.
☐ **2.** Delusions or hallucinations.
☐ **3.** Suicidal thoughts.
☐ **4.** Onset of symptoms within a 2-week period.
☐ **5.** Symptoms that occur in the winter and resolve in spring.
☐ **6.** Appetite disturbance.

Answer: 1, 3, 6

Rationale: Dysthymia is a mild, but chronic, form of depression. Sleep and appetite disturbances and suicidal thoughts can appear in clients with dysthymia or major depressive disorders. Onset of symptoms are gradual and may appear over weeks or months. Delusions and other psychotic symptoms may occur in major depression but do not occur in dysthymia. Episodes of depression occurring solely in the winter are indicative of seasonal affective disorder.

Test-taking strategy: Analyze to determine what information the question asks for, which is characteristics of dysthymia. "Select all that apply" questions require considering each option to decide its merit. Recall that the key point of dysthymia is mild depression; thus, consider options of an altered mood. Review the defining characteristics of dysthymia if you had difficulty answering this question.

Client needs category: Psychosocial integrity

Client needs subcategory: None

Cognitive level: Applying

---

3. A nurse is developing a care plan for a client with acute mania. Place the following behaviors according to the order in which they progress in a client with acute mania. Use all of the options.

| **1.** Has delusions of grandeur. |
| **2.** Uses relevant, calm speech patterns. |
| **3.** Shows high productivity and competitive attitude in work and leisure activities. |
| **4.** Becomes easily irritated. |
| **5.** Demonstrates poor judgment and impulse control. |

Answer: 2, 3, 4, 5, 1

Rationale: Mania is an abnormally elated mental state, typically characterized by feelings of euphoria, lack of inhibition, racing thoughts, risk taking, and irritability. Relevant and calm speech patterns are indicative of normal behavior. An early sign of dysphoria at the beginning of a manic episode is the client's lack of sleep. Since sleep is not a priority, the client soon begins displaying a high level of productivity and competitiveness in work and leisure activities. As the mania increases, the client becomes more easily irritated and requires medication. The client demonstrates poor judgment and impulse control; therefore, client safety becomes a major concern. Lastly, the client becomes psychotic and has grandiose ideas that evolve into delusions of grandeur.

Test-taking strategy: Analyze to determine what information the question asks for, which is progression of symptoms in a client with acute mania. Note that as symptoms progress, they typically progress from minor symptoms to potentially dangerous or debilitating conditions. Review the progression of behaviors of mania from mild to major if you had difficulty answering this question.

Client needs category: Psychosocial integrity

Client needs subcategory: None

Cognitive level: Analyzing

4. A nurse is caring for a client displaying extreme mood swings with suicidal tendencies. A physician prescribes lithium (Eskalith) and diagnoses the client with bipolar disorder. When teaching the client, which statements, verbalized by the client, indicate a good understanding of the teaching session? Select all that apply.

☐ **1.** "I understand that there is a potential for addiction."

☐ **2.** "The signs and symptoms of drug toxicity include blurred vision and ringing in the ears."

☐ **3.** "There are no concerns with pregnancy and Lithium administration."

☐ **4.** "I will need to be on a low-tyramine diet."

☐ **5.** "I will need to consistently monitor blood levels."

☐ **6.** "There is an amount of time needed for mood changes to occur."

Answer: 2, 5, 6

Rationale: Client education should cover the signs and symptoms of drug toxicity, which include blurred vision and ringing in the ears. It is important to report toxicity to the physician immediately. There is also a need for regular monitoring of drug blood levels. Therapeutic blood levels are between 0.8 and 1.2 mEq/L. The nurse should also inform the client that mood changes may not be apparent for 7 to 21 days after treatment is initiated. Lithium does not have addictive properties and can be harmful to an unborn fetus. Birth control should be initiated for sexually active females. There is no need to be on a low-tyramine diet. Tyramine is a potential concern to clients who are also taking monoamine oxidase (MAO) inhibitors.

Test-taking strategy: Analyze to determine what information the question asks for, which is correct statements following a client teaching session. "Select all that apply" questions require considering each option to decide its merit. Recall that lithium is a potent medication with a narrowed therapeutic index. Review teaching considerations of lithium if you had difficulty answering this question.

Client needs category: Physiological integrity

Client needs subcategory: Pharmacological therapies

Cognitive level: Applying

---

5. After interviewing a client diagnosed with recurrent depression, a nurse determines the client's potential to commit suicide. Which factors listed below might contribute to the client's risk of suicide? Select all that apply.

☐ **1.** Psychomotor retardation.

☐ **2.** Impulsive behaviors.

☐ **3.** Overwhelming feelings of guilt.

☐ **4.** Chronic, debilitating illness.

☐ **5.** Decreased physical activity.

☐ **6.** Repression of anger.

Answer: 2, 3, 4, 6

Rationale: Recurrent depression represents a major consideration in suicide prevention due to its high prevalence. Impulsive behavior, overwhelming guilt, chronic illness, and repressed anger are factors that contribute to suicide potential. Psychomotor retardation and decreased physical activity are symptoms of depression, but these do not typically lead to suicide because the client does not have the energy and cognitive abilities to harm himself.

Test-taking strategy: Analyze to determine what information the question asks for, which is factors that contribute to client suicide. Consider that the nurse must be aware of the client's feelings, thoughts, and behaviors as they may indicate the likelihood of suicide. Review the risk factors for suicide if you had difficulty answering this question.

Client needs category: Psychosocial integrity

Client needs subcategory: None

Cognitive level: Analyzing

6. A nurse is assessing a client who talks freely about feeling depressed. During the interaction, the nurse hears the client state, "Things will never change." What other indications of hopelessness should the nurse look for? Select all that apply.

☐ **1.** Bouts of anger.
☐ **2.** Periods of irritability.
☐ **3.** Preoccupation with delusions.
☐ **4.** Feelings of worthlessness.
☐ **5.** Self-destructive behaviors.
☐ **6.** Auditory hallucinations.

Answer: 1, 2, 4, 5

Rationale: Clients who are depressed and feeling hopeless are often irritable and express inappropriate anger, feelings of worthlessness, and suicidal thoughts. In addition, they may demonstrate self-destructive behaviors. Preoccupation with delusions and auditory hallucinations is generally seen in clients with schizophrenia or other psychotic disorders rather than in those expressing hopelessness.

Test-taking strategy: Analyze to determine what information the question asks for, which is indications of hopelessness. "Select all that apply" questions require considering each option to decide its merit. Recall that many people consider suicide but most people decide to live as they realize that the crisis is temporary and death is permanent. Hopelessness, unfortunately, makes the client feel that their situation is permanent and they act out feeling angry, irritable, worthless, etc. Review behaviors associated with hopelessness and depression if you had difficulty answering this question.

Client needs category: Psychosocial integrity

Client needs subcategory: None

Cognitive level: Analyzing

7. A nurse interviews the family of a client hospitalized with severe depression and suicidal ideation. What family assessment information is essential to know when formulating an effective plan of care? Select all that apply.

☐ **1.** Physical pain.
☐ **2.** Personal responsibilities.
☐ **3.** Employment skills.
☐ **4.** Communication patterns.
☐ **5.** Role expectations.
☐ **6.** Current family stressors.

Answer: 4, 5, 6

Rationale: When working with the family of a depressed client, it is helpful for the nurse to be aware of the family's communication style, role expectations, and current family stressors. This information can help identify family difficulties and teaching points that could benefit the client and the family. Information concerning physical pain, personal responsibilities, and employment skills would not be helpful because these areas are not directly related to their experience of having a depressed family member.

Test-taking strategy: Analyze to determine what information the question asks for, which is family assessment information essential to planning care. "Select all that apply" questions require considering each option to decide its merit. The key words are "family assessment," meaning that it is information about family relations. It is important to answer the question that is asked. Review the family assessment, not assessment of the client if you had difficulty answering this question.

Client needs category: Psychosocial integrity

Client needs subcategory: None

Cognitive level: Analyzing

8. A client is prescribed sertraline (Zoloft), a selective serotonin reuptake inhibitor. Which adverse effects would the nurse review when creating a medication teaching plan? Select all that apply.

- ☐ **1.** Agitation.
- ☐ **2.** Agranulocytosis.
- ☐ **3.** Sleep disturbance.
- ☐ **4.** Intermittent tachycardia.
- ☐ **5.** Dry mouth.
- ☐ **6.** Seizures.

Answer: 1, 3, 5

Rationale: Sertraline (Zoloft) is used to treat depression, obsessive-compulsive disorder, and panic and anxiety disorders. Common adverse effects of sertraline are agitation, sleep disturbance, and dry mouth. Agranulocytosis, intermittent tachycardia, and seizures are adverse effects of clozapine (Clozaril).

Test-taking strategy: Analyze to determine what information the question asks for, which is the adverse effects of Zoloft. "Select all that apply" questions require considering each option to decide its merit. Recall that many select serotonin reuptake inhibitors affect the rapid eye movement sleep causing insomnia. Also, adverse effects may have an opposite effect than the therapeutic effect anticipated. Review the side effects of serotonin reuptake inhibitors if you had difficulty answering this question.

Client needs category: Physiological integrity

Client needs subcategory: Pharmacological therapies

Cognitive level: Applying

---

9. A nurse is assessing a client for dementia. What history findings would the nurse anticipate while talking with the client and family? Select all that apply.

- ☐ **1.** The progression of symptoms has been slow.
- ☐ **2.** The client admits to feelings of sadness.
- ☐ **3.** The client acts apathetic and pessimistic.
- ☐ **4.** The family cannot determine when the symptoms first appeared.
- ☐ **5.** The client has been exhibiting basic personality changes.
- ☐ **6.** The client has great difficulty paying attention to others.

Answer: 1, 4, 5, 6

Rationale: Dementia is the loss of brain function. It can affect memory, thinking, language, judgment, and behavior. Dementia is characterized by a slow onset of symptoms, which makes it difficult to determine when symptoms first occurred. It progresses to noticeable changes in the individual's personality and impaired ability to pay attention to other people. Sadness, apathy, and pessimism are symptoms of depression.

Test-taking strategy: Analyze to determine what information the question asks for, which is past history of symptoms of dementia. "Select all that apply" questions require considering each option to decide its merit. Recall clinical manifestations of dementia and relate to the options. Consider the insidious nature of the disease and the symptoms that appear over time. Review the signs and symptoms of dementia if you had difficulty answering this question.

Client needs category: Health promotion and maintenance

Client needs subcategory: None

Cognitive level: Analyzing

10. A client has been diagnosed with an adjustment disorder with mixed anxiety and depression. What are the primary nursing diagnoses the nurse would associate with this type of adjustment disorder? Select all that apply.

☐ **1.** Activity intolerance.
☐ **2.** Impaired social interaction.
☐ **3.** Risk for situational low self-esteem.
☐ **4.** Disturbed personal identity.
☐ **5.** Acute confusion.
☐ **6.** Impaired memory.

Answer: 2, 3

Rationale: Adjustment disorder occurs when an individual is unable to adjust or cope with a particular stressor such as a major life event. A client with an adjustment disorder is likely to exhibit *impaired social interaction* and *risk for situational low self-esteem.* Primary nursing diagnosis would not include the others as the client is able to participate in activities, if desired, and has no deficits in cognition or personal identity.

Test-taking strategy: Analyze to determine what information the question asks for, which is selecting primary nursing diagnoses for a client with adjustment disorder. "Select all that apply" questions require considering each option to decide its merit. The one key is understanding that adjustment disorder occurs from a major life event, not a disease process. Also, to select a "primary" nursing diagnosis, look to the cause and effect of the relationship of major events to psychosocial diagnoses. Review the defining characteristics of adjustment disorder, if you had difficulty answering this question.

Client needs category: Psychosocial integrity
Client needs subcategory: None
Cognitive level: Analyzing

11. A nurse is preparing discharge instructions for a client with resistant depression who was prescribed a new medication regimen that includes phenelzine (Nardil). If the teaching was successful, what foods should the client state that he/she needs to avoid? Select all that apply.

☐ **1.** Aged cheese.
☐ **2.** Cottage cheese.
☐ **3.** Milk.
☐ **4.** Wine.
☐ **5.** Salami.
☐ **6.** Fruit.

Answer: 1, 4, 5

Rationale: Phenelzine is an MAO inhibitor. MAO is an enzyme responsible for metabolizing neurotransmitters, serotonin and norepinephrine. This drug requires being on a tyramine-free diet to avoid hypertensive crisis. Aged cheese, salami, and wine will cause vasoconstriction and a rise in blood pressure. Cottage cheese, milk, and fruit are allowed on a tyramine-free diet.

Test-taking strategy: Analyze to determine what information the question asks for, which is food selections that a client should avoid when prescribed phenelzine. "Select all that apply" questions require considering each option to decide its merit. First, it is essential to identify that phenelzine is an MAO inhibitor. Once completed, select options that contain tyramine such as are noted above. Review the pharmacologic effects of MAO inhibitors if you had difficulty answering this question.

Client needs category: Physiological integrity
Client needs subcategory: Pharmacological therapies
Cognitive level: Applying

1. A nurse is assessing a new client and notices clang associations in the speech pattern. From this assessment finding, the nurse begins to evaluate for the potential of which psychiatric conditions? Select all that apply.

☐ **1.** Dissociative identity disorder.
☐ **2.** Schizophrenia.
☐ **3.** Narcolepsy.
☐ **4.** Mania.
☐ **5.** Organic disorders.
☐ **6.** Intermittent explosive disorder.

Answer: 2, 4, 5

Rationale: This speech pattern, characterized by meaningless rhymes, is found most commonly in clients with schizophrenia but may also be present in those with bipolar disorder (during the manic phase) and organic disorders. It is not characteristic of dissociative identity disorders, narcolepsy, or explosive disorders.

Test-taking strategy: Analyze to determine what information the question asks for, which is psychiatric conditions that contain clang associations. "Select all that apply" questions require considering each option to decide its merit. Recall that clang associations are a component of disorganized thinking and even psychosis. Choose options that are characterized by periods of disorganized thinking. Review clang associations related to disease processes if you had difficulty answering this question.

Client needs category: Psychosocial integrity

Client needs subcategory: None

Cognitive level: Analyzing

2. A nurse is monitoring a client who appears to be hallucinating. The client is gesturing at a figure on the television and appears agitated with speech containing paranoid content. Which nursing interventions are appropriate at this time? Select all that apply.

☐ **1.** In a firm voice, instruct the client to stop the behavior.
☐ **2.** Reassure the client that there is no danger.
☐ **3.** Acknowledge the presence of the hallucinations.
☐ **4.** Instruct other team members to ignore the client's behavior.
☐ **5.** Immediately implement physical restraints.
☐ **6.** Give simple commands in a calm voice.

Answer: 2, 3, 6

Rationale: Hallucinations are false or distorted sensory perceptions that appear to be real. Using a calm voice and giving simple commands, the nurse should reassure the client of safety. The nurse should not challenge the client; rather, acknowledge the hallucinatory experience. It is not appropriate to ask the client to stop the behavior. Ignoring behavior will not reduce the client's agitation. Implementing restraints is not warranted at this time. Although the client is agitated, he does not appear to be at risk for harm.

Test-taking strategy: Analyze to determine what information the question asks for, which is nursing interventions when a client is experiencing hallucinations. "Select all that apply" questions require considering each option to decide its merit. Recall that the nurse must facilitate conversation, validate that hallucinations are occurring, and calmly reassure. Review nursing interventions when a client is experiencing hallucinations if you had difficulty answering this question.

Client needs category: Psychosocial integrity

Client needs subcategory: None

Cognitive level: Applying

3. The nurse is monitoring a client with schizophrenia who is prescribed clozapine (Clozaril). During a multidisciplinary mental health team meeting, which signs and symptoms should be brought to the psychiatrist's attention? Select all that apply.

- ☐ **1.** Sore throat.
- ☐ **2.** Pill-rolling movements.
- ☐ **3.** Polyuria.
- ☐ **4.** Fever.
- ☐ **5.** Polydipsia.
- ☐ **6.** Orthostatic hypotension.

Answer: 1, 4, 6

Rationale: Sore throat, fever, and the sudden onset of other flu-like symptoms are signs of agranulocytosis, an adverse effect of clozapine that should be brought to the psychiatrists' attention. The condition is caused by a deficiency of granulocytes (a type of white blood cell), which causes the individual to be susceptible to infection. The client's white blood cell count should be monitored at least weekly during clozapine treatment. Orthostatic hypotension may occur with initial use of the drug. Dizziness upon standing with or without fainting can also occur during clozapine treatment. Extrapyramidal effects (such as pill-rolling) either does not occur or occur at a much lesser rate with the atypical antipsychotic medications. Polydipsia (excessive thirst) and polyuria (increased urination) are common adverse effects of lithium.

Test-taking strategy: Analyze to determine what information the question asks for, which is adverse effects of clozapine. "Select all that apply" questions require considering each option to decide its merit. Recall that, although unknown, clozapine is thought to use an immune mechanism that causes the agranulocytosis with subsequent symptoms. Review the adverse effects of antipsychotic medications, especially clozapine, if you had difficulty answering this question.

Client needs category: Physiological integrity
Client needs subcategory: Pharmacological therapies
Cognitive level: Applying

---

4. A delusional client says to a nurse "I am the Easter bunny," and insists that the nurse refer to him/her as such. The belief appears to be fixed and unchanging. Which nursing interventions should the nurse implement when working with this client? Select all that apply.

- ☐ **1.** Consistently use the client's name in interactions.
- ☐ **2.** Smile at the humor of the situation.
- ☐ **3.** Agree that the client is the Easter bunny.
- ☐ **4.** Logically point out why the client could not be the Easter bunny.
- ☐ **5.** Provide an as-needed medication.
- ☐ **6.** Provide the client with structured activities.

Answer: 1, 6

Rationale: This client needs continuous reality-based orientation, so the nurse should use the client's name in all interactions. Structured activities can help the client refocus and resolve this delusion. The nurse should not contribute to the delusion by smiling at the comment or agreeing with the client. Logical arguments and an as-needed medication are not likely to change the client's beliefs.

Test-taking strategy: Analyze to determine what information the question asks for, which is nursing interventions appropriate in working with a delusional client. "Select all that apply" questions require considering each option to decide its merit. Recall that clients with delusions require similar interventions as those with hallucinations. Among those, include a need for safety and security, divert focus back to reality, and teach cognitive strategies recognition strategies. Review nursing interventions when caring for a client with delusion if you had difficulty answering this question.

Client needs category: Psychosocial integrity
Client needs subcategory: None
Cognitive level: Applying

5. A physician prescribes haloperidol (Haldol) 1 mg t.i.d. When assessing the client for extrapyramidal adverse effects, which nursing measures should be initiated? Select all that apply.

☐ **1.** Review subcutaneous injection technique.
☐ **2.** Closely monitor vital signs, especially temperature.
☐ **3.** Observe for increased pacing and restlessness.
☐ **4.** Monitor blood glucose levels.
☐ **5.** Provide the client with hard candy.
☐ **6.** Monitor for signs and symptoms of urticaria.

Answer: 2, 3, 5

Rationale: Neuroleptic malignant syndrome is a life-threatening extrapyramidal adverse effect of antipsychotic medications such as haloperidol. It is associated with a rapid increase in temperature. The most common extrapyramidal adverse effect, akathisia, is a form of psychomotor restlessness that is often exhibited as pacing. Haloperidol and the anticholinergic medications that are provided to alleviate its extrapyramidal effects can result in dry mouth. Providing the client with hard candy to suck on can help alleviate this problem. Haloperidol is not given subcutaneously and does not affect blood glucose levels. Urticaria is not usually associated with haloperidol administration.

Test-taking strategy: Analyze to determine what information the question asks for, which is nursing measures for assessment of extrapyramidal adverse effects when taking Haldol. "Select all that apply" questions require considering each option to decide its merit. Choose the options that foreshadow the beginning of extrapyramidal symptoms. Consider the data of which each nursing measure could provide. Review Haldol administration and extrapyramidal adverse effects if you had difficulty answering this question.

Client needs category: Physiological integrity
Client needs subcategory: Pharmacological therapies
Cognitive level: Analyzing

---

6. When teaching a group of students in a psychiatric assistant class about the use of antipsychotic medications, the nurse advises them that certain symptoms can occur within the first few weeks of treatment. Which symptoms are likely to occur? Select all that apply.

☐ **1.** Acute dystonic reactions.
☐ **2.** Akathisia.
☐ **3.** Tardive dyskinesia.
☐ **4.** Neuroleptic malignant syndrome.
☐ **5.** Hearing loss.
☐ **6.** Orthostatic hypotension.

Answer: 1, 2, 4, 6

Rationale: Acute dystonia, akathisia, neuroleptic malignant syndrome, and orthostatic hypotension can occur during the first few weeks of treatment with antipsychotic drugs. Tardive dyskinesia does not typically occur until at least 6 months after starting treatment. Hearing loss is not an adverse effect of antipsychotic drugs.

Test-taking strategy: Analyze to determine what information the question asks for, which is early onset side effects of antipsychotic medications. "Select all that apply" questions require considering each option to decide its merit. The key words are "first few weeks of treatment," indicating a more minor side effect than those with later side effects. Note that an early effect includes motor disturbances due to medication effects in the motor control center of the brain. Review the adverse effects of the different classes of antipsychotic medications if you had difficulty answering this question.

Client needs category: Psychosocial integrity
Client needs subcategory: None
Cognitive level: Analyzing

7. A nurse is working with a schizophrenic client who suddenly begins experiencing auditory hallucinations. Place the following interventions in the order that best prevents exacerbation of the client's anxiety. Use all of the options.

1.	Ask the client, "What are you experiencing right now?"

2.	Encourage the client to relate the history of the hallucinations.

3.	Tell the client, "I'd like to spend time with you to discuss your hallucinations. Is that okay with you?"

4.	Ask the client if he/she has recently taken any drugs or alcohol.

Answer: 3, 1, 4, 2

Rationale: Asking the client about discussing the hallucinations promotes trust, an essential first step in communicating with hallucinating clients. When the client relates the hallucinations, the nurse should observe for nonverbal cues, such as the client's eyes looking around the room. Asking the client about these observations will help promote understanding of the symptoms, increase trust, and decrease the client's perception that the nurse can read his/her mind. Asking the client of recent drug or alcohol activity helps determine the source of the current experience. Once trust is established, the client will be more comfortable discussing the history of the hallucinations, such as when the voices started. This step will be beneficial in helping him/her manage in the present.

Test-taking strategy: Analyze to determine what information the question asks for, which is ordering interventions to prevent exacerbation of the client's anxiety. "Select all that apply" questions require considering each option to decide its merit. Identify the first as asking for permission, which is essential for communication/trust and decreases anxiety. Note that the last option would be relating the history of hallucinations as the nurse would move from present symptoms to history. Lastly, order the remaining two options. Review options to decrease client anxiety when experiencing auditory hallucinations if you had difficulty answering this question.

Client needs category: Psychosocial integrity

Client needs subcategory: None

Cognitive level: Applying

8. A client who is taking medication to control schizophrenia asks the nurse to explain the causes of the disorder. The nurse knows that an overactive dopamine system in the brain is one of the leading causes of schizophrenia and tells the client that excessive dopamine activity is responsible for symptoms. Which symptoms is the nurse referring to? Select all that apply.

- ☐ **1.** Hallucinations.
- ☐ **2.** Withdrawn behavior.
- ☐ **3.** Grandiosity.
- ☐ **4.** Delusional thinking.
- ☐ **5.** Excessive tearfulness.
- ☐ **6.** Hypotension.

Answer: 1, 3, 4

Rationale: Hallucinations, grandiosity, and delusional thinking are attributable to the effects of excessive dopamine activity. Withdrawn behavior is not associated with dopamine. Excessive tearfulness and hypotension are not commonly associated with schizophrenia or dopamine activity.

Test-taking strategy: Analyze to determine what information the question asks for, which is symptoms of schizophrenia related to dopamine activity. "Select all that apply" questions require considering each option to decide its merit. Consider that dopamine, a neurotransmitter, is excitable in the structurally changed schizophrenic brain. Recall that when drugs block the dopamine receptors the symptoms of schizophrenia are reduced. Review the effects of dopamine on the brain, and signs and symptoms of schizophrenia if you had difficulty answering this question.

Client needs category: Psychosocial integrity

Client needs subcategory: None

Cognitive level: Analyzing

---

9. A client with a diagnosis of undifferentiated schizophrenia is admitted to the inpatient unit after developing water intoxication. Which nursing interventions are appropriate? Select all that apply.

- ☐ **1.** Medicate the client at night.
- ☐ **2.** Provide gum for the client.
- ☐ **3.** Lock the unit's kitchen and bathroom.
- ☐ **4.** Weigh the client every day.
- ☐ **5.** Monitor the client's intake and output.
- ☐ **6.** Maintain a structured environment.

Answer: 2, 4, 5, 6

Rationale: Water intoxication is a potentially fatal disturbance in brain functions that results when the normal balance of electrolytes is outside of safe limits by overhydration. It is appropriate for the nurse to monitor intake and output, weigh the client daily, and encourage the client to chew gum rather than drink water. The nurse also provides a structured environment as a way to distract and divert the client away from obtaining fluids. Medicating the client at night and locking the unit's kitchen and bathroom should not be necessary.

Test-taking strategy: Analyze to determine what information the question asks for, which is nursing interventions for a schizophrenic client who has developed water intoxication. "Select all that apply" questions require considering each option to decide its merit. Consider options that monitor the electrolyte status and fluid volume and provide structure for the schizophrenic client. Review water intoxication for a schizophrenic client if you had difficulty answering this question.

Client needs category: Physiological integrity

Client needs subcategory: Reduction of risk potential

Cognitive level: Applying

Substance Abuse, Eating Disorders, and Impulse Control Disorders

1. During the nurse's assessment of a client who has been diagnosed with bulimia nervosa, the nurse evaluates certain characteristics that accompany binge eating. Which characteristics are most applicable. Select all that apply.

- ☐ **1.** Guilt.
- ☐ **2.** Dental caries.
- ☐ **3.** Self-induced vomiting.
- ☐ **4.** Weight loss.
- ☐ **5.** Normal weight.
- ☐ **6.** Introverted behavior.

Answer: 1, 2, 3, 5

Rationale: Bulimia nervosa is an eating disorder in which individuals binge on food and then begins to make up for it by purging, taking laxatives, and starving themselves. Guilt, dental caries, self-induced vomiting, and normal weight are associated with bulimia nervosa. Weight loss and introverted behavior are associated with anorexia nervosa.

Test-taking strategy: Analyze to determine what information the question asks for, which is characteristics of a client with bulimia nervosa and binge eating. "Select all that apply" questions require considering each option to decide its merit. Recall consequences from ingesting and then eliminating food from the body. Consider each option to the effects of gastric contents being eliminated. Review bulimia nervosa, binge eating, and the client's bodily effects if you had difficulty answering this question.

Client needs category: Psychosocial integrity

Client needs subcategory: None

Cognitive level: Analyzing

2. A nurse is employed at an outpatient rehabilitation facility caring for the client with opioid addiction who is in withdrawal. When assessing clients who present for their counseling session, which signs and symptoms would be commonly observed? Select all that apply.

- ☐ **1.** Abdominal cramps.
- ☐ **2.** Dry, warm skin.
- ☐ **3.** Rhinorrhea.
- ☐ **4.** Dilated pupils.
- ☐ **5.** Hypersomnia.
- ☐ **6.** Feelings of hunger.

Answer: 1, 3, 4

Rationale: Opioid withdrawal refers to the wide range of symptoms that occur stopping or dramatically reducing opiate drugs. Opioid withdrawal commonly manifests as abdominal cramps, rhinorrhea, dilated pupils, and anorexia (not hunger). Insomnia (not hypersomnia) and diaphoresis (not dry, warm skin) are also common.

Test-taking strategy: Analyze to determine what information the question asks for, which is common signs of opioid withdrawal. "Select all that apply" questions require considering each option to decide its merit. Recall that when withdrawing from opioids, the body needs time to recover from the physical dependence. Many times the client will experience flu-like symptoms. Review the withdrawal effects of opioids on the various body systems if you had difficulty answering this question.

Client needs category: Physiological integrity

Client needs subcategory: Pharmacological therapies

Cognitive level: Analyzing

3. During the nurse's shift in the emergency department, a nurse assesses a client who is suspected of being under the influence of amphetamines. Which symptoms are indicative of amphetamine use? Select all that apply.

☐ **1.** Depressed effect.
☐ **2.** Diaphoresis.
☐ **3.** Shallow respirations.
☐ **4.** Hypotension.
☐ **5.** Tremors.
☐ **6.** Dilated pupils.

Answer: 2, 3, 5, 6

Rationale: A client under the influence of amphetamines may present with euphoria, diaphoresis, shallow respirations, dilated pupils, dry mouth, anorexia, tachycardia, hypertension, hyperthermia, tremors, seizures, and altered mental status. Depressed affect and hypotension are not associated with amphetamine use.

Test-taking strategy: Analyze to determine what information the question asks for, which is symptoms of amphetamine use. "Select all that apply" questions require considering each option to decide its merit. Recall the overall effect of amphetamines as body stimulant. Note the exaggerated effect on the body. Review amphetamine administration and abuse if you had difficulty answering this question.

Client needs category: Physiological integrity
Client needs subcategory: Pharmacological therapies
Cognitive level: Applying

---

4. A nurse is caring for an anorexic client with a nursing diagnosis of *imbalanced nutrition: less than body requirements related to dysfunctional eating patterns*. Which interventions would be supportive for this client? Select all that apply.

☐ **1.** Provide small, frequent meals.
☐ **2.** Monitor weight gain.
☐ **3.** Allow the client to skip meals until the antidepressant levels are therapeutic.
☐ **4.** Encourage the client to keep a journal.
☐ **5.** Monitor the client during meals and for 1 hour afterward.
☐ **6.** Encourage the client to eat three substantial meals per day.

Answer: 1, 2, 4, 5

Rationale: Anorexia nervosa is an eating disorder characterized by excessive food restriction and irrational fear of gaining weight. Because the clients are engaged in self-starvation, clients with anorexia rarely can tolerate large meals three times per day. Small, frequent meals may be tolerated better and they provide a way to gradually increase daily caloric intake. The nurse should monitor the client's weight carefully because a client with anorexia may try to hide the weight loss. The nurse should also monitor the client during meals and for 1 hour afterward to ensure that the client consumes all of the food and does not attempt to purge. The client may be afraid to express feelings; keeping a journal can serve as an outlet for these feelings, which can assist recovery. A client with anorexia is already underweight and should not be permitted to skip meals.

Test-taking strategy: Analyze to determine what information the question asks for, which is nursing interventions for an anorexic client with a nursing diagnosis of imbalanced nutrition. "Select all that apply" questions require considering each option to decide its merit. Focus on the key words of anorexia and nursing diagnosis of imbalanced nutrition and eating patterns. Always answer what the question is asking. Note the relation between the correct answers and the nursing diagnosis. Review nursing interventions for the anorexic client if you had difficulty answering this question.

Client needs category: Psychosocial integrity
Client needs subcategory: None
Cognitive level: Analyzing

---

5. When assessing a client diagnosed with impulse control disorder, the nurse observes violent, aggressive, and assaultive behavior. Which assessment data is the nurse also likely to find? Select all that apply.

☐ **1.** The client functions well in other areas of life.
☐ **2.** The degree of aggressiveness is out of proportion to the stressor.
☐ **3.** The violent behavior is usually justified by a stressor.
☐ **4.** The client has a history of parental alcoholism and a chaotic, abusive family life.
☐ **5.** The client has no remorse about the inability to control behavior.

Answer: 1, 2, 4

Rationale: A client with an impulse control disorder who displays violent, aggressive, and assaultive behavior generally functions well in other areas of life. The degree of aggressiveness is out of proportion to the stressor, and there is frequently a history of parental alcoholism and a chaotic family life. The client often verbalizes sincere remorse and guilt for the aggressive behavior.

Test-taking strategy: Analyze to determine what information the question asks for, which is data typically found when assessing a client with impulse control disorder. "Select all that apply" questions require considering each option to decide its merit. Recall that individuals with impulse control disorders cannot resist the urge to do something harmful to themselves or others. Consider that psychological factors are associated with this disorder and remorse is frequently seen. Review the clinical manifestations of impulse control disorder if you had difficulty answering this question.

Client needs category: Psychosocial integrity
Client needs subcategory: None
Cognitive level: Applying

---

6. A nurse is caring for a client with borderline personality disorder. Which interventions are appropriate for clients with this disorder? Select all that apply.

☐ **1.** Providing antianxiety medications.
☐ **2.** Providing emotional consistency.
☐ **3.** Exploring anger in appropriate ways.
☐ **4.** Encouraging independence as soon as possible.
☐ **5.** Promoting gradual separation and individuation.
☐ **6.** Ensuring the client's safety.

Answer: 2, 3, 5, 6

Rationale: In clients with borderline personalities, the primary goal is to ensure a safe environment. As the client begins to learn how to manage his/her behavior, suicide still remains a risk. A key intervention includes providing emotional support that is consistent. The client needs to learn how to manage anger effectively and typically begins needing less support as he/she separates and develops individual coping behaviors. Antianxiety drugs are reserved for clinical emergencies.

Test-taking strategy: Analyze to determine what information the question asks for, which is nursing interventions for a client with borderline personality disorder. "Select all that apply" questions require considering each option to decide its merit. Recall that with borderline personality disorder how the client views himself/herself is distorted, making the client feel worthless and emotional instability leading to anger, stress, and other problems. Consider each option in relation to clinical manifestations. Review the nursing interventions necessary when caring for a client with borderline personality disorder if you had difficulty answering this question.

Client needs category: Psychosocial integrity
Client needs subcategory: None
Cognitive level: Applying

7. A client is prescribed chlordiazepoxide (Librium) as needed to control the symptoms of alcohol withdrawal. Which symptoms may indicate the need for an additional dose of this medication? Select all that apply.

- ☐ **1.** Tachycardia.
- ☐ **2.** Mood swings.
- ☐ **3.** Elevated blood pressure and temperature.
- ☐ **4.** Piloerection.
- ☐ **5.** Tremors.
- ☐ **6.** Increasing anxiety.

Answer: 1, 3, 5, 6

Rationale: Benzodiazepines such as chlordiazepoxide are usually administered based on elevations in heart rate, blood pressure, and temperature, as well as on the presence of tremors and increasing anxiety. Mood swings are expected during the withdrawal period and are not an indication for further medication administration. Piloerection (goosebumps, or a feeling of hair of the skin standing on end) is not a symptom of alcohol withdrawal.

Test-taking strategy: Analyze to determine what information the question asks for, which is symptoms of uncontrolled alcohol withdrawal. "Select all that apply" questions require considering each option to decide its merit. Consider symptom management of alcohol withdrawal and therapeutic Librium effects. Recall that Librium is used to relieve anxiety and control agitation. Review the clinical manifestations of alcohol withdrawal and Librium use if you had difficulty answering this question.

Client needs category: Physiological integrity

Client needs subcategory: Pharmacological therapies

Cognitive level: Analysis

---

8. The nurse is assessing a client who is a polysubstance abuser, with cocaine being one of the drugs most frequently used. Which physiological symptom is suggestive of cocaine intoxication? Select all that apply.

- ☐ **1.** Respiratory depression.
- ☐ **2.** Psychomotor agitation.
- ☐ **3.** Cardiac arrhythmias.
- ☐ **4.** Dilated pupils.
- ☐ **5.** Projectile vomiting.
- ☐ **6.** Slurred speech.

Answer: 1, 2, 3, 4

Rationale: A polysubstance abuser is an individual who abuses at least three. Caffeine and nicotine are not included substances. When assessing for cocaine intoxication, the most common physiological symptoms observed are respiratory depression, cardiac arrhythmias, psychomotor agitation, and dilated pupils. Projectile vomiting and slurred speech are not associated with cocaine intoxication.

Test-taking strategy: Analyze to determine what information the question asks for, which is suggestive symptoms of cocaine intoxication. "Select all that apply" questions require considering each option to decide its merit. Recall that cocaine tends to affect the central nervous system. An exaggerated effect would be noted with intoxication. Review the clinical manifestations of cocaine intoxication and the effects on body systems if you had difficulty answering this question.

Client needs category: Physiological integrity

Client needs subcategory: Physiological adaptation

Cognitive level: Analyzing

PART SEVEN

Comprehensive Test

1. A client arrives at the emergency department with chest and stomach pain and a report of black, tarry stools for several months. Which order should the nurse anticipate?

☐ **1.** Cardiac monitor, oxygen, creatine kinase, and lactate dehydrogenase (LD) levels.
☐ **2.** Prothrombin time (PT), partial thromboplastin time (PTT), fibrinogen, and fibrin split product values.
☐ **3.** ECG (electrocardiogram), complete blood count, testing for occult blood, and comprehensive serum metabolic panel.
☐ **4.** EEG (electroencephalogram), alkaline phosphatase and aspartate aminotransferase levels, and basic serum metabolic panel.

Answer: 3

Rationale: An ECG evaluates the complaint of chest pain, laboratory tests determine anemia, and the test for occult blood determines blood in the stool. Cardiac monitoring, oxygen, and creatine kinase and LD levels are appropriate for a primary cardiac problem. A basic metabolic panel and alkaline phosphatase and aspartate aminotransferase levels assess liver function. PT, PTT, fibrinogen, and fibrin split products are measured to verify bleeding dyscrasias. An EEG evaluates brain electrical activity.

Test-taking strategy: Analyze to determine what information the question asks for, which is anticipated laboratory testing for a client with complaints of chest and stomach pain. Select the option that reflects laboratory/diagnostic testing that would address client symptoms. Review cardiac and gastrointestinal (GI) diagnostic testing if you had difficulty answering this question.

Client needs category: Physiological integrity

Client needs subcategory: Reduction of risk potential

Cognitive level: Analyzing

2. The family of a client, stung by a bee, rushed the client to the emergency room. The client is experiencing hives and redness at the site. Upon arrival, the client states, "I feel a lump in my throat and I am sweating. I can't breathe! I think I am going to die!" The nurse anticipates which emergency treatment next?

☐ **1.** Administer Lopressor 50 mg b.i.d.
☐ **2.** Administer Albuterol 2 puffs stat.
☐ **3.** Administer an injection of epinephrine stat.
☐ **4.** Have the client in high Fowler's position in the bed.

Answer: 3

Rationale: Symptoms of hives and redness at the bee sting site coupled with a progression of symptoms including respiratory difficulty and an impending feeling of doom indicate anaphylaxis. Emergency treatment of anaphylaxis is an injection of epinephrine. Bronchodilators may help but are not the primary treatment. β-Adrenergic blockers are not indicated in the management of anaphylaxis because they may cause bronchospasm. Having the client in high Fowler's position is appropriate but not emergency treatment.

Test-taking strategy: Analyze to determine what information the question asks for, which is emergency treatment for a client in respiratory distress. Analyze the symptoms to conclude that the client is having an anaphylactic reaction. Remember the ABCs (airway, breathing, and circulation) of emergency care and recall that epinephrine (adrenaline) reduces the body's allergic response. If unsure, consider that an injection enters the blood stream rapidly. Review emergency treatment of anaphylaxis if you had difficulty answering this question.

Client needs category: Physiological integrity

Client needs subcategory: Physiological adaptation

Cognitive level: Analyzing

3. A nurse is providing nutritional teaching for a client with a family history of colon cancer. Which food choice by the client demonstrates an understanding of the correct diet to follow?

- ☐ **1.** Vegetarian chili.
- ☐ **2.** Hot dogs and sauerkraut.
- ☐ **3.** Egg salad on rye bread.
- ☐ **4.** Spaghetti and meat sauce.

Answer: 1

Rationale: A high-fiber, low-fat food, such as vegetarian chili, increases gastric motility and decreases the chance of constipation, helping to reduce the risk of colon cancer. The other choices are not representative of a high-fiber, low-fat diet.

Test-taking strategy: Analyze to determine what information the question asks for, which is nutritional choice for a client with a family history of colon cancer. Recall that most studies state that a plant-based diet rich in fruits, vegetables, legumes, and whole grains are associated with a lower risk of a number of common cancers. Recall dietary guidelines for preventing colon cancer if you had difficulty answering this question.

Client needs category: Health promotion and maintenance

Client needs subcategory: None

Cognitive level: Applying

---

4. A nurse has a four-patient assignment in the medical step-down unit. When planning care for the clients, which client would have the following treatment goals: fluid replacement, vasopressin replacement, and correction of underlying intracranial pathology?

- ☐ **1.** The client with diabetes mellitus.
- ☐ **2.** The client with diabetes insipidus.
- ☐ **3.** The client with diabetic ketoacidosis.
- ☐ **4.** The client with syndrome of inappropriate antidiuretic hormone (SIADH) secretion.

Answer: 2

Rationale: Maintaining adequate fluid, replacing vasopressin, and correcting underlying intracranial problems (typically lesions, tumors, or trauma affecting the hypothalamus or pituitary gland) are the main objectives in treating diabetes insipidus. Diabetes mellitus does not involve vasopressin deficiencies or an intracranial disorder, but rather a disturbance in the production or use of insulin. Diabetic ketoacidosis results from severe insulin insufficiency. An excess of vasopressin leads to SIADH, causing the client to retain fluid.

Test-taking strategy: Analyze to determine what information the question asks for, which is selecting the client with a specific treatment plan. Discriminate through the options to select the disease process which includes a disruption in fluid status, lack of vasopressin that is normally secreted by the pituitary gland, and having an intracranial disorder. Review endocrine disorders and their treatment plans if you had difficulty answering this question.

Client needs category: Physiological integrity

Client needs subcategory: Physiological adaptation

Cognitive level: Analyzing

5. A nurse, working on a community disaster response team, is teaching about the cause and effects of anthrax. The nurse is most correct to include which routes of anthrax transmission in the teaching? Select all that apply.

☐ **1.** Inhalation of anthrax substance
☐ **2.** Sexual contact with an infected person
☐ **3.** Physical contact with an infected person
☐ **4.** Being coughed on by an infected person
☐ **5.** Gastrointestinal ingestion of anthrax
☐ **6.** Touching a surface where anthrax is present

Answer: 1, 5, 6

Rationale: Anthrax is caused by the *Bacillus anthracis*. A common route of infection is through the skin, which causes an ugly sore that usually goes away without treatment. Humans and animals can ingest anthrax. Ingestion of anthrax can cause serious, sometimes fatal disease. The most deadly form is inhalation anthrax. If the spores of anthrax are inhaled, they migrate to lymph glands in the chest where they proliferate, spread, and produce toxins that often cause death. Anthrax is not spread from person to person.

Test-taking strategy: Analyze to determine what information the question asks for, which is route of anthrax transmission. Recall that contamination occurs between a person and the anthrax, eliminating person-to-person transmission. Review transmission of anthrax if you had difficulty answering this question.

Client needs category: Safe and effective care environment

Client needs subcategory: Safety and infection control

Cognitive level: Analyzing

---

6. The nurse is working at the local family planning clinic doing family education. When devising a teaching plan, in which client group would the nurse stress the importance of an annual Papanicolaou test?

☐ **1.** Clients with a history of recurrent candidiasis.
☐ **2.** Clients who were pregnant before age 20.
☐ **3.** Clients infected with the human papillomavirus (HPV).
☐ **4.** Clients with a long history of oral contraceptive use.

Answer: 3

Rationale: Annual Papanicolaou testing is a screening to detect potential precancerous and cancerous cells in the endocervical canal of the female reproductive system. HPV causes genital warts, which are associated with an increased incidence of cervical cancer. Recurrent candidiasis, pregnancy before age 20, and use of oral contraceptives do not increase the risk of cervical cancer.

Test-taking strategy: Analyze to determine what information the question asks for, which is client group that would most benefit from annual Papanicolaou testing. Recall the diagnostic findings associated with a Papanicolaou test and relate to the risk factors noted in each option. Review the benefits associated with annual Papanicolaou testing if you had difficulty answering this question.

Client needs category: Health promotion and maintenance

Client needs subcategory: None

Cognitive level: Analyzing

7. The nurse is caring for an infant diagnosed with thrush. Which instruction should the nurse give to a client's mother who will be administering nystatin (Mycostatin) oral solution?

☐ **1.** Administer the drug right after meals by swabbing the mouth.

☐ **2.** Administer the drug right before meals by using a gauze pad.

☐ **3.** Mix the drug with small amounts of formula in bottle.

☐ **4.** Administer half the dose before and half after a feeding.

Answer: 1

Rationale: Nystatin oral solution is an antifungal medication used to treat fungal or yeast infections. Nystatin oral solution should be swished around the mouth after eating for the best contact with mucous membranes. Taking the drug before or with meals does not allow for optimal contact with mucous membranes.

Test-taking strategy: Analyze to determine what information the question asks for, which is instructions for a mother administering Nystatin oral solution. Recall that the action of the medication needs contact with the mucous membranes. Options 2 and 4 are eliminated as eating after administration removes the medication and splitting the dosage before provides an incorrect dosage. Option 3 violates the standard of not putting medication in a bottle. Review Nystatin administration if you had difficulty answering this question.

Client needs category: Physiological integrity

Client needs subcategory: Pharmacological therapies

Cognitive level: Applying

---

8. A client at 42 weeks of gestation is 3 cm dilated and 30% effaced, with membranes intact and the fetus at +2 station. Fetal heart rate (FHR) is 140 beats/minute. After 2 hours, the nurse notes that, for the past 10 minutes, the external fetal monitor has been displaying a FHR of 190 beats/minute. The client states that her baby has been extremely active. Uterine contractions are strong, occurring every 3 to 4 minutes and lasting 40 to 60 seconds. Which finding would indicate fetal hypoxia?

☐ **1.** Abnormally long uterine contractions.

☐ **2.** Abnormally strong uterine intensity.

☐ **3.** Excessively frequent contractions, with rapid fetal movement.

☐ **4.** Excessive fetal activity and fetal tachycardia.

Answer: 4

Rationale: Fetal tachycardia and excessive fetal activity are the first signs of fetal hypoxia. The duration of uterine contractions is within normal limits. Uterine intensity can be mild to strong yet still within normal limits. The frequency of contractions is within normal limits for the active phase of labor.

Test-taking strategy: Analyze to determine what information the question asks for, which is signs of fetal hypoxia. Sift through the data to interpret abnormalities and then relate to a correlation with fetal hypoxia. Recall that restlessness and agitation are key features in hypoxia which would lead to the correct answer. Review the signs of fetal hypoxia and relate them to FHR if you had difficulty answering this question.

Client needs category: Physiological integrity

Client needs subcategory: Reduction of risk potential

Cognitive level: Analyzing

9. The nurse is caring for a 3-day-old neonate born to an opioid-dependent mother. When attempting to interact with the neonate experiencing drug withdrawal, the nurse recognizes which behavior as a sign of the neonate's willingness to interact?

☐ **1.** Gaze aversion.
☐ **2.** Hiccups.
☐ **3.** Quiet, alert state.
☐ **4.** Yawning.

Answer: 3

Rationale: When caring for a neonate experiencing drug withdrawal, the nurse needs to be alert for signs of distress from the neonate. Stimuli should be introduced one at a time when the neonate is in a quiet, alert state. Gaze aversion, yawning, sneezing, hiccups, and body arching are distress signals that the neonate cannot handle stimuli at that time.

Test-taking strategy: Analyze to determine what information the question asks for, which is signs of willingness to interact. Recall that "willingness to interact" includes behaviors of a more relaxed state without agitation. In this state, the neonate is able to accept stimuli, including positive stimuli of touch, soothing vocalization, and eye contact. Review characteristics of drug withdrawal in the neonate if you had difficulty answering this question.

Client needs category: Psychosocial integrity

Client needs subcategory: None

Cognitive level: Analyzing

---

10. A nurse is caring for a client recovering from cardiac revascularization surgery of 3 days ago. Upon analysis of lab reports, the nurse notes the client's platelet count decreased from 230,000 to 5,000 μL? Which condition is suspected?

☐ **1.** Pancytopenia.
☐ **2.** Idiopathic thrombocytopenic purpura (ITP).
☐ **3.** Disseminated intravascular coagulation (DIC).
☐ **4.** Heparin-associated thrombosis and thrombocytopenia (HATT).

Answer: 4

Rationale: HATT may occur after cardiac revascularization surgery due to heparin use during surgery. Pancytopenia is a reduction in all blood cells. Although ITP and DIC cause platelet aggregation and bleeding, neither is common in a client after revascularization surgery.

Test-taking strategy: Analyze to determine what information the question asks for, which are conditions causing a noted drop in platelet count. Recall that HATT is an immune system complication of using heparin therapy, resulting in devastating throboembolitic outcomes. Review complications of cardiac revascularization surgery and heparin use if you had difficulty answering this question.

Client needs category: Physiological integrity

Client needs subcategory: Physiological adaptation

Cognitive level: Applying

11. The nurse is caring for a comatose client who needs a nasopharyngeal airway for suctioning. After the airway is inserted, the client gags and coughs. Which action should the nurse take?

- ☐ **1.** Remove the airway and insert a shorter one.
- ☐ **2.** Reposition the airway.
- ☐ **3.** Leave the airway in place until the client gets used to it.
- ☐ **4.** Remove the airway and attempt suctioning without it.

Answer: 1

Rationale: If the client gags or coughs after nasopharyngeal airway placement, the tube may be too long. The nurse should remove it and insert a shorter one. Simply repositioning the airway will not solve the problem. The client will not get used to the tube because it is the wrong size. Suctioning without a nasopharyngeal airway causes trauma to the natural airway.

Test-taking strategy: Analyze to determine what information the question asks for, which is correct procedure for placing a nasopharyngeal airway. Recall the symptoms in relation to the anatomy of the respiratory system indicating a problem. Eliminate options 1 and 2 as not correcting the problem. Eliminate option 4 as inappropriate nursing care. Review the procedure for nasopharyngeal airway placement and suctioning if you had difficulty answering this question.

Client needs category: Physiological integrity

Client needs subcategory: Reduction of risk potential

Cognitive level: Applying

---

12. A nurse is caring for a young adult client recently diagnosed with Bell's palsy. The client just began a new job and moved to an area away from family. When the nurse is prioritizing nursing diagnoses from greatest to least, in what order would the nurse arrange these?

1. Low self-esteem related to disfigurement from facial drooping
2. Imbalanced nutrition: Less than body requirements related to loss of muscle tone
3. Deficient knowledge related to new diagnosis
4. Risk for loneliness related to living away from family
5. Anxiety related to physical disfigurement

Answer: 3, 2, 5, 1, 4

Rationale: The highest priority is the knowledge deficit in understanding the disease process and care. The nurse must instruct on the disease process, including signs and symptoms and care. The next priority would be imbalanced nutrition, as the disease process affects the ability to chew. Anxiety is the next priority, as the client may be anxious related to job situation and physical deformity. Low self-esteem is a psychosocial nursing diagnosis more than likely exacerbated by the lack of family support. Lastly is the risk for loneliness, in which the nurse identifies a potential problem.

Test-taking strategy: Analyze to determine what information the question asks for, which is priority of nursing diagnoses for a client newly diagnosed with Bell's palsy. Consider the priority of information needed in providing self-care and avoiding side effects associated with Bell's palsy. Note that the psychosocial diagnosis and "risk for" diagnosis are of a lesser priority. Review priorities for Bell's palsy if you had difficulty answering this question.

Client needs category: Safe and effective care environment

Client needs subcategory: Coordinated care

Cognitive level: Analyzing

13. The orthopedic nurse is providing discharge instruction to a surgical client. Which action, by the client, would demonstrate proper touchdown weight bearing?

☐ **1.** Bearing full weight on the affected extremity.
☐ **2.** Bearing 30% to 50% of weight on the affected extremity.
☐ **3.** Bearing no weight on the extremity but allowing the extremity to touch the floor.
☐ **4.** Bearing no weight on the extremity and keeping the extremity elevated at all times.

Answer: 3

Rationale: Touchdown weight bearing involves bearing no weight on the extremity but allowing the affected extremity to touch the floor. Full weight bearing allows for full weight to be put on the affected extremity. Partial weight bearing allows for 30% to 50% weight bearing on the affected extremity. Non-weight bearing refers to bearing no weight on the affected extremity.

Test-taking strategy: Analyze to determine what information the question asks for, which is the correct procedure for touchdown weight bearing. Use the terminology "touchdown" which suggests very little weight bearing, to provide a clue. Review the term *touchdown*, and guidelines for the amount of weight bearing and extremity activity allowed if you had difficulty answering this question.

Client needs category: Safe and effective care environment

Client needs subcategory: Coordinated care

Cognitive level: Applying

---

14. A medication nurse is preparing to administer 9 a.m. medications to a client with liver cancer. Which consideration is the nurse's highest priority?

☐ **1.** Frequency of the medication.
☐ **2.** Purpose of the medication.
☐ **3.** Necessity of the medication.
☐ **4.** Metabolism of the medication.

Answer: 4

Rationale: The rate and ability of the liver to metabolize medications will be altered in a client with liver cancer. Therefore, it is essential to understand how each medication is metabolized. The other considerations are important but not as vital.

Test-taking strategy: Analyze to determine what information the question asks for, which is nursing priority in administering medications to a client with liver cancer. The key word is "liver" as the liver plays a key role in medication metabolism. If unsure, use the key words in the options of frequency, purpose, necessity, and metabolism to guide your priority selection. Review normal drug metabolism and the pathophysiology of liver cancer as it relates to medication administration if you had difficulty answering this question.

Client needs category: Physiological integrity

Client needs subcategory: Reduction of risk potential

Cognitive level: Analyzing

15. A nurse is caring for a client diagnosed with Cushing's syndrome. When considering fluid balance, sodium and water retention contribute to which common disorder?

- ☐ **1.** Hypoglycemia and dehydration.
- ☐ **2.** Hypotension and hyperglycemia.
- ☐ **3.** Pulmonary edema and dehydration.
- ☐ **4.** Hypertension and heart failure.

Answer: 4

Rationale: In Cushing's syndrome, increased mineralocorticoid activity results in sodium and water retention, which commonly contributes to hypertension and heart failure. Hypoglycemia and dehydration are uncommon in a client with Cushing's syndrome. Diabetes mellitus and hyperglycemia may develop, but hypotension is not part of the disease process. Pulmonary edema and dehydration also are not complications of Cushing's syndrome.

Test-taking strategy: Analyze to determine what information the question asks for, which is a common disorder effecting sodium and water retention. The key word is "retention." Eliminate options 1, 2, and 3 as each has a component of dehydration and hypotension, common in fluid loss. Review the effects of water and sodium retention on various body systems if you had difficulty answering this question.

Client needs category: Physiological integrity

Client needs subcategory: Physiological adaptation

Cognitive level: Analyzing

---

16. The nurse is preparing to assess a school-aged child with abdominal discomfort. Place the following assessment skills in order of when the nurse would use them. Use all of the following:

1. Palpation
2. Auscultation
3. Percussion
4. Inspection

Answer: 4, 2, 3, 1

Rationale: When caring for a school-aged child with abdominal pain, the nurse must consider the child's developmental level and assess the abdomen starting with the least traumatic assessment. Inspection requires no physical contact by the nurse. The nurse evaluates the look of the abdomen, posture of the child, and whether the child demonstrates any guarding. The nurse then auscultates bowel sound patterns and percusses for tones. Lastly, the nurse palpates for pertinent information regarding any abnormal abdominal masses or specific area of pain.

Test-taking strategy: Analyze to determine what information the question asks for, which is order of assessment techniques when caring for a school-aged child. Recall that standard practice guidelines dictate beginning with the least traumatic assessment technique. Because it may cause client anxiety, end with palpation of the abdomen for pertinent information. Palpation may also cause the most discomfort. Review assessment techniques if you had difficulty answering this question.

Client needs category: Safe and effective care environment

Client needs subcategory: Coordinated care

Cognitive level: Applying

17. The Women's Clinic nurse is instructing a client on the proper use of an applicator to instill vaginal cream. Which of the following instructions is applicable when teaching a client about vaginal medication insertion?

- ☐ **1.** Insert the nozzle about 3" (8 cm) into the vagina.
- ☐ **2.** Direct the tip of the applicator toward the sacrum.
- ☐ **3.** Instill the cream slowly over 5 minutes.
- ☐ **4.** Sterilize the applicator in boiling water to prepare for next use.

Answer: 2

Rationale: The normal position of the vagina slants up and back toward the sacrum. Directing the tip of the applicator toward the sacrum allows it to follow the normal slant of the vagina and minimizes tissue trauma. The applicator should be inserted about 2" (5 cm). The medication can be administered by placing continuous pressure until the tip of the plunger until it hits the applicator, taking 10 to 15 seconds. This eliminates the medication from the applicator placing it in the vagina. Should the applicator need to be reused, the applicator may be washed thoroughly and placed on a towel to dry.

Test-taking strategy: Analyze to determine what information the question asks for, which is correct application of vaginal medication. Consider the location and condition of the vagina when discriminating through the options. Review the anatomy of the female reproductive system and clean versus sterile technique if you had difficulty answering this question.

Client needs category: Safe and effective care environment

Client needs subcategory: Safety and infection control

Cognitive level: Applying

---

18. The licensed practical nurse is collecting a wound culture from a client's gaping surgical incision. Which of the following would the nurse consider to ensure proper culture collection?

- ☐ **1.** Thoroughly irrigate the wound with normal saline before collecting the culture.
- ☐ **2.** Use a sterile swab to wipe the crusty area around the outside of the wound.
- ☐ **3.** Gently roll a sterile swab from the center of the wound outward to collect drainage.
- ☐ **4.** Use one sterile swab to collect drainage from several possible infected sites along the incision.

Answer: 3

Rationale: Rolling a swab from the center outward is the correct way to culture a wound. Irrigating the wound washes away drainage, debris, and many of the microorganisms colonizing or infecting the wound. The outside of the wound may be colonized with microorganisms from this wound or another wound, or from normal microorganisms found on the client's skin. These may grow in culture and confuse the interpretation of results. All of the sources of drainage from an incision or a surgical wound may not be infected, or they may be infected with different microorganisms; consequently, each swab should be used on only one site.

Test-taking strategy: Analyze to determine what information the question asks for, which is the correct procedure to obtain a surgical wound culture. Visualize the procedure and consider ways to obtain drainage from the surgical site. Focus on obtaining drainage at the site of any crusting, redness, or drainage. Review standard procedure for obtaining a surgical wound culture if you had difficulty answering this question.

Client needs category: Safe and effective care environment

Client needs subcategory: Safety and infection control

Cognitive level: Applying

19. A mental health nurse in an outpatient clinic is caring for a client who is newly diagnosed with phobic disorder. Which individual counseling approach is best to assist the client in daily activities?

☐ **1.** Have the client keep a daily journal.
☐ **2.** Help the client identify the source of the anxiety.
☐ **3.** Teach the client effective ways to problem-solve.
☐ **4.** Develop strategies to prevent the client from using substances.

Answer: 2

Rationale: By understanding the source of the anxiety, the client will understand how this anxiety has been displaced as a phobic response. Keeping a journal is an effective method in many situations; however, its use is limited in the treatment of phobias. Problem solving is a more useful technique for clients with obsessive-compulsive disorder than for clients with phobias. People with phobias do not tend to self-medicate like clients with other psychiatric disorders.

Test-taking strategy: Analyze to determine what information the question asks for, which is approach to assist the client in daily activities. Consider that phobias are fears and is a type of anxiety disorder. Review the defining characteristics of phobic disorders and focus on the optimal therapeutic approach if you had difficulty answering this question.

Client needs category: Psychosocial integrity

Client needs subcategory: None

Cognitive level: Applying

---

20. A client with antisocial personality disorder is trying to manipulate the health care team. Which strategy is most important for the staff to use?

☐ **1.** Focus on how to teach the client more effective behaviors for meeting basic needs.
☐ **2.** Help the client verbalize underlying feelings of hopelessness and learn coping skills.
☐ **3.** Remain calm and do not emotionally respond to the client's manipulative actions.
☐ **4.** Help the client eliminate the intense desire to have everything in life turn out perfectly.

Answer: 3

Rationale: The best strategy to use with a client trying to manipulate staff is to stay calm and refrain from responding emotionally. Negative reinforcement of inappropriate behavior increases the chance it will be repeated. Later, it may be possible to address how to meet the client's basic needs. Clients with antisocial personality disorder do not tend to experience feelings of hopelessness or to desire life events to turn out perfectly. In most cases, these clients negate responsibility for their behavior.

Test-taking strategy: Analyze to determine what information the question asks for, which is a strategy to use with an antisocial personality who is manipulative. Recall that manipulation is a client attempt for control. Focus on the strategy that does not reinforce the client's behavior. Review how to interact with manipulative clients if you had difficulty answering this question.

Client needs category: Psychosocial integrity

Client needs subcategory: None

Cognitive level: Analyzing

21. A child is admitted to the hospital for an asthma exacerbation. The nursing history reveals this client was exposed to varicella (chickenpox) 1 week ago. When, if at all, would this client require isolation?

☐ **1.** Isolation is not required at this time.
☐ **2.** Immediate isolation is required in a private room.
☐ **3.** Isolation would be required 10 days after exposure.
☐ **4.** Isolation would be required 12 days after exposure.

Answer: 2

Rationale: The incubation period for varicella (chickenpox) is 2 to 3 weeks, usually 13 to 17 days. A client is commonly isolated 1 week after exposure to avoid the risk of an earlier breakout. A person is infectious from 1 day before eruption of lesions to 6 days after the vesicles have formed crusts.

Test-taking strategy: Analyze to determine what information the question asks for, which is when isolation is necessary after chickenpox exposure. Recall the communicable nature and incubation period for chickenpox and relate this to the timing of isolation. If unsure, also consider the immunocompromised status of hospital clients and the need to protect. Review isolation precautions especially related to communicable diseases if you had difficulty answering this question.

Client needs category: Safe and effective care environment

Client needs subcategory: Safety and infection control

Cognitive level: Applying

22. The school nurse is monitoring the diet of a child with cystic fibrosis. Which type of diet would be stressed to the family?

☐ **1.** Fat restricted.
☐ **2.** High calorie.
☐ **3.** Low protein.
☐ **4.** Sodium restricted.

Answer: 2

Rationale: A well-balanced high-calorie, high-protein diet is recommended for a child with cystic fibrosis due to the impaired intestinal absorption. Fat restriction is not required because digestion and absorption of fat in the intestine are impaired. The child usually increases enzyme intake along with the consumption of high-fat foods. Low-sodium foods can lead to hyponatremia; therefore, high-sodium foods are recommended, especially during hot weather or when the child has a fever.

Test-taking strategy: Analyze to determine what information the question asks for, which is dietary recommendation for a client with cystic fibrosis. Recall that clients with cystic fibrosis need to ingest 50% more calories due to malabsorption. Also, clients who are in a good nutritional state are able to fight off infections and viruses. Review the disease process of cystic fibrosis in relation to children's nutritional needs if you had difficulty answering this question.

Client needs category: Safe and effective care environment

Client needs subcategory: Coordinated care

Cognitive level: Applying

23. The nurse is caring for an infant who is receiving I.V. therapy. The physician orders D5NS 400-mL to infuse in 8 hours. How much I.V. solution would the nurse place in the buretrol?

- ☐ **1.** 30-mL
- ☐ **2.** 50-mL
- ☐ **3.** 100-mL
- ☐ **4.** 150-mL

Answer: 2

Rationale: When calculating the mL/hour, divide 400-mL by 8 hours to get 50-mL/hour. When caring for an infant, only place one hour's worth of fluid into the buretrol to be infused.

Test-taking strategy: Analyze to determine what information the question asks for, which is amount of I.V. fluid to place in an infant's buretrol. Recall that the purpose of a buretrol is to protect the infant from fluid overload. Calculate the mL/hour of I.V. fluid to be infused and place that amount of fluid into the buretrol. Review I.V. calculations and rationale for buretrol use if you had difficulty answering this question.

Client needs category: Physiological integrity

Client needs subcategory: Pharmacological therapies

Cognitive level: Applying

---

24. A child has just returned to the pediatric unit following ventriculoperitoneal shunt placement for hydrocephalus. Which intervention should a nurse perform first?

- ☐ **1.** Assess intake and output.
- ☐ **2.** Place the child on the side opposite the shunt.
- ☐ **3.** Offer fluids because the child has a dry mouth.
- ☐ **4.** Administer pain medication by mouth as ordered.

Answer: 2

Rationale: Following shunt placement surgery, the child should be placed on the side opposite of the surgical site to prevent pressure on the shunt valve. Intake and output will also need to be assessed, but that is not the nurse's priority. The child is usually on nothing-by-mouth status until the nasogastric (NG) tube is removed and bowel sounds return. Pain medication should be administered by an I.V. route initially postoperatively.

Test-taking strategy: Analyze to determine what information the question asks for, which is postoperative priority for a client with shunt placement. Consider safety needs following surgery and immediate nursing care. Review nursing care in the immediate postoperative period if you had difficulty answering this question.

Client needs category: Physiological integrity

Client needs subcategory: Basic care and comfort

Cognitive level: Applying

25. The nurse is caring for a client in the diagnostic studies area of the hospital. Which information should a nurse provide to the parents of a child undergoing testing for muscular dystrophy?

☐ **1.** Genitals will be covered by a lead apron.
☐ **2.** Local anesthetic will be used for the test.
☐ **3.** Electrode wires will be attached to the scalp.
☐ **4.** A fiber-optic endoscope will be inserted into a joint.

Answer: 2

Rationale: A muscle biopsy, used to confirm the diagnosis of muscular dystrophy, shows the degeneration of muscle fibers and infiltration of fatty tissue. It is typically performed using a local anesthetic. Genitals are covered by a lead apron during an X-ray examination, which is used to detect osseous, not muscular, problems. Electrode wires are attached to the scalp during an electro-encephalography to observe brain wave activity; this test is not used to diagnose muscular dystrophy. Arthroscopy, also not used to test for muscular dystrophy, involves the insertion of a fiber-optic scope into a joint.

Test-taking strategy: Analyze to determine what information the question asks for, which is information to provide parents on diagnostic testing for muscular dystrophy. Recall that muscular dystrophy involves analysis of nerve fibers obtained invasively leading to the answer of local anesthetic. Eliminate options 1, 3, and 4 as these diagnostic testing sites include areas not used in muscle fiber testing. Review definite testing for muscular dystrophy if you had difficulty answering this question.

Client needs category: Physiological integrity

Client needs subcategory: Basic care and comfort

Cognitive level: Applying

---

26. A nurse is caring for a 7-month-old who has just had surgical repair of a cleft palate. Which instruction should be included in the discharge teaching to the parents?

☐ **1.** Continue a normal diet.
☐ **2.** Continue using arm restraints at home.
☐ **3.** Do not allow the child to drink from a cup.
☐ **4.** Establish good mouth care and proper brushing.

Answer: 2

Rationale: Cleft palate is a congenital deformity that, if not treated, causes speech problems, feeding difficulty, and maxillofacial growth and dentition deviations. Surgical repair is suggested before the client is 1 year old. Discharge instructions include arm restraints used at home to keep the child's hands away from the mouth until the palate is healed. A soft diet is recommended; no food harder than mashed potatoes can be eaten. Fluids are best taken from a cup. Proper mouth care is encouraged after the palate is healed.

Test-taking strategy: Analyze to determine what information the question asks for, which is discharge instruction following cleft palate repair. Recall the nature and placement of cleft palate including special care needs for the areas inside and coming in contact with the mouth. Eliminate options 1 and 4 as appropriate for a normal oral cavity. Eliminate option 3 as the cup is acceptable following repair. Review the child's age and immediate home care needs, and recall postoperative interventions following cleft palate repair if you had difficulty answering this question.

Client needs category: Physiological integrity

Client needs subcategory: Physiological adaptation

Cognitive level: Applying

27. In teaching a group of parents about monitoring for urinary tract infection (UTI) in preschoolers, the nurse should mention which finding as most indicative of the need to have a child evaluated?

- ☐ **1.** The child voids only twice in any 6-hour period.
- ☐ **2.** The child exhibits incontinence after being toilet trained.
- ☐ **3.** The child has difficulty sitting still for more than a 30-minute period.
- ☐ **4.** The child's urine smells strongly of ammonia after standing for more than 2 hours.

Answer: 2

Rationale: A child who exhibits incontinence after being toilet trained should be evaluated for UTI. Most urine smells strongly of ammonia after standing for more than 2 hours, so this does not necessarily indicate UTI. The other options are not reasons for parents to suspect problems with their child's urinary system.

Test-taking strategy: Analyze to determine what information the question asks for, which is indications of a UTI in preschoolers. Consider the common signs and symptoms of UTI and relate to a preschool-age child. Recall that in the adult, UTI symptoms include urinary frequency and relate to incontinence to the preschooler. Review signs of UTI in pediatrics if you had difficulty answering this question.

Client needs category: Safe and effective care environment

Client needs subcategory: Coordinated care

Cognitive level: Applying

---

28. A nurse is evaluating essential nutrition for a burn client. Which statement best describes the nutritional needs?

- ☐ **1.** A child needs 100 cal/kg during hospitalization.
- ☐ **2.** The hypermetabolic state after a burn injury leads to poor healing.
- ☐ **3.** Caloric needs can be lowered by controlling environmental temperature.
- ☐ **4.** Maintaining a hypermetabolic rate will lower the child's risk of infection.

Answer: 2

Rationale: A burn injury causes a hypermetabolic state that leads to protein and lipid catabolism, which affects wound healing. Caloric intake should be 1½ to 2 times the basal metabolic rate, with a minimum of 1.5 to 2 g/kg of body weight of protein daily. Keeping the temperature within a normal range lets the body function efficiently and use calories for healing and normal physiological processes. If the temperature is too warm or cold, energy must be used for warming or cooling, taking energy away from tissue repair. High metabolic rates increase the risk of infection

Test-taking strategy: Analyze to determine what information the question asks for, which is the nutritional needs of a burn client. Consider the increased nutritional needs related to metabolism and wound healing. Without the essential nutrients in the diet, healing and growth and development may be compromised. Review the nutritional needs of the burn client if you had difficulty answering this question.

Client needs category: Physiological integrity

Client needs subcategory: Basic care and comfort

Cognitive level: Analyzing

29. The nurse is providing anticipatory guidance to a 16-year-old female at her well checkup. Which topics would be included in the discussion? Select all that apply.

☐ **1.** Menstrual period irregularities
☐ **2.** Driving responsibilities
☐ **3.** Protection from sexually transmitted infections
☐ **4.** Anxiety related to career choices
☐ **5.** Childhood diseases
☐ **6.** Vaccination records

Answer: 2, 3, 4

Rationale: Anticipatory guidance is provided to the client to discuss future activities related to growth and development. Driving, sexual development, and career choices are the next stage in development for a 16-year-old. The client typically would have had a menstrual period for a few years already. Childhood diseases and vaccination records are past occurrences.

Test-taking strategies: Analyze to determine what information the question asks for, which is appropriate anticipatory guidance topics. The key word is "anticipatory," meaning anticipated or in the future. Select the topics that are typical in the next stage of development or in young adulthood. Review anticipatory guidance topics and growth and development if you had difficulty answering this question.

Client needs category: Health promotion and maintenance

Client needs subcategory: None

Cognitive level: Applying

---

30. A healthy client comes to the clinic for a routine examination. When auscultating lower lung lobes, the nurse anticipates which type of breath sound?

☐ **1.** Bronchial.
☐ **2.** Tracheal.
☐ **3.** Vesicular.
☐ **4.** Bronchovesicular.

Answer: 3

Rationale: Vesicular breath sounds are soft, low-pitched sounds normally heard over the lower lobes of the lung. They are prolonged on inhalation and shortened on exhalation. Bronchial breath sounds are loud, high-pitched sounds normally heard next to the trachea; they are discontinuous and loudest during exhalation. Tracheal breath sounds are harsh, discontinuous sounds heard over the trachea during inhalation or exhalation. Bronchovesicular breath sounds are medium-pitched, continuous sounds that occur during inhalation or exhalation and are best heard over the upper third of the sternum and between the scapulae.

Test-taking strategy: Analyze to determine what information the question asks for, which is anticipated breath sounds in a healthy client. Memorization and recognition of normal breath sounds are essential to answer this question. Review the anatomy of the lungs and breath sound characteristics if you had difficulty answering this question.

Client needs category: Health promotion and maintenance

Client needs subcategory: None

Cognitive level: Applying

31. The nurse is preparing to do a 12-lead ECG on a client. Indicate the correct area where the V₂ electrode should be placed on the figure below.

Answer:

Rationale: The V₂ electrode should be placed over the fourth intercostal space, at the left sternal border.

Test-taking strategy: Analyze to determine what information the question asks for, which is placement of the V₂ electrode during ECG monitoring. Recall that V₂ is one of the six precordial leads. Review the anatomy of chest, and correct placement of electrodes for a 12-lead ECG if you had difficulty answering this question.

Client needs category: Safe and effective care environment

Client needs subcategory: Coordinated care

Cognitive level: Applying

---

32. A client is ready to be discharged after arthroscopic knee surgery. Which information would the nurse expect the physician to write on the discharge instructions?

☐ **1.** "Ice and elevate the extremity for 12 hours after discharge."

☐ **2.** "Infection should not be a problem because of the small incision size."

☐ **3.** "Swelling and coolness of the joint and limb are normal right after surgery."

☐ **4.** "Take acetaminophen with codeine every 4 hours as necessary for pain relief."

Answer: 4

Rationale: Mild to moderate pain is normal after this type of surgery and can be relieved by oral opioid analgesics. To minimize swelling, the client should ice and elevate the extremity for at least 24 hours after surgery. Infection is a potential problem after an invasive procedure, regardless of the incision size. Swelling and coolness of the joint and limb may indicate complications from tourniquet use during surgery.

Test-taking strategy: Analyze to determine what information the question asks for, which is anticipated discharge instructions. Consider that pain is a priority concern after a surgical procedure. Review postoperative management, and the potential complications of arthroscopy if you had difficulty answering this question.

Client needs category: Physiological integrity

Client needs subcategory: Basic care and comfort

Cognitive level: Applying

33. The nurse is caring for an elderly resident with a cough. The resident has standing orders for guaifenesin syrup 200 mg, P.O., every 4 hours. The nurse has a dosage of 100-mg/5-mL. Mark on the medicine cup the amount of syrup the nurse would pour.

Answer:

Rationale: Use the formula

$$\frac{\text{Desired}}{\text{Have}} \times \text{Quantity} = \frac{200\,\text{mg}}{100\,\text{mg}} \times 5\,\text{mL} = \frac{1000\,\text{mg/mL}}{100\,\text{mg}} = 10\,\text{mL}$$

Test-taking strategy: Analyze to determine what information the question asks for, which is dosage of guaifenesin syrup to pour for a correct dose. Use knowledge of dosage calculations to arrive at the correct dose. Also, for this dosage, use of mental math is appropriate, since 200 mg is double the proportion in the ratio of mg per mL; thus, doubling 100 to 200 mg means doubling 5 to 10 mL. Recall that 1 mL = 1 cc. Review dosage calculations if you had difficulty answering this question.

Client needs category: Physiological integrity

Client needs subcategory: Pharmacological therapies

Cognitive level: Applying

---

34. The nurse is caring for a client with possible Cushing's syndrome undergoing diagnostic testing. The physician orders lab work and a dexamethasone suppression test. Which parameter is measured with the dexamethasone suppression test?

☐ **1.** The amount of dexamethasone in the system.
☐ **2.** Cortisol levels after the system is challenged.
☐ **3.** Changes in certain body chemicals, which are altered in depression.
☐ **4.** Cortisol levels before and after the system is challenged with a synthetic steroid.

Answer: 4

Rationale: The dexamethasone suppression test measures cortisol levels before and after the system is challenged with a synthetic steroid. The dexamethasone suppression test does not measure dexamethasone or body chemicals altered in depression. Dexamethasone is used to challenge the cortisol level.

Test-taking strategy: Analyze to determine what information the question asks for, which is the parameter measured in a dexamethasone suppression test. The key word is "suppression" indicating a reduction. Recall that dexamethasone is an exogenous steroid that provides negative feedback to the pituitary to suppress the secretion of adrenocorticotropic hormone. A normal result in the decrease is cortisol level. Review the dexamethasone suppression test if you had difficulty answering this question.

Client needs category: Health promotion and maintenance

Client needs subcategory: None

Cognitive level: Applying

35. During a routine physical examination, a firm mass is palpated in the right breast of a 35-year-old female client. Which assessment or client history finding would suggest breast cancer rather than fibrocystic disease?

☐ **1.** History of early menarche.
☐ **2.** Cyclic change in mass size.
☐ **3.** History of anovulatory cycles.
☐ **4.** Increased vascularity of the breast.

Answer: 4

Rationale: Increase in breast size or vascularity is consistent with breast cancer. Early menarche as well as late menopause or a history of anovulatory cycles is associated with fibrocystic disease. Masses associated with fibrocystic disease of the breast are firm, most commonly located in the upper outer quadrant of the breast, and increase in size prior to menstruation. They may be bilateral in a mirror image and are typically well demarcated and freely movable.

Test-taking strategy: Analyze to determine what information the question asks for, which is assessment or history finding associated with breast cancer. Recall that cancer has an increased blood supply and feeds the cancer. Research studies have confirmed that whole breast vascularity indicated growth and metastatic potential of a breast cancer. Review the pathophysiology and clinical manifestations of breast cancer and fibrocystic disease if you had difficulty answering this question.

Client needs category: Health promotion and maintenance

Client needs subcategory: None

Cognitive level: Applying

---

36. The licensed practical nurse (LPN) is coassigned with a registered nurse (RN) who is administering I.V. hydrocortisone (Solu-Cortef); 40 mg b.i.d. Which laboratory value would the nurses expect to be elevated as a result of this medication regimen?

☐ **1.** Calcium.
☐ **2.** Glucose.
☐ **3.** Magnesium.
☐ **4.** Potassium.

Answer: 2

Rationale: Hydrocortisone (Solu-Cortef) is used in the treatment of a variety of disease processes mainly for the medication's anti-inflammatory immunosuppressant activity. Corticosteroids increase blood sugar and tend to lower serum potassium and calcium levels. Their effect on magnesium is not substantial.

Test-taking strategy: Analyze to determine what information the question asks for, which is anticipated lab value elevation following I.V. hydrocortisone administration. Consider the action of corticosteroids within the body and also that illness effects blood glucose levels. Review the action of corticosteroids in the body, and laboratory values if you had difficulty answering this question.

Client needs category: Physiological integrity

Client needs subcategory: Pharmacological therapies

Cognitive level: Analyzing

37. When caring for a client on the medical unit, which precaution, unique to phenytoin (Dilantin), must be taken when administering to a client with an NG tube for feeding?

☐ **1.** Check the phenytoin level after giving the drug to monitor for toxicity.

☐ **2.** Elevate the head of the bed before giving phenytoin through the NG tube.

☐ **3.** Give phenytoin 1 hour before or 2 hours after NG tube feedings to ensure absorption.

☐ **4.** Verify proper placement of the NG tube by placing the end of the tube in a glass of water and observing for bubbles.

Answer: 3

Rationale: Nutritional supplements and milk interfere with the absorption of phenytoin, decreasing its effectiveness. Phenytoin levels are typically checked before giving the drug, and the drug is withheld for elevated levels to avoid compounding toxicity. The head of the bed should be elevated when giving any drug or solution, so this is not specific to phenytoin administration. The nurse verifies NG tube placement by checking for stomach contents before giving drugs and feedings.

Test-taking strategy: Analyze to determine what information the question asks for, which is precautions when administering phenytoin via an NG tube. Consider both (1) precautions when giving the medication through the NG tube and (2) normal considerations of the medication use. Consider phenytoin considerations the same as oral administration. Review safety precautions specific to NG tubes and phenytoin administration if you had difficulty answering this question.

Client needs category: Physiological integrity

Client needs subcategory: Pharmacological therapies

Cognitive level: Applying

---

38. A client is undergoing peritoneal dialysis. The dialysate dwell time is completed, and the clamp is opened to allow the dialysate to drain. The nurse notes that drainage has stopped and that only 500 mL has drained; the amount of dialysate instilled was 1,500 mL. Which intervention should be done first?

☐ **1.** Change the client's position.

☐ **2.** Call the physician.

☐ **3.** Check the catheter for kinks or obstruction.

☐ **4.** Clamp the catheter and instill more dialysate at the next exchange time.

Answer: 3

Rationale: The first intervention should be to check for kinks and obstructions because that could be preventing drainage. After checking for kinks, have the client change position to promote drainage. Do not give the next scheduled exchange until the dialysate is drained because abdominal distention will occur, unless the output is within the parameters set by the physician. If unable to get more output despite checking for kinks and changing the client's position, the nurse should then call the physician to determine the proper intervention.

Test-taking strategy: Analyze to determine what information the question asks for, which is nursing action when peritoneal dialysate drainage has stopped. Note the key word as "first" intervention, indicating that other choices could be correct but completed at a later time. Focus on the most obvious causes of lack of dialysate drainage and use the process of elimination to select the answer. Review care for peritoneal dialysis if you had difficulty answering this question.

Client needs category: Physiological integrity

Client needs subcategory: Reduction of risk potential

Cognitive level: Analyzing

39. A client has been hospitalized with a diagnosis of conversion disorder blindness. Which statement best explains this manifestation?

☐ **1.** The client is suppressing true feelings.
☐ **2.** The client's anxiety has been relieved through physical symptoms.
☐ **3.** The client is acting indifferent because he/she does not want to show actual fear.
☐ **4.** The client's needs are being met, so he/she does not need to be anxious.

Answer: 2

Rationale: Conversion accomplishes anxiety reduction through the production of a physical symptom symbolically linked to an underlying conflict. The client is not aware of the internal conflict. Hospitalization does not remove the source of the conflict.

Test-taking strategy: Analyze to determine what information the question asks for, which is explanation of conversion disorder. Recall that conversion disorder is an anxiety disorder. Also, note that conversion means changing in form or function. Discriminate between options 2 and 4 as they are the only options dealing with anxiety. Eliminate option 4 as client needs are not being met. Review conversion disorders if you had difficulty answering this question.

Client needs category: Psychosocial integrity

Client needs subcategory: None

Cognitive level: Analyzing

---

40. The licensed practical nurse (LPN) unit manager is planning clinical assignments at a skilled rehabilitation unit. The nurse realizes that a new client with herpes zoster has been placed on the unit. Which staff members are able to be assigned to the client? Select all that apply.

☐ **1.** A nurse who has a negative rubella titer
☐ **2.** A nurse who has never had chickenpox
☐ **3.** A nurse who is positive to a tuberculin (TB) test
☐ **4.** A nurse who obtains yearly influenza vaccines
☐ **5.** A nurse who never received the varicella-zoster vaccine

Answer: 1, 3, 4

Rationale: Many facilities require a varicella titer on hire to document staff immune status. The unit manager assigns staff members who have either been exposed to varicella (by having the chickenpox) or received the varicella-zoster vaccine. A staff member who has a negative rubella titer will need a rubella injection but is able to care for a client with herpes zoster. Those with a positive TB test will have a chest x-ray to confirm no active disease process. Yearly influenza vaccines are encouraged.

Test-taking strategy: Use the process of elimination to relate the herpes zoster condition to the status of each staff member. Consider the ability of the herpes zoster client to infect the staff member, which could potentially spread the communicable disease. Recall that herpes zoster is caused by the reactivation of the varicella-zoster virus. Review the relationship between the herpes zoster virus and chickenpox if you had difficult answering this question.

Client needs category: Safe and effective care environment

Client needs subcategory: Safety and infection control

Cognitive level: Analyzing

41. A pediatric nurse is providing discharge instructions for the family of a school-age child with idiopathic thrombocytopenia. Which activity should be restricted until further notice?

☐ **1.** Swimming.
☐ **2.** Bicycle riding.
☐ **3.** Computer games.
☐ **4.** Exposure to large crowds.

Answer: 2

Rationale: When routine blood counts reveal the platelet level is 100,000/mm³ or less, the child should not engage in contact sports, bicycle or scooter riding, climbing, or other activities that could lead to injury (especially to the head). Swimming releases energy, builds muscle, and allows the child to compete without risking injury, as long as the child follows normal safety precautions. Computer games do not cause physical injury. It is not necessary for this child to avoid large crowds because idiopathic thrombocytopenia does not suppress the immune system.

Test-taking strategy: Analyze to determine what information the question asks for, which is activity restriction for a pediatric client with idiopathic thrombocytopenia. Recall the definition of thrombocytopenia as an abnormal drop in platelet count. Select the option that could include possible bruising or bleeding. Review idiopathic thrombocytopenia if you had difficulty answering this question.

Client needs category: Safe and effective care environment

Client needs subcategory: Safety and infection control

Cognitive level: Applying

42. A toddler in respiratory distress is admitted to the pediatric intensive care unit. When the toddler refuses to keep the oxygen face mask on, the mother tries to help. Which action by the nurse is most appropriate?

☐ **1.** Giving the child a favorite toy to play with.
☐ **2.** Asking the mother to read the child's favorite book.
☐ **3.** Administering a strong sedative so the child will sleep.
☐ **4.** Telling the child that the face mask will help with breathing.

Answer: 2

Rationale: Having the mother read the child's favorite book will ease anxiety and provide comfort to the child. Although giving the child a favorite toy is also appropriate, the child needs the mother's comfort because the face mask is frightening. Sedation is contraindicated because it can mask signs of respiratory distress. A toddler is too young to understand that something will make him/her feel better.

Test-taking strategy: Analyze to determine what information the question asks for, which is nursing action most appropriate when attempting to get a toddler to wear a face mask. Recall that toddlers are fearful of strange surroundings and strangers. Consider that the mother might be most successful in getting the toddler to comply. Review the child's age and the circumstances surrounding hospitalization, with ways to obtain cooperation if you had difficulty answering this question.

Client needs category: Safe and effective care environment

Client needs subcategory: Coordinated care

Cognitive level: Applying

43. The nurse is caring for a 30-month-old client in the pediatrician's office. The client is being assessed for autism spectrum disorder. While assessing the client with the physician, which clinical characteristics does the nurse anticipate documenting in the medical record? Select all that apply.

- ☐ **1.** Talking with an imaginary playmate
- ☐ **2.** Sitting on the lap of the office staff
- ☐ **3.** Avoiding eye-to-eye contact with others
- ☐ **4.** Using repetitive behaviors throughout session
- ☐ **5.** Displaying separation anxiety when the parent leaves the room

Answer: 3, 4

Rationale: Autism spectrum disorder is a group of complex disorders of brain development. These disorders are characterized, in varying degrees, by difficulties in social interaction, verbal and nonverbal communication, and repetitive behaviors. When assessing for symptoms of autism spectrum disorder, the nurse would anticipate documenting avoiding eye-to-eye contact and using the repetitive behaviors. Talking with an imaginary playmate, sitting on the lap of office staff, and experiencing separation anxiety are common characteristics in the toddler/early preschooler age.

Test-taking strategy: Analyze to determine what information the question asks for, which is the characteristics of autism spectrum disorder. Analyze the responses for age-appropriate characteristics and recall that children with autism have difficulty with social interaction. Review the characteristics of autism if you had difficulty answering this question.

Client needs category: Physiological integrity

Client needs subcategory: Physiological adaptation

Cognitive level: Analyzing

---

44. A 6-year-old boy is admitted to a pediatric unit for the treatment of osteomyelitis. The nurse knows that the peak incidence in children is between ages 1 and 12 and that boys are affected two to three times more commonly than girls. Which organism most commonly causes osteomyelitis?

- ☐ **1.** *Staphylococcus epidermidis.*
- ☐ **2.** *Escherichia coli* O157.H7.
- ☐ **3.** *Pneumocystis carinii.*
- ☐ **4.** *S. aureus.*

Answer: 4

Rationale: S. aureus is the most common causative pathogen of osteomyelitis; the usual source of the infection is an upper respiratory infection (URI) or skin lesion. *S. epidermidis* is a microorganism found on the skin of healthy individuals. *E. coli* O157:H7, which is in uncooked meat, can cause a severe case of diarrhea. *P. carinii* causes pneumonia in clients with human immunodeficiency virus (HIV) or acquired immunodeficiency syndrome but does not normally cause healthy individuals to become ill.

Test-taking strategy: Analyze to determine what information the question asks for, which is causative pathogen of osteomyelitis. Recall that osteo (meaning bone) and myelitis (meaning infection) and consider possible sources of the bone infection. Eliminate options 1, 2, and 3 as either causative organisms for other disorders or normal to healthy individuals. Review osteomyelitis sources if you had difficulty answering this question.

Client needs category: Physiological integrity

Client needs subcategory: Physiological adaptation

Cognitive level: Applying

45. The nurse is preparing to teach a client about the prescribed medication spironolactone (Aldactone) and to monitor for adverse effects of the drug. The nurse should instruct the client about which adverse effects? Select all that apply.

- ☐ **1.** Confusion.
- ☐ **2.** Fatigue.
- ☐ **3.** Hypertension.
- ☐ **4.** Leg cramps.
- ☐ **5.** Weakness.
- ☐ **6.** Urinary retention.

Answer: 1, 2, 5

Rationale: Spironolactone (Aldactone) is used to treat hypertension and edema by removing excess fluid. Aldactone is known as a potassium-sparing diuretic. Confusion, fatigue, and weakness are signs of hyperkalemia, an adverse effect of spironolactone. Spironolactone is used to treat hypertension, so it would not produce this effect. Leg cramps are an adverse effect of hypokalemia. Urinary retention is a side effect of anticholinergics.

Test-taking strategy: Analyze to determine what information the question asks for, which is adverse effects of spironolactone. Consider the action of the medication and its potassium-sparing quality. Recall that adverse effects can be an extension of a therapeutic effect. Review spironolactone (Aldactone) actions and adverse effects if you had difficulty answering this question.

Client needs category: Physiological integrity

Client needs subcategory: Pharmacological therapies

Cognitive level: Analyzing

---

46. A client presents to the emergency room with abdominal pain and blood in the stool. The client is sweating and appears to be in moderate distress. Which nursing action would be a priority at this time?

- ☐ **1.** Obtain vital signs.
- ☐ **2.** Document history of the symptoms.
- ☐ **3.** Assess bowel sounds and abdominal tenderness.
- ☐ **4.** Insert an NG tube and connect to suction.

Answer: 1

Rationale: The priority nursing action is vital signs. Vital signs provide valuable information on the internal body system. Symptoms of shock, such as low blood pressure, a rapid weak pulse, cold clammy skin, and restlessness, can be monitored. Assessing bowel sounds and abdominal tenderness can provide useful data but is not a priority. Documentation is a lower priority and a physician's order is needed for an NG tube placement.

Test-taking strategy: Analyze to determine what information the question asks for, which is a priority action for a client with abdominal pain and an upper GI bleed. The key word is "priority" which indicates that one action occurs before another. Use the ABCs to determine priority with vital sign focus. Review symptoms of upper GI bleeding and priority nursing actions if you had difficulty answering this question.

Client needs category: Physiological integrity

Client needs subcategory: Physiological adaptation

Cognitive level: Analyzing

47. A client has received dietary instructions as part of the treatment plan for diabetes type 1. Which statement by the client should alert the nurse of needing additional instructions?

- ☐ **1.** "I'll need a bedtime snack because I take an evening dose of NPH insulin."
- ☐ **2.** "I can eat whatever I want as long as I cover the calories with sufficient insulin."
- ☐ **3.** "I can have an occasional low-calorie drink as long as I include it in my meal plan."
- ☐ **4.** "I should eat meals as scheduled, even if I'm not hungry, to prevent hypoglycemia."

Answer: 2

Rationale: Diabetes mellitus is a chronic condition associated with abnormally high glucose in the blood. The goal of dietary therapy in diabetes mellitus is to attain and maintain ideal body weight. Each client is prescribed a specific caloric intake and insulin regimen to help accomplish this goal. The other statements are correct.

Test-taking strategy: Analyze to determine what information the question asks for, which is nursing statement alerting the nurse that additional client teaching on dietary therapy is needed. The key words are "additional teaching," indicating that the statement is incorrect. Recall that dietary management of diabetes mellitus requires regular monitoring of diet along with blood sugar readings. Review the goals of dietary therapy for type 1 diabetes mellitus if you had difficulty answering this question.

Client needs category: Physiological integrity

Client needs subcategory: Basic care and comfort

Cognitive level: Analyzing

---

48. The nurse is caring for a 3-year-old diagnosed with a Wilms' tumor. If both kidneys are affected, the nurse should understand that treatment prior to surgery might include which of the following?

- ☐ **1.** Peritoneal dialysis.
- ☐ **2.** Abdominal gavage.
- ☐ **3.** Radiation and chemotherapy.
- ☐ **4.** Antibiotics and I.V. fluid therapy.

Answer: 3

Rationale: If both kidneys are involved, the child may be treated with radiation therapy or chemotherapy preoperatively to shrink the tumor, allowing more conservative therapy. Peritoneal dialysis would be needed only if the kidneys are not functioning. Abdominal gavage would not be indicated. Antibiotics are not needed because Wilms' tumor is not an infection.

Test-taking strategy: Analyze to determine what information the question asks for, which is treatment when a Wilms' tumor involves both kidneys. Recall that a Wilms' tumor is the most common cause of kidney cancer in children. Option 3 is the only option dealing with cancer treatment. Review Wilms' tumor nursing care and treatment if you had difficulty answering this question.

Client needs category: Safe and effective care environment

Client needs subcategory: Coordinated care

Cognitive level: Applying

49. The nurse is caring for a client on the neurological unit who is diagnosed with a T2 spinal cord injury secondary to a fall. When completing the plan of care, which priority nursing interventions are included? Select all that apply.

☐ **1.** Initiate a bowel/bladder regimen.
☐ **2.** Instruct to cough and deep breathe.
☐ **3.** Obtain blood pressure every 4 hours.
☐ **4.** Encourage family visitation daily.
☐ **5.** Consult a social worker for long-term planning.

Answer: 2, 3, 4

Rationale: In the immediate postinjury period, nursing interventions include coughing and deep breathing, as respirations and the airway are a priority due to the thoracic region site of injury. Also, vital signs, including blood pressure, reflect information on body system functioning. Family visitation is encouraged for client support in this difficult and anxious time. It is too early to initiative a bowel/bladder regimen and begin long-term planning, as the client's functional level may change.

Test-taking strategy: Analyze to determine what information the question asks for, which is priority nursing interventions for a client with a T2 spinal cord injury. Consider implications of trauma to the thoracic region and changing neurological status as the client gains treatment for an injury in this acute injury time frame. Review care of the client with a thoracic spinal cord injury if you had difficulty answering this question.

Client needs category: Physiological integrity
Client needs subcategory: Physiological adaptation
Cognitive level: Analyzing

50. Topical treatment with 2.5% hydrocortisone (Cortane) is prescribed for a 6-month-old infant with eczema. The mother is instructed to use the cream for no longer than 1 week. Why is this time limit appropriate?

☐ **1.** The drug loses its efficacy after prolonged use.
☐ **2.** This reduces adverse effects, such as skin atrophy and fragility.
☐ **3.** If no improvement is seen after 1 week, a stronger concentration will be prescribed.
☐ **4.** If no improvement is seen after 1 week, an antibiotic will be prescribed.

Answer: 2

Rationale: Eczema is a chronic skin disorder which involves scaly and itchy rashes. Hydrocortisone cream helps to soothe dry, itchy, or healing patches but should be used for brief periods to decrease such adverse effects as atrophy of the skin. The drug does not lose efficacy after prolonged use. A stronger concentration may not be prescribed if no improvement is seen, and an antibiotic would be inappropriate in this instance.

Test-taking strategy: Analyze to determine what information the question asks for, which is treatment protocol of hydrocortisone cream for eczema. Recall that hydrocortisone is a synthetic steroid with adverse effects in which benefits can outweigh risks. Review the use of hydrocortisone cream for eczema and the effects on various body systems if you had difficulty answering this question.

Client needs category: Physiological integrity
Client needs subcategory: Pharmacological therapies
Cognitive level: Applying

51. A 23-year-old client develops cardiac tamponade when the car hits a telephone pole; the client was not wearing seatbelt. The nurse helps the physician perform pericardiocentesis. Which outcome would indicate that pericardiocentesis has been effective?

☐ **1.** Neck vein distention.
☐ **2.** Pulsus paradoxus.
☐ **3.** Increased blood pressure.
☐ **4.** Muffled heart sounds.

Answer: 3

Rationale: Cardiac tamponade is associated with decreased cardiac output, which in turn reduces blood pressure. By removing a small amount of blood, pericardiocentesis increases blood pressure. Neck vein distention, pulsus paradoxus, and muffled heart sounds indicate persistent cardiac tamponade, meaning pericardiocentesis has not been effective.

Test-taking strategy: Analyze to determine what information the question asks for, which is signs that pericardiocentesis has been effective. Consider options that would include improved cardiac output, improved vital signs, and normalization of heart sounds. Review the disease process of cardiac tamponade with treatment results if you had difficulty answering this question.

Client needs category: Physiological integrity

Client needs subcategory: Physiological adaptation

Cognitive level: Analyzing

---

52. The nurse is caring for a child with history of strep throat. Upon current assessment, the child states abdominal pain and joint achiness. Which laboratory data would the nurse communicate with the physician immediately?

☐ **1.** Leukocytosis.
☐ **2.** Anemia.
☐ **3.** Low hemoglobin level.
☐ **4.** Normal erythrocyte sedimentation rate.

Answer: 1

Rationale: Leukocytosis can be seen as an immune response triggered by colonization of the pharynx with group A streptococci. This finding is expected in a client with rheumatic fever. Laboratory data indicating anemia or a low hemoglobin level will need to be addressed but are not critical and associated with the current disease process. A normal erythrocyte sedimentation rate would be communicated on the laboratory report.

Test-taking strategy: Analyze to determine what information the question asks for, which is laboratory data which need to be brought to the physician's attention. Recall that a history of strep throat can lead to serious complications. Analyze current symptoms and which lab data could confirm a new diagnosis, such as rheumatic fever. Review complications of strep throat and associated laboratory data if you had difficulty answering this question.

Client needs category: Physiological integrity

Client needs subcategory: Pharmacological therapies

Cognitive level: Analyzing

53. A nurse is caring for a client newly diagnosed with multiple myeloma. Which substance is associated with abnormal values early in the disease process?

- ☐ **1.** Immunoglobulins.
- ☐ **2.** Platelets.
- ☐ **3.** Red blood cells (RBCs).
- ☐ **4.** WBCs.

Answer: 1

Rationale: Multiple myeloma is characterized by malignant plasma cells that produce an increased amount of immunoglobulin that is not functional. As more malignant plasma cells are produced, there is less space in the bone marrow for RBC production. In late stages, platelets and WBCs are reduced as the bone marrow is infiltrated by malignant plasma cells.

Test-taking strategy: Analyze to determine what information the question asks for, which is abnormal blood characteristics early in the disease process. The key word is "early," indicating a change from the later stages of the disease. Review the pathophysiology of multiple myeloma and the effect on various cells of the body if you had difficulty answering this question.

Client needs category: Physiological integrity

Client needs subcategory: Reduction of risk potential

Cognitive level: Analyzing

---

54. The nurse is instructing the client prior to a colonoscopy. At which location along the colon would the nurse explain that semifluid stool turns into a mush-style stool?

Answer:

Rationale: Semifluid stool becomes a mushy, soft stool along the transverse colon prior to becoming more solid in the descending colon to the rectum.

Test-taking strategy: Analyze to determine what information the question asks for, which is where there is a change in consistency from a semifluid stool to a mushy stool. Recall that water is absorbed from the stool as the bowel contents advance along the colon to the rectum. A mushy stool occurs between the ascending and descending colon segments. Review the progression of bowel contents along the colon if you had difficulty answering this question.

Client needs category: Physiological integrity

Client needs subcategory: Reduction of risk potential

Cognitive level: Applying

55. A 20-year-old client with cystic fibrosis is being discharged with a high-frequency chest wall oscillating vest. Which statement by the client indicates an understanding of how to use the vest?

- ☐ **1.** "I'll wear the vest for 5 minutes each time a treatment is due."
- ☐ **2.** "I'll lie down to use the vest."
- ☐ **3.** "I'll require help in applying the vest."
- ☐ **4.** "I can be in any position to use the vest."

Answer: 4

Rationale: The high-frequency chest wall oscillating vest offers airway clearance treatment for individuals with cystic fibrosis. The vest system does not require special positioning or breathing to be effective. In most cases, treatments last 15 to 20 minutes and clients can manage therapy without any assistance.

Test-taking strategy: Analyze to determine what information the question asks for, which is correct statement indicating understanding of vest usage. Analyze each option for a correct statement. Review the purpose and correct use of the vest if you had difficulty answering this question.

Client needs category: Physiological integrity

Client needs subcategory: Basic care and comfort

Cognitive level: Analyzing

56. A rehabilitation nurse in an extended care setting is caring for a client injured in a swimming accident. Which intervention is most appropriate to include in a bladder program for a client in rehabilitation for a spinal cord injury?

- ☐ **1.** Insert an indwelling urinary catheter.
- ☐ **2.** Schedule intermittent catheterization every 2 to 4 hours.
- ☐ **3.** Perform a straight catheterization every 8 hours while the client is awake.
- ☐ **4.** Perform Credé's maneuver to the lower abdomen before the client voids.

Answer: 2

Rationale: Intermittent catheterization should begin every 2 to 4 hours early in treatment. When residual volume is less than 400 mL, the schedule may advance to every 4 to 6 hours. Indwelling catheters may predispose the client to infection and are removed as soon as possible. Credé's maneuver is applied after voiding to enhance bladder emptying.

Test-taking strategy: Analyze to determine what information the question asks for, which is nursing interventions to include in a bladder program. Analyze each option for the best possible method for urinary elimination. Eliminate option 4 as not relating to urinary elimination. Discriminate between the remaining three options as to which best meets the goal. Review the bladder programs if you had difficulty answering this question.

Client needs category: Physiological integrity

Client needs subcategory: Basic care and comfort

Cognitive level: Applying

57. The nurse is caring for a client on the urinary unit. When providing report to the next shift, it is noted that the client has osteopenia and history of renal calculi. Which of the following disorders would the nurse suspect?

☐ **1.** Hyperparathyroidism.
☐ **2.** Hypoparathyroidism.
☐ **3.** Hypopituitarism.
☐ **4.** Hypothyroidism.

Answer: 1

Rationale: Hyperparathyroidism is characterized by osteopenia and renal calculi secondary to over-production of parathyroid hormone. The hallmark symptom of hypoparathyroidism is tetany from hypocalcemia. Hypopituitarism presents with extreme weight loss and atrophy of all endocrine glands. Symptoms of hypothyroidism include hair loss, weight gain, and cold intolerance.

Test-taking strategy: Analyze to determine what information the question asks for, which is disorder characterized by osteopenia and renal calculi. Focus on the pathophysiology of the disorders mentioned and review the clinical manifestations of each. Review the endocrine disorders if you had difficulty answering this question.

Client needs category: Physiological integrity

Client needs subcategory: Physiological adaptation

Cognitive level: Applying

---

58. A client arrives to the emergency department with suspected appendicitis. The admitting nurse performs an assessment. Order the following steps according to the sequence in which they are performed. Use all of the options.

1. Percuss all four abdominal quadrants.
2. Obtain a health history.
3. Inspect the abdomen, noting the shape, contours, and any visible peristalsis or pulsations.
4. Auscultate bowel sounds in all four quadrants.
5. Gently palpate all four quadrants, saving the painful area for last.

Answer: 2, 3, 4, 1, 5

Rationale: The first step in the data collection process is to obtain a health history. Then, the nurse should visually inspect the abdomen. Of the three remaining steps, it is important to auscultate before percussing or palpating the client's abdomen. Touching or palpating the abdomen before listening may actually change the bowel sounds, leading to faulty data.

Test-taking strategy: Analyze to determine what information the question asks for, which is sequence of actions with suspected appendicitis. Always begin with questioning for data collection. Second, begin the abdominal-focused assessment progressing from least contact to most contact. Review basic assessment techniques if you had difficulty answering this question.

Client needs category: Physiological integrity

Client needs subcategory: Physiological adaptation

Cognitive level: Analyzing

59. The nurse is evaluating the client's knowledge after gastric bypass surgery. Which statement, made by the client, indicates a good understanding of nutritional needs? Select all that apply.

☐ **1.** "I will eat 3 small meals daily."
☐ **2.** "I will consume a high-protein diet."
☐ **3.** "I will limit my fluid intake to 1,300 mL/day."
☐ **4.** "I will drink milk to increase my calcium intake."
☐ **5.** "I will need a vitamin B$_{12}$ injection to be given."

Answer: 2, 4, 5

Rationale: The client indicates a good understanding of dietary requirements following gastric bypass surgery by stating that a high-protein diet minimizes rapid stomach emptying and the dumping syndrome. Calcium deficiency and vitamin B$_{12}$ deficiency are late complications of surgery. Additional calcium-rich foods in the diet and life-long vitamin B$_{12}$ supplementation may be necessary. Both the frequency of meals and amount of fluid intake need increase following surgery.

Test-taking strategy: Analyze to determine what information the question asks for, which is evaluation of client knowledge regarding gastric bypass surgery. Consider that gastric bypass surgery makes changes to the digestive system requiring lifestyle changes in nutrition and eating habits. Review changes in behavior and nutritional requirements following gastric bypass surgery if you had difficulty answering this question.

Client needs category: Physiological integrity

Client needs subcategory: Basic care and comfort

Cognitive level: Analyzing

60. A mother infected with HIV asks the nurse about the possibility of breast-feeding her neonate. Which response by the nurse would be most appropriate?

☐ **1.** "Breast-feeding isn't an option."
☐ **2.** "Breast-feeding would be best for your baby."
☐ **3.** "Breast-feeding is only an option if the mother is taking zidovudine (Retrovir)."
☐ **4.** "Breast-feeding is an option if milk is expressed and fed by a bottle."

Answer: 1

Rationale: Mothers infected with HIV are unable to breast-feed because the virus has been isolated in breast milk and could be transmitted to the infant. Taking zidovudine does not prevent transmission. The risk of breast-feeding is not associated with direct contact with the breast but with the possibility of the HIV contained in the breast milk.

Test-taking strategy: Analyze to determine what information the question asks for, which is correct information regarding HIV transmission in breast milk. Recall how HIV is transmitted and that HIV has been found in breast milk. If unsure, eliminate options 2 and 4 as essentially the same. Eliminate option 3 as medication does not eliminate the virus completely. Review breast-feeding and HIV transmission if you had difficulty answering this question.

Client needs category: Health promotion and maintenance

Client needs subcategory: None

Cognitive level: Applying

61. When a 6-month-old infant is admitted for intestinal obstruction, which assessment finding should alert the nurse to a potential problem?

☐ **1.** Presence of the Moro reflex.
☐ **2.** The child's playing with his/her feet.
☐ **3.** Eruption of the first tooth.
☐ **4.** Rolling from the stomach to back.

Answer: 1

Rationale: By 6 months of age, the Moro (startle) reflex should no longer be observed. Playing with the feet, eruption of the first tooth, and rolling from the stomach to back are all normal for a 6-month-old infant.

Test-taking strategy: Analyze to determine what information the question asks for, which is an assessment finding that is inconsistent with 6 months of age. Note that there is no relation to the diagnosis needed. Recall developmental milestones. If unsure, recall that the Moro reflex is assessed at birth. Review the infant's age and developmental milestones if you had difficulty answering this question.

Client needs category: Health promotion and maintenance

Client needs subcategory: None

Cognitive level: Analyzing

---

62. The medication nurse is administering noon medications. Which assessment finding should alert the nurse to change the intranasal route for vasopressin administration?

☐ **1.** Mucous membrane irritation.
☐ **2.** Severe coughing.
☐ **3.** Nosebleeds.
☐ **4.** Pneumonia.

Answer: 1

Rationale: Mucous membrane irritation caused by a cold or allergy renders the intranasal route unreliable. Severe coughing, pneumonia, or nosebleeds should not interfere with the intranasal route.

Test-taking strategy: Analyze to determine what information the question asks for, which is assessment finding requiring a change from intranasal route. Focus on nasal structures that eliminate options 2 and 4. Recall the route of administration and consider which assessment finding would interfere with the drug's absorption. Review the intranasal route of administration if you had difficulty answering this question.

Client needs category: Physiological integrity

Client needs subcategory: Pharmacological therapies

Cognitive level: Applying

63. A nurse is developing a teaching plan for a client who will undergo a stapedectomy for the treatment of otosclerosis. Which instruction should the plan include?

- ☐ **1.** Ringing in the ears is common after surgery.
- ☐ **2.** Vertigo and dizziness are common after surgery.
- ☐ **3.** Hearing should return immediately after surgery.
- ☐ **4.** Excessive drainage is common after surgery.

Answer: 2

Rationale: Vertigo is the most common complication of stapedectomy. The client should move slowly to avoid triggering or worsening vertigo and should ask for assistance with ambulation. Ringing in the ears (tinnitus) rarely follows this surgery and should be reported to the physician. Hearing typically decreases after surgery because of ear packing and tissue swelling, but commonly returns over the next 2 to 6 weeks. Usually, postoperative drainage and pain are minimal; excessive drainage should be reported.

Test-taking strategy: Analyze to determine what information the question asks for, which is instruction included in the teaching plan. Recall the physiology and function of the stapes which are impacted by the surgery. Also consider that the middle ear is essential in the function of balance. Review complication from a stapedectomy if you had difficulty answering this question.

Client needs category: Physiological integrity

Client needs subcategory: Reduction of risk potential

Cognitive level: Applying

64. When providing discharge teaching for a client with uric acid calculi, the nurse should include an instruction to avoid which type of diet?

- ☐ **1.** Low calcium.
- ☐ **2.** Low oxalate.
- ☐ **3.** High oxalate.
- ☐ **4.** High purine.

Answer: 4

Rationale: To control uric acid calculi, the client should follow a low-purine diet, which excludes high-purine foods such as organ meats. The other diets do not control uric acid calculi.

Test-taking strategy: Analyze to determine what information the question asks for, which is dietary instruction for a client with uric acid calculi. Recall the cause of uric acid calculi and dietary guidelines of a low-purine diet as uric acids are the waste product of purines. Review a low-purine diet if you had difficulty answering this question.

Client needs category: Physiological integrity

Client needs subcategory: Reduction of risk potential

Cognitive level: Applying

65. The nurse is caring for a client diagnosed with angina pain who underwent a cardiac catheterization. When assessing the postprocedural dressing at the left femoral access site, the nurse sees bloody drainage soaking through the dressing. Identify the site where the nurse should apply steady, consistent pressure until clotting occurs.

Answer:

Rationale: The X is placed approximately 2 inches above the femoral artery access site, where the femoral artery is punctured. Steady pressure assists the body in diminishing bleeding and improving clotting.

Test-taking strategy: Analyze to determine what information the question asks for, which is pressure site to slow/stop bleeding of the femoral artery following puncture. Use knowledge of medical terminology (femoral = femur) and anatomical position (left from right). Review care following cardiac catheterization if you had difficulty answering this question.

Client needs category: Physiological integrity

Client needs subcategory: Reduction of risk potential

Cognitive level: Applying

---

66. The nurse is caring for a client who has been placed on phenobarbital 30 mg daily for newly diagnosed seizure activity. Which instruction should be included in client teaching specifically related to anticonvulsant drug efficacy?

☐ **1.** Wear a medical identification bracelet.
☐ **2.** Maintain a seizure frequency chart.
☐ **3.** Avoid potentially hazardous activities.
☐ **4.** Discontinue the drug immediately if adverse effects are suspected.

Answer: 2

Rationale: Ongoing evaluation of therapeutic effects can be accomplished by maintaining a seizure frequency chart that indicates the date, time, and nature of all seizure activities. These data may be helpful in making dosage alterations and specific drug selection. Avoidance of hazardous activities and wearing a medical identification bracelet are ways to minimize dangers related to seizure activity, but these factors do not affect drug efficacy. Anticonvulsant drugs should never be discontinued abruptly because of the risk of developing status epilepticus.

Test-taking strategy: Analyze to determine what information the question asks for, which is instruction specifically related to drug efficacy. The key words are "drug efficacy," which means amount of drug to produce the drug effect. The option that would reflect the therapeutic effect is to maintain tracking of seizure activity. Review the therapeutic activity of anticonvulsants if you had difficulty answering this question.

Client needs category: Physiological integrity

Client needs subcategory: Pharmacological therapies

Cognitive level: Applying

67. The nurse is triaging phone calls at a local pediatrician's office. Which statement by the parent of a child being treated for pinworms indicates that further teaching is needed?

- [ ] **1.** "I'll make my child wash his/her hands well before meals."
- [ ] **2.** "I'll warn my child to avoid sharing hairbrushes and hats to prevent spreading pinworms to others."
- [ ] **3.** "I'll give my child only one dose of medication."
- [ ] **4.** "I'll keep my child's nails short."

Answer: 2

Rationale: Sharing hairbrushes and hats reduces the spread of lice, not pinworms. Hands should be washed well before food preparation and eating to avoid ingesting eggs that may be under the fingernails from scratching the itchy infested perianal area. Only a single dose of medication, such as mebendazole, is needed to treat pinworms. Keeping the fingernails short reduces the risk of carrying eggs under the nails.

Test-taking strategy: Analyze to determine what information the question asks for, which is parent statements that need further instruction. The key words are "need further instruction" indicating an incorrect statement. Analyze each option for an incorrect statement related to pinworms. Recall the cause and location of pinworms which will lead to the correct answer. Review nursing instruction of pinworms if you had difficulty answering this question.

Client needs category: Safe and effective care environment

Client needs subcategory: Safety and infection control

Cognitive level: Applying

---

68. The nurse is caring for a homeless client with pneumonia. Laboratory testing reveals the following results: blood urea nitrogen (BUN) 180 mg/dL, creatinine 30 mg/dL, potassium 6.2 mEq/L, and hemoglobin 6.2%. Based on the physician's order below, which drug order should the nurse question?

Physician Orders	
12/21/10 0900	Gentamicin 180 mg I.V. piggyback every 8 hours
	Erythropoietin 50 units/kg subcutaneously Monday, Wednesday, and Friday
	Aluminum hydroxide gel 500 mg P.O. four times daily
	Ferrous sulfate 325 mg P.O. three times daily ———————— Garry Reynolds, MD

- [ ] **1.** Gentamicin.
- [ ] **2.** Erythropoietin.
- [ ] **3.** Aluminum hydroxide gel.
- [ ] **4.** Ferrous sulfate.

Answer: 1

Rationale: Based on the high BUN, creatinine, and potassium levels, the client is in renal failure. Gentamicin is nephrotoxic and can exacerbate the renal failure. Ferrous sulfate and erythropoietin would be given to treat the client's anemia. Aluminum hydroxide gel would also be appropriate because it binds with phosphate, which is elevated in renal failure.

Test-taking strategy: Analyze to determine what information the question asks for, which is drug order to be questioned. The key word is "questioned" indicating a problem. Analyze each option for correct dosage, adverse effects, etc., in relation to the laboratory information provided in the question. Review the laboratory results and medication contraindications if you had difficulty answering this question.

Client needs category: Physiological integrity

Client needs subcategory: Reduction of risk potential

Cognitive level: Analyzing

69. The nurse is working in an internal medicine office. A daughter brings her elderly mother to the doctor's appointment. Upon reviewing the medication list, the daughter states, "Which medication is prescribed to prevent a stroke?" The nurse is correct to answer which medication?

☐ **1.** Allopurinol (Zyloprim).
☐ **2.** Claritin (Loratadine).
☐ **3.** Ticlopidine (Ticlid).
☐ **4.** Methylprednisolone (Medrol).

Answer: 3

Rationale: Ticlopidine inhibits platelet aggregation by interfering with adenosine diphosphate release in the coagulation cascade and, therefore, is used to prevent thromboembolic stroke. Allopurinol is an antigout medication used to reduce uric acid. Claritin is an over-the-counter allergy medication. Methylprednisolone, a steroid with anticoagulant properties, is not used to treat thromboembolic stroke.

Test-taking strategy: Analyze to determine what information the question asks for, which is medication prescribed to prevent a stroke. Consider each option for the action and property of the medication. Review the indications for the medications listed if you had difficulty answering this question.

Client needs category: Physiological integrity

Client needs subcategory: Pharmacological therapies

Cognitive level: Applying

---

70. The nurse is caring for a client admitted to the hospital from home with a stage 3 ulcer. When describing the status of the wound, the nurse would note the deepest layer of the wound at which location?

Answer:

Rationale: The stage 3 pressure ulcer is a full-thickness skin loss extending to the subcutaneous tissue level. The subcutaneous level is below the dermis and epidermis and above the muscle layer.

Test-taking strategy: Analyze to determine what information the question asks for, which is the deepest layer affected by a stage 3 pressure ulcer. Recall that a stage 1 ulcer affects the outer layer of the skin and a stage 2 ulcer affects skin loss of the epidermis, the dermis, or both. Stage 3 then extends to the subcutaneous layer. Review pressure ulcer staging if you had difficulty answering this question.

Client needs category: Physiological integrity

Client needs subcategory: Basic care and comfort

Cognitive level: Applying

71. The nurse is volunteering at a camp for children with various medical conditions. In planning for the event, a parent asks, "What causes an acquired immune deficiency?" Which is correct for the nurse to answer?

- ☐ **1.** Age.
- ☐ **2.** Genetics.
- ☐ **3.** Environment.
- ☐ **4.** Medical treatments.

Answer: 4

Rationale: Immune deficiencies may result from medical treatments, such as medications, radiation, and transplants. Immune function may decline with age, but it is not considered the cause of acquired immune deficiency. Genetics and environment have not been shown to be factors in acquired immune deficiency.

Test-taking strategy: Analyze to determine what information the question asks for, which is the cause of acquired immune deficiency. Focus on the word *acquired* when considering the answer. Review the causes of acquired immune deficiency if you had difficulty answering this question.

Client needs category: Physiological integrity

Client needs subcategory: Physiological adaptation

Cognitive level: Applying

---

72. A nurse teaches a group of police officers about the spread of TB. Which statement by an officer indicates that teaching has been effective?

- ☐ **1.** "I could get TB by being in close proximity for a brief time with someone who has the disease."
- ☐ **2.** "I could get TB if I inhale infected droplets when an infected individual coughs."
- ☐ **3.** "I could get TB if I search the home of someone infected with TB."
- ☐ **4.** "I could get TB if I come in contact with blood from an infected person."

Answer: 2

Rationale: TB infection typically occurs from inhaling infected droplets after a person with TB coughs. Transmission usually requires close, frequent, and prolonged contact. HIV, not TB, is spread through contact with an infected person's blood.

Test-taking strategy: Analyze to determine what information the question asks for, which is correct statement related to TB transmission. Recall the transmission precautions for TB as airborne requiring inhalation for transmission. Review transmission-based precautions if you had difficulty answering this question.

Client needs category: Safe and effective care environment

Client needs subcategory: Safety and infection control

Cognitive level: Analyzing

73. The emergency room nurse is caring for a client who fell breaking the tibia. The nurse determines that a client understands the risk of compartment syndrome when knowing to report which early symptom following treatment?

☐ **1.** Heat.
☐ **2.** Paresthesia.
☐ **3.** Skin pallor.
☐ **4.** Swelling.

Answer: 2

Rationale: Compartment syndrome is the compression of the nerves, blood vessels, and muscle inside a closed space. Paresthesia is the earliest sign of compartment syndrome. Pain, heat, and swelling are also signs but occur after paresthesia. Skin pallor is not a sign of compartment syndrome.

Test-taking strategy: Analyze to determine what information the question asks for, which is an early symptom of compartment syndrome. Consider that compartment = compression. Recall the structures that compartment syndrome effects (nerves), which lead to the correct answer. Review the signs of compartment syndrome if you had difficulty answering this question.

Client needs category: Physiological integrity

Client needs subcategory: Physiological adaptation

Cognitive level: Analyzing

---

74. The nurse is teaching a client how to change an ostomy appliance via a step-by-step outline. Place the instructions in ascending chronological order.

1.	Add 1/16 to 1/8 inch to the size of the stoma.
2.	Wash stoma area and pat dry.
3.	Apply thin layer of paste around stoma.
4.	Cut stoma opening into wafer.
5.	Apply pouch.
6.	Measure the stoma site

Answer: 2, 6, 1, 4, 3, 5

Rationale: Standards of practice exist for changing ostomy appliances. Clients are taught independent care of the ostomy by changing the ostomy appliance. Adhesive remover is used to promote skin integrity when removing the old pouch. After washing, the skin must be gently but thoroughly dried. Once the stoma size is measured, an area of 1/16 to 1/8 inch is added so that the stoma is independent of any barrier. A thin layer of paste is used to help maintain the pouch seal. Pouches can remain in place for up to 7 days if the seal is unbroken.

Test-taking strategy: Analyze to determine what information the question asks for, which is correct procedure for caring for an ostomy. Critically think through the steps of the procedure beginning with cleansing/preparing the skin, measuring the stoma and then preparing the wafer, affixing the wafer, and applying the pouch. Visualize the procedure while instructing. Review ostomy appliance care if you had difficulty answering this question.

Client needs category: Health promotion and maintenance

Client needs subcategory: None

Cognitive level: Applying

75. A client presents to the outpatient center for a gastroscopy which revealed redness and inflammation of the stomach indicating acute gastritis. Which action should be included in the immediate management?

☐ **1.** Advising the client to reduce work-related stress.
☐ **2.** Preparing the client for gastric resection.
☐ **3.** Treating the underlying cause of disease.
☐ **4.** Administering enteral tube feedings.

Answer: 3

Rationale: Discovering and treating the cause of gastritis is the most beneficial approach in the immediate management phase. Reducing the amount of stress and reducing or eliminating oral intake until the symptoms are gone are important in the recovery phase. A gastric resection is considered only when serious erosion has occurred.

Test-taking strategy: Analyze to determine what information the question asks for, which is immediate management for acute gastritis. The key word is *"immediate."* Recall the acute nature of the situation. The goal of treatment and management is to reduce the redness and irritation which leads to the correct answer. Review the management of acute gastritis if you had difficulty answering this question.

Client needs category: Safe and effective care environment

Client needs subcategory: Safety and infection control

Cognitive level: Analyzing

---

76. A client comes to the emergency department complaining of dull, deep bone pain that is unrelated to movement. The nurse eliminates the diagnosis of a possible fracture based on which assessment finding?

☐ **1.** The client has the classic symptoms of a fracture.
☐ **2.** Fracture pain is sharp and related to movement.
☐ **3.** Fracture pain is sharp and unrelated to movement.
☐ **4.** Fracture pain is dull, deep, and related to movement.

Answer: 2

Rationale: Fracture pain is sharp and related to movement. Pain that is dull, deep, and unrelated to movement is not typical of a fracture, eliminating a fracture as an option.

Test-taking strategy: Analyze to determine what information the question asks for, which is assessment finding not consistent with that of a fracture. Focus on the client's specific symptoms and review the pathophysiology of a fracture, particularly with respect to pain. Review signs and symptoms of a fracture if you had difficulty answering this question.

Client needs category: Health promotion and maintenance

Client needs subcategory: None

Cognitive level: Analyzing

77. A physician and nurse are discussing treatment options with a client diagnosed with severe ulcerative colitis symptoms. Which potential complication requires frequent assessment?

☐ **1.** Gastritis.
☐ **2.** Bowel herniation.
☐ **3.** Bowel outpouching.
☐ **4.** Bowel perforation.

Answer: 4

Rationale: Bowel perforation, obstruction, or hemorrhage and toxic megacolon are common complications of ulcerative colitis that may require surgery. Gastritis and herniation are not associated with irritable bowel diseases, and outpouching of the bowel wall is diverticulosis.

Test-taking strategy: Analyze to determine what information the question asks for, which is surgical interventions to treat a complication of ulcerative colitis. Recall the pathophysiology of severe ulcerative colitis and analyze each option for potential complications. Recall that ulcerative colitis is comprised of ulcers and open sores which could lead to a perforation. Review complications of ulcerative colitis if you had difficulty answering this question.

Client needs category: Safe and effective care environment

Client needs subcategory: Safety and infection control

Cognitive level: Applying

---

78. A nurse is reviewing the medication regimen with a client who was recently discharged from the hospital. The nurse noted that the client was started on metformin (Glucophage) and glyburide (DiaBeta). Which symptoms does the nurse anticipate that the client would have initially displayed?

☐ **1.** Polydipsia, polyuria, and weight loss.
☐ **2.** Weight gain, tiredness, and bradycardia.
☐ **3.** Irritability, diaphoresis, and tachycardia.
☐ **4.** Diarrhea, abdominal pain, and weight loss.

Answer: 1

Rationale: Symptoms of hyperglycemia include polydipsia, polyuria, and weight loss. Metformin and sulfonylureas are commonly ordered medications. Weight gain, tiredness, and bradycardia are symptoms of hypothyroidism. Irritability, diaphoresis, and tachycardia are symptoms of hypoglycemia. Symptoms of Crohn's disease include diarrhea, abdominal pain, and weight loss.

Test-taking strategy: Analyze to determine what information the question asks for, which is signs indicating the need for Metformin (Glucophage) and Metformin (DiaBeta). Recall that these medications are used for the management of type 2 diabetes and may be used with diet, insulin, or other sulfonylurea/oral hypoglycemics to control blood sugar. To require these medications, blood sugar would need to be elevated. Review the signs of hyperglycemia if you had difficulty answering this question.

Client needs category: Physiological integrity

Client needs subcategory: Reduction of risk potential

Cognitive level: Analyzing

79. The nurse is caring for a client diagnosed with cancer of the cervix. When instructing on intracavitary radiation which explanation best explains the importance of emptying the bowel?

- [ ] **1.** Feces in the bowel increase the risk of ileus.
- [ ] **2.** An empty bowel allows the applicator to be positioned with little or no discomfort.
- [ ] **3.** Bowel movements increase the risk of inadvertent contamination of the vagina and urethra.
- [ ] **4.** Pressure changes in the pelvis associated with bowel movements can alter the position of the applicator and the radiation source.

Answer: 4

Rationale: A position change of the radioactive implant could deliver more radiation to healthy tissue and less to the malignant lesion. This increases the risk of injury to healthy tissue and decreases the effectiveness of treatment on the cancer. Feces in the bowel increase the likelihood of a bowel movement, which can change the position of the applicator and radiation source. Feces in the bowel do not increase the risk of ileus or inadvertent contamination of the vagina and urethra from a bowel movement. Applicators are usually inserted under anesthesia in the operating room.

Test-taking strategy: Analyze to determine what information the question asks for, which is best explanation of the importance of emptying the bowel prior to radioactive implant placement. Consider the goal of radioactive implant therapy which is to insert a radioactive source into a hollow organ to deliver a high radiation dose to the lesion while sparing the surrounding tissue. To accomplish the goal, it is best for there to be limited fecal matter for bowel movements. Review radioactive implants and intracavitary radiation for cervical cancer if you had difficulty answering this question.

Client needs category: Physiological integrity

Client needs subcategory: Reduction of risk potential

Cognitive level: Analyzing

---

80. The nurse is reviewing client documentation before receiving shift report. After reading the selection below, which stage of labor will the nurse plan upcoming care for the client?

Progress notes	
7/3/06 0135	Client experienced spontaneous rupture of membranes. Fluid is odorless and clear. Contractions are 50 seconds long and occur every 4 minutes. See flow sheet for details. Client is 4 cm dilated. ———————————————————A. Wilkens, LPN

- [ ] **1.** Stage 1, latent stage
- [ ] **2.** Stage 2
- [ ] **3.** Stage 1, active phase
- [ ] **4.** Stage 1, transition stage

Answer: 3

Rationale: During the active phase of stage 1 labor, membranes may rupture spontaneously. Contractions last about 40 to 60 seconds and recur every 3 to 5 minutes, and the cervix dilates from about 3 to 7 cm. During the latent phase of stage 1, contractions last 20 to 40 seconds and occur every 5 to 30 minutes, and the cervix dilates from 0 to 30 cm. During stage 2 of labor, the cervix is fully dilated and effaced and the neonate is born. During the transition phase of stage 1, contractions last 60 to 90 seconds, and occur every 2 to 3 minutes, and the cervix dilates from 7 cm to a fully dilated 10 cm.

Test-taking strategy: Analyze to determine what information the question asks for, which is stage of labor documented in a nurse note. Analyze the note to determine key information such as rupture of membranes and contractions that allow the nurse to determine stage of labor. Review stages of labor if you had difficult answering this question.

Client needs category: Health promotion and maintenance

Client needs subcategory: None

Cognitive level: Applying

81. The assessment of a client on the first day after a thoracotomy shows a temperature of 100°F (37.8°C); heart rate, 96 beats/minute; blood pressure, 136/86 mm Hg; and shallow respirations at 24 breaths/minute, with rhonchi at the bases. The client complains of incisional pain. Which nursing action has priority?

☐ **1.** Medicate the client for pain.
☐ **2.** Help the client get out of bed.
☐ **3.** Give ibuprofen (Motrin) as ordered to reduce the fever.
☐ **4.** Encourage the client to cough and deep breathe.

Answer: 1

Rationale: Although the interventions are incorporated in the client's care plan, the priority is to relieve the client's pain and make him/her comfortable. This would give the client energy and stamina to achieve the other objectives.

Test-taking strategy: Analyze to determine what information the question asks for, which is priority nursing action following a thoracotomy. First, analyze the data given and prioritize actions according to abnormalities. Note shallow breathing, rhonchi, and pain. Recall that pain impedes the client's desire to ambulate and cough and deep breath, which are essential to diminish the presenting symptoms. Review nursing actions that prioritize interventions according to the most beneficial to the client symptoms if you had difficulty answering this question.

Client needs category: Physiological integrity

Client needs subcategory: Basic care and comfort

Cognitive level: Applying

---

82. The nurse is working in a psychiatric facility on an anxiety disorder unit. The unit is locked and clients have scheduled group and family therapy sessions. Which other standard is maintained on this unit for a client diagnosed with panic disorder?

☐ **1.** Clients may come and go as they desire.
☐ **2.** Clients may eat anything that is facility prepared.
☐ **3.** Suicide precautions are instituted.
☐ **4.** A security guard is present at the door.

Answer: 3

Rationale: Clients with anxiety disorders including panic disorder are at risk for suicide because they can be impulsive. Unit standards include maintaining suicide precautions. Nutritional problems do not typically accompany panic disorder and family can bring in client requests. Clients, depending on their status, typically remain on the unit; however, while there is facility security, there is no guard at the unit door.

Test-taking strategy: Analyze to determine what information the question asks for, which is unit standards of care for a panic disorder. Consider that every client is individual but there are priority standard precautions for safety and client behavior. Review nursing precautions for a client with panic disorder if you had difficulty answering this question.

Client needs category: Psychosocial integrity

Client needs subcategory: None

Cognitive level: Applying

83. A client recovering from alcohol addiction asks the nurse how he should talk to his children about the impact of his addiction on them. Which response is most appropriate?

☐ **1.** "Try to limit references to the addiction, and focus on the present."

☐ **2.** "Talk about all the hardships you've had in working to remain sober."

☐ **3.** "Tell them you're sorry, and emphasize that you're doing so much better now."

☐ **4.** "Talk to them by acknowledging the difficulties and pain your drinking caused."

Answer: 4

Rationale: Part of the healing process for the family is to acknowledge the pain, embarrassment, and overall difficulties the client's drinking problem caused to family members. The first option facilitates the client's ability to deny the problem. The second option prevents the client from acknowledging the difficulties the children endured. The third option might lead the client to believe that only a simple apology is needed. The addiction must be addressed, and the children's pain acknowledged.

Test-taking strategy: Analyze to determine what information the question asks for, which is nursing guidance on facilitating therapeutic communication between the parent and the child. Consider therapeutic communication in an open environment and which statement will be most helpful in the healing process of the family. Review therapeutic communication if you had difficulty answering this question.

Client needs category: Psychosocial integrity

Client needs subcategory: None

Cognitive level: Applying

---

84. The nurse is instructing the client at 24 weeks of gestation regarding a glucose tolerance test to screen for gestational diabetes. The client asks, "What will be done if I have this disorder?" The nurse is correct to state that gestational diabetes is managed by which therapy?

☐ **1.** Dietary control of carbohydrates, fats, and proteins.

☐ **2.** Metformin (Glucophage).

☐ **3.** Ultra-lente (long-acting) insulin.

☐ **4.** Metformin (Glucophage) and ultra-lente (long-acting) insulin.

Answer: 1

Rationale: Clients with gestational diabetes are usually managed by dietary control of carbohydrates, fats, and proteins alone to control their glucose intolerance. Oral hypoglycemic drugs such as Metformin are contraindicated in pregnancy and are considered teratogenic. Long-acting insulin such as ultra-lente usually is not needed for blood glucose control in the client with gestational diabetes.

Test-taking strategy: Analyze to determine what information the question asks for, which is management of gestational diabetes. Consider the term "gestational" as typically a temporary condition and during pregnancy. Recall that dietary management would be the first step in controlling the high glucose levels. Review the management of gestational diabetes if you had difficulty answering this question.

Client needs category: Health promotion and maintenance

Client needs subcategory: None

Cognitive level: Applying

85. The nurse is instructing a prenatal class in the progression of postpartum behaviors. The nurse is expecting to observe which behavior in a client on the fourth postpartum day?

☐ **1.** The client asks many questions about the baby's care.

☐ **2.** The client wants to relate her birth experience.

☐ **3.** The client asks the nurse to select her meals for her.

☐ **4.** The client asks the nurse to help her bathe herself.

Answer: 1

Rationale: The taking-hold phase usually lasts from days 3 to 10 postpartum. During this stage, the mother strives for independence and autonomy; she also becomes curious and interested in the care of the baby and is most ready to learn. During the taking-in phase, which usually lasts 2 to 3 days, the mother is passive and dependent and expresses her own needs. During this taking-in phase, the client may ask the nurse to help her with self-care, wants to talk about the birth experience, and lets others make decisions for her.

Test-taking strategy: Analyze to determine what information the question asks for, which is behaviors by the client on the fourth postpartum day. Consider the mother's behavior of focusing on herself and the birth experience to focusing on the newborn and his/her needs. Review the transition phases of the postpartum period and when each phase occurs if you had difficulty answering this question.

Client needs category: Psychosocial integrity

Client needs subcategory: None

Cognitive level: Applying

---

86. The client is being seen in the endocrinologist's office and scheduled for an outpatient thyroid scan. Which nursing instructions help to prepare the client for the scan? Select all that apply.

☐ **1.** Eliminate iodized salt and/or iodized salt substitutes 1 week prior to the scan.

☐ **2.** Refrain from all seafood 1 week prior to the scan.

☐ **3.** Take nothing by mouth after midnight before the scan.

☐ **4.** Hold prescription thyroid medication the day of the scan.

☐ **5.** Hold thyroid medication until notified about scan results.

Answer: 1, 2, 4

Rationale: A thyroid scan visualizes the distribution of radioactive dye in the thyroid gland. Instructions before the exam include stopping the ingestion of iodine, which is found in iodized salt, salt substitutes, and seafood. Any medications that would interfere with the scan should not be taken. The client may have food/fluids, because the dye is administered intravenously. Routinely prescribed medications can be taken after the scan.

Test-taking strategy: Analyze to determine what information the question asks for, which is instructions given prior to a thyroid scan. Consider the nature of the thyroid scan and what interactions, among salt, seafood, and medications, may interfere with the results. Review instructions prior to a thyroid scan if you had difficulty answering this question.

Client needs category: Physiological integrity

Client needs subcategory: Reduction of risk potential

Cognitive level: Applying

87. A 29-week gestation client arrives in the labor and delivery suite for an emergency cesarean section. The neonate is born and exogenous surfactant is administered. Which action best explains the main function and goal of surfactant use?

- ☐ **1.** Assists with ciliary body maturation in the upper airways eliminating mucous.
- ☐ **2.** Helps maintain a rhythmic breathing pattern reducing tachypnea.
- ☐ **3.** Promotes mucus production lubricating the respiratory tract.
- ☐ **4.** Helps lungs remain expanded after the initiation of breathing improving oxygenation.

Answer: 4

Rationale: Surfactant works by reducing surface tension in the lung. It allows the lung to remain slightly expanded, decreasing the amount of work required for inspiration. Improved oxygenation, as determined by arterial blood gases, is noted. Surfactant has not been shown to influence ciliary body maturation, regulate the neonate's breathing pattern, or lubricate the respiratory tract.

Test-taking strategy: Analyze to determine what information the question asks for, which is function and goal of surfactant in a premature neonate. Recall that surfactant is given to promote lung maturity, resulting in more efficient respirations and improving oxygenation. Review complications of prematurity if you had difficulty answering this question.

Client needs category: Health promotion and maintenance

Client needs subcategory: None

Cognitive level: Applying

---

88. A nurse is assisting a gastroenterologist in caring for a client with complaints of epigastric pain. The nurse is explaining the role of the gastric glands in the fundus and body of the stomach which secrete intrinsic factor and hydrochloric acid. The nurse is correct when stating which of these substances as those needed in the GI tract. Select all that apply.

- ☐ **1.** Vitamin B_{12} absorption.
- ☐ **2.** Emulsifying fats.
- ☐ **3.** Dissolving food fibers.
- ☐ **4.** Killing microorganisms.
- ☐ **5.** Activating the enzyme pepsin.
- ☐ **6.** Vitamin B_6 absorption.

Answer: 1, 3, 4, 5

Rationale: Intrinsic factor is needed for vitamin B_{12} absorption, and hydrochloric acid is needed for dissolving food fibers, killing microorganisms, and activating the enzyme pepsin. Vitamin B_6, an essential nutrient, must be replaced daily because it is water soluble and eliminated in urine. Bile is the substance secreted from the gallbladder to emulsify fats as they are consumed.

Test-taking strategy: Analyze to determine what information the question asks for, which is rationale for intrinsic factor and hydrochloric acid use in the stomach. Recall the action of the stomach and needs for digestion. Review the anatomy and physiology of the GI system if you had difficulty answering this question.

Client needs category: Physiological integrity

Client needs subcategory: Physiological adaptation

Cognitive level: Analyzing

89. The nurse is caring for a client with a ventricular septal repair receiving dopamine (Intropin) postoperatively. Which response indicates a therapeutic response of the medication?

☐ **1.** Decreased heart rate.
☐ **2.** Decreased urine output.
☐ **3.** Increased cardiac output.
☐ **4.** Decreased cardiac contractility.

Answer: 3

Rationale: Dopamine stimulates β1- and β2-adrenergic receptors. It is a selective cardiac stimulant that increases cardiac output, heart rate, and cardiac contractility. Urine output increases in response to dilation of the blood vessels leading to the mesentery and kidneys.

Test-taking strategy: Analyze to determine what information the question asks for, which is identifying the therapeutic response of dopamine. Consider that dopamine is frequently prescribed in client with heart surgery and heart failure to increase perfusion. Also, in analyzing the options, option 3 is the only one which is increasing cardiac response rather than decreasing it. Recall the action of the medication in relation to the cardiovascular system if you had difficulty answering this question.

Client needs category: Physiological integrity
Client needs subcategory: Pharmacological therapies
Cognitive level: Evaluating

90. A child with status asthmaticus is admitted to the pediatric unit and begins to receive intermittent treatment with albuterol, given by nebulizer. Which adverse effect is common with this drug?

☐ **1.** Bradycardia.
☐ **2.** Lethargy.
☐ **3.** Tachycardia.
☐ **4.** Tachypnea.

Answer: 3

Rationale: Albuterol is a rapid-acting bronchodilator. Common adverse effects include tachycardia, nervousness, tremors, insomnia, irritability, and headache.

Test-taking strategy: Analyze to determine what information the question asks for, which is an adverse effect from an albuterol nebulizer treatment. Consider the type of medication and common side effects. Review the action and adverse effects of albuterol if you had difficulty answering this question.

Client needs category: Physiological integrity
Client needs subcategory: Pharmacological therapies
Cognitive level: Applying

91. A nurse is percussing a client's abdomen during a well checkup. The nurse assesses liver dullness in which anatomical location?

Answer:

Rationale: The liver is located on the upper right side of the abdomen, just below the diaphragm. To hear liver dullness, the nurse should percuss the abdomen at the right midclavicular line, starting at a level below the umbilicus (in an area of tympany, not dullness) and continuing upward toward the liver.

Test-taking strategy: Analyze to determine what information the question asks for, which is the area where liver dullness is assessed. Consider that dullness is heard over liver tissue denoting the size of the liver. Noting the size of the liver through percussion can be helpful in determining the health of the liver. Review anatomy of the gastrointestinal system and techniques for assessing the liver if you had difficulty answering this question.

Client needs category: Health promotion and maintenance

Client needs subcategory: None

Cognitive level: Applying

---

92. The school nurse is assessing the diabetic status of a 15-year-old athlete. Which physiologic change should the nurse anticipate as a diabetic teenager becomes more physically active during the day?

☐ **1.** Increased need for food.
☐ **2.** Decreased need for food.
☐ **3.** Decreased risk of insulin shock.
☐ **4.** Increased risk of hyperglycemia.

Answer: 1

Rationale: If a child is more active at one time of the day than another, food intake or insulin can be adjusted to meet this increased activity pattern. Ideally, food intake should be increased, typically with a snack, when a diabetic teen is more physically active. The child would have an increased risk of insulin shock and a decreased risk of hyperglycemia when more physically active.

Test-taking strategy: Analyze to determine what information the question asks for, which is anticipated changes as a diabetic teen becomes more active throughout the day. Consider the relationship between blood glucose, calories, and exercise. Recall that food is the source of energy which needs to be metabolized to be available in the teen's system. Review diabetic management throughout the day if you had difficulty answering this question.

Client needs category: Safe and effective care environment

Client needs subcategory: Coordinated care

Cognitive level: Applying

93. A teenager asks advice from a nurse about getting a tattoo. When the nurse is providing education, which statement about tattoos is a common misconception?

☐ **1.** Human immunodeficiency syndrome (HIV) is a possible risk factor.
☐ **2.** Hepatitis B is a possible risk factor.
☐ **3.** Tattoos are easily removed with laser surgery.
☐ **4.** Allergic response to pigments is a possible risk factor.

Answer: 3

Rationale: A common misconception regarding tattoos is that tattoos can be removed. Removing a tattoo is not an easy process, and most people are left with a significant scar. Also, the cost is expensive and not covered by insurance. Because of the moderate amount of bleeding with a tattoo, both hepatitis B and HIV are potential risks if proper techniques are not followed. Allergic reactions are possible when establishments do not use Food and Drug Administration-approved pigments for tattoo coloring. Reactions can also occur in clients who are hypersensitive to the pigments or tools used.

Test-taking strategy: Analyze to determine what information the question asks for, which is a common misconception regarding tattoo use. The key word is "misconception," meaning that the statement is inaccurate. Review facts about tattoos if you had difficulty answering this question.

Client needs category: Health promotion and maintenance

Client needs subcategory: None

Cognitive level: Analyzing

---

94. The nurse is teaching a client about the pathophysiology of asthma. Place in chronological order the sequence of an asthma attack. Use all of the options.

| **1.** Inflammation. |
| **2.** Mucus production. |
| **3.** Airflow limitation. |
| **4.** Trigger by stimulus. |
| **5.** Acute asthma attack. |
| **6.** Breathlessness. |

Answer: 4, 1, 2, 3, 6, 5

Rationale: Asthma is triggered by a stimulus. The stimulus may be environmental, stress related, or medication related. Inflammation in the airways occurs as a response to the stimulus, followed by an increase in mucus production. The presence of inflammation and mucus narrow the bronchi, causing limited airflow. At this point, the client experiences breathlessness, chest tightness, and wheezing—all symptoms of an acute asthma attack.

Test-taking strategy: Analyze to determine what information the question asks for, which is sequence of an asthma attack. First, place option 4 (trigger) and option 5 (attack) as the first and last in the sequence. Next, take the remaining four and place them in order moving from the beginning symptoms present until option 6 (breathlessness) occurs. Review the causes and pathophysiology of asthma if you had difficulty answering this question.

Client needs category: Physiological integrity

Client needs subcategory: Physiological adaptation

Cognitive level: Applying

95. A nurse is reviewing diagnostic information on a newly admitted client. A chest X-ray shows a client's lungs to be clear. The Mantoux test is positive, with 10 mm of induration. The previous test was negative. Upon analysis of the data, the nurse is able to provide which information on shift report?

☐ **1.** The client had TB in the past and no longer has it.

☐ **2.** The client was successfully treated for TB, but skin tests always stay positive.

☐ **3.** The client is a seroconverter, meaning the TB has gotten to the bloodstream.

☐ **4.** The client is a tuberculin converter, meaning the client has been exposed to TB since the last skin test.

Answer: 4

Rationale: A tuberculin converter's skin test will be positive, meaning the client has been exposed to and infected with TB and now has a cell-mediated immune response to the skin test. The client's blood and X-ray results may stay negative. It does not mean the infection has advanced to the active stage. Because the X-ray is negative, he/she should be monitored every 6 months to see if he/she develops changes in the chest X-ray or pulmonary examination. Being a seroconverter does not mean the TB has gotten into the bloodstream; it means it can be detected by a blood test.

Test-taking strategy: Analyze to determine what information the question asks for, which is the correct analysis of a diagnostic test. Eliminate options 1 (client has had TB), 2 (treated for TB), and 3 (TB in bloodstream) as all stating that the client has had TB. Review the purpose of the Mantoux test and the disease course following exposure to TB if you had difficulty answering this question.

Client needs category: Physiological integrity

Client needs subcategory: Physiological adaptation

Cognitive level: Analyzing

---

96. A client at the eye clinic is newly diagnosed with glaucoma. The nurse should stress the need to take medication as prescribed because noncompliance may lead to which condition?

☐ **1.** Diplopia.

☐ **2.** Permanent vision loss.

☐ **3.** Progressive loss of peripheral vision.

☐ **4.** Pupillary constriction.

Answer: 2

Rationale: Without treatment, glaucoma may progress to irreversible blindness. Treatment will not restore visual damage but will halt disease progression. Blurred or foggy vision, not diplopia, is typical in glaucoma. Central vision loss, not peripheral loss, is typical in glaucoma. Miotics, which constrict the pupil, are used in the treatment of glaucoma to permit the outflow of aqueous humor.

Test-taking strategy: Analyze to determine what information the question asks for, which is consequence of noncompliance with glaucoma treatment. Focus on the pathophysiology of glaucoma as the deterioration will continue without treatment. Review signs and treatment options of glaucoma if you had difficulty answering this question.

Client needs category: Physiological integrity

Client needs subcategory: Pharmacological therapies

Cognitive level: Applying

97. A client with newly diagnosed chronic obstructive pulmonary disease (COPD) comes to the clinic for a routine examination. The nurse teaches the client strategies for preventing airway irritation and infection. Which statement by the client indicates that teaching was successful?

☐ **1.** "I should avoid enclosed, crowded areas during the summer."
☐ **2.** "I'm glad I only need to get the flu vaccine."
☐ **3.** "I should use products with aerosol sprays."
☐ **4.** "I should avoid using powders."

Answer: 4

Rationale: A client with COPD should avoid exposure to powders, dust, and smoke from cigarettes, pipes, and cigars. The client should stay indoors when the humidity, temperature, and pollen counts are high; and should avoid aerosol sprays. The client should also obtain immunizations against pneumococcal pneumonia as well as influenza.

Test-taking strategy: Analyze to determine what information the question asks for, which is correct statement regarding prevention of COPD. The key words are "successful teaching," indicating that the client statement is correct. Analyze each option for accuracy. Review essential teaching for a client newly diagnosed with COPD if you had difficulty answering this question.

Client needs category: Health promotion and maintenance

Client needs subcategory: None

Cognitive level: Analyzing

98. A histamine (H2) receptor antagonist is prescribed for a client with recurrent gastrointestinal discomfort. The nurse is instructing the client from a medication pamphlet and highlights which medications in this classification? Select all that apply.

☐ **1.** Cimetidine (Tagament)
☐ **2.** Ranitidine (Zantac)
☐ **3.** Nizatidine (Axid)
☐ **4.** Famotidine (Pepcid)
☐ **5.** Esomeprazole (Nexium)

Answer: 1, 2, 3, 4

Rationale: H2 receptor antagonists suppress secretion of gastric action, alleviate symptoms of heartburn, and help to prevent peptic ulcer disease. Esomeprazole is a proton pump inhibitor.

Test-taking strategy: Analyze to determine what information the question asks for, which is medications that are classified as H2 receptor antagonists. Review all medications listed and note that four end in "dine," which correctly suggests that they fall in the same classification. Review medications listed as H2 receptor antagonists if you had difficulty answering this question.

Client needs category: Physiological integrity

Client needs subcategory: Pharmacological therapies

Cognitive level: Applying

99. The home health nurse is instructing a client and spouse on helpful recommendations to manage symptoms of multiple sclerosis (MS). Which measure would be included in teaching to avoid exacerbation of the disease?

☐ **1.** Patching the affected eye.
☐ **2.** Sleeping 8 hours each night.
☐ **3.** Taking hot baths for relaxation.
☐ **4.** Drinking 1½ to 2 qt (1.5 to 2 L) of fluid daily.

Answer: 2

Rationale: MS is exacerbated by exposure to stress, fatigue, and heat. Clients should balance activity with rest. Patching the affected eye may result in improvement in vision and balance but will not prevent exacerbation of the disease. Adequate hydration will help prevent UTIs secondary to a neurogenic bladder.

Test-taking strategy: Analyze to determine what information the question asks for, which is measure to prevent exacerbation of the disease. Always answer what the question is asking or an option related to exacerbation of the disease. Note that only option 2 is preventative. Review the pathophysiology of MS if you had difficulty answering this question.

Client needs category: Physiological integrity

Client needs subcategory: Reduction of risk potential

Cognitive level: Applying

---

100. During a multidisciplinary team conference, a nurse and dietitian discuss the best diet for a client recovering from a fracture. A high-protein diet was recommended to the physician for which reason?

☐ **1.** Protein promotes gluconeogenesis.
☐ **2.** Protein has anti-inflammatory properties.
☐ **3.** Protein promotes cell growth and bone union.
☐ **4.** Protein decreases pain medication requirements.

Answer: 3

Rationale: High-protein intake promotes cell growth and bone union. Protein does not promote gluconeogenesis, exert anti-inflammatory properties, or decrease pain medication requirements.

Test-taking strategy: Analyze to determine what information the question asks for, which is rationale to recommend a high-protein diet for a client with a fracture. Recall that protein, along with calcium and vitamin D, is an important nutrient in the formation of bone tissue. Review the benefits of protein in the diet if you had difficulty answering this question.

Client needs category: Physiological integrity

Client needs subcategory: Basic care and comfort

Cognitive level: Applying

101. The victim of a motor vehicle accident is brought into the trauma center with substernal injuries and in a great deal of pain. The nurse assesses the client's pain level as a 9 on 0-to-10 pain scale and notifies the physician, who orders *morphine sulfate gr ½ I.M. stat.* The only available morphine is morphine sulfate in a 20-mL vial, labeled 15 mg/mL. How many milliliters of pain medication should the nurse administer? Record your answer using a whole number.

_____ mL

Answer: 2

Rationale: Calculate the dosage by converting grains to milligrams:

$$1 \text{ gr} : 60 \text{ mg} :: \tfrac{1}{2} \text{ gr} : X \text{ mg} = 30 \text{ mg}.$$

Then, use the ratio-and-proportion method to determine the amount of milliliters to administer:

$$15 \text{ mg} : 1 \text{ mL} :: 30 \text{ mg} : X \text{ mL}$$

$$\frac{15 \times X}{15} = \frac{30}{15}$$

$$X = 2 \text{ mL}.$$

Test-taking strategy: Analyze to determine what information the question asks for, which is how many milliliters of pain medications should be administered. Use the above formula entering known data and solving for *X*. Proofread the math calculation. Review dosage calculations using ratios and proportions, and review equivalents for the apothecaries' system if you had difficulty answering this question.

Client needs category: Physiological integrity

Client needs subcategory: Pharmacological therapies

Cognitive level: Applying

---

102. A nurse is working in the office of a gastroenterologist. When reviewing the list of clients to be seen for the day, the nurse notes the following disease processes. With which client would the nurse instruct on signs of rectal cancer?

☐ **1.** Adenomatous polyps.
☐ **2.** Diverticulitis.
☐ **3.** Hemorrhoids.
☐ **4.** Peptic ulcer disease.

Answer: 1

Rationale: A client with adenomatous polyps has a higher risk for developing rectal cancer than others do. Clients with diverticulitis are more likely to develop colon cancer. Hemorrhoids do not increase the chance of any type of cancer. Clients with peptic ulcer disease have a higher incidence of gastric cancer.

Test-taking strategy: Analyze to determine what information the question asks for, which is disease process that contains a risk of rectal cancer. Recall the adenomatous polyps (benign) can signal a potential for cancer throughout the colon to the rectum; thus, the term colorectal cancer. Screening with a colonoscopy is essential. Review the signs of rectal cancer if you had difficulty answering this question.

Client needs category: Health promotion and maintenance

Client needs subcategory: None

Cognitive level: Analyzing

103. The nurse is preparing to administer pediatric eye drops to a 9-month-old. Which of the following interventions would be in the nurse's plan of care? Select all that apply.

☐ **1.** Have the child sit on the parent's lap.
☐ **2.** Wash hands.
☐ **3.** Place the drop in the conjunctival sac.
☐ **4.** Massage the eye after instillation.
☐ **5.** Put on gloves.
☐ **6.** Pull the lower lid down.

Answer: 2, 3, 5, 6

Rationale: To administer eye medications to an infant, the infant is placed supine on a flat surface to steady the head. The nurse washes hands and puts on gloves. The nurse lowers the lid against the cheek bone and instills one drop into the conjunctival sac. The eye is not massaged after instillation.

Test-taking strategy: Analyze to determine what information the question asks for, which is standards of care when administering eye drops to a pediatric client. Consider the client's age and ability to follow directions when selecting position for procedure. Also consider placement of medication. Review the procedure for administering eye drops if you had difficulty answering this question.

Client needs category: Physiological integrity

Client needs subcategory: Pharmacological therapies

Cognitive level: Applying

104. The enterostomal therapy nurse is caring for a client with a newly placed ileal conduit. Which instruction about skin care at the stoma site should be given?

☐ **1.** Change the appliance at bedtime.
☐ **2.** Leave the stoma open to air while changing the appliance.
☐ **3.** Clean the skin around the stoma with mild soap and water, and dry it thoroughly.
☐ **4.** Cut the faceplate or wafer of the appliance no more than 4 mm larger than the stoma.

Answer: 3

Rationale: Cleaning the skin around the stoma with mild soap and water and drying it thoroughly helps keep the area clean from urine, which can irritate the skin. The appliance should be changed early in the morning, when urine output is less, to decrease the amount of urine in contact with the skin. The stoma should be covered with a gauze pad when changing the appliance to prevent seepage of urine onto the skin. The faceplate or wafer of the appliance should not be more than 3 mm larger than the stoma to reduce the skin area in contact with urine.

Test-taking strategy: Analyze to determine what information the question asks for, which is instruction regarding ileal conduit stoma care. Consider that the stoma is new and the surrounding skin needs meticulous care as it heals. Urine on the sensitive skin can cause breakdown. Simple soap and water care is effective in cleansing the area. Review care of a ileal conduit, stoma, and surrounding skin if you had difficulty answering this question.

Client needs category: Physiological integrity

Client needs subcategory: Basic care and comfort

Cognitive level: Applying

105. A client with facial lacerations requires wound care, I.V. antibiotics, and hospitalization for 1 week. During the assessment on the third admission day, the nurse notes scabs on the wounds. This finding corresponds to which phase of the normal wound healing.

☐ **1.** Contraction phase.
☐ **2.** Inflammatory phase.
☐ **3.** Proliferative phase.
☐ **4.** Remodeling phase.

Answer: 3

Rationale: During the proliferative phase of wound healing, which lasts from the 4th to 21st day after injury, granulation tissue appears (scabs form) and the wound edges start to pull together. Contraction, the third phase of wound healing, may begin around the 7th day and involves a significant decrease in the wound surface. The inflammatory phase, the first healing phase, immediately follows the injury and lasts 4 to 6 days; it involves control of bleeding and release of chemicals needed for healing. The remodeling phase, the final phase, may lead to scar flattening and correction of any deformities that occurred during the third phase.

Test-taking strategy: Analyze to determine what information the question asks for, which is the phase of wound healing with scab formation. Recall what occurs during the different phases of wound healing. If unsure, consider that proliferative comes from proliferation, meaning the growth or production of cells. Review the phases of wound healing if you had difficulty answering this question.

Client needs category: Physiological integrity

Client needs subcategory: Basic care and comfort

Cognitive level: Applying

106. The nurse is documenting a prenatal history of *gravida 4, para 2 on the* woman's clinic paperwork. The paperwork is sent to the birthing center for review. Upon the expectant mother's admission to the birthing center, the admission nurse is most correct to confirm which prenatal history?

☐ **1.** A client has been pregnant four times and had two miscarriages.
☐ **2.** A client has been pregnant four times and had two children born after 20 weeks of gestation.
☐ **3.** A client has been pregnant four times and had two cesarean deliveries.
☐ **4.** A client has been pregnant four times and had two spontaneous abortions.

Answer: 2

Rationale: Gravida refers to the number of times a client had been pregnant; *para* refers to the number of viable children born after 20 weeks of gestation. Therefore, the client who is gravida 4, para 2 has been pregnant four times and had two live-born children.

Test-taking strategy: Analyze to determine what information the question asks for, which is specific prenatal history. Focus on the meaning of the terms *gravida* and *para* as noted above. Review documentation of prenatal history using the terms gravida and para if you had difficulty answering this question.

Client needs category: Health promotion and maintenance

Client needs subcategory: None

Cognitive level: Applying

107. The nurse assists the client to the operating room table and supervises the operating room technician preparing the sterile field. Which action, completed by the surgical technician, indicates to the nurse that a sterile field has been contaminated?

- ☐ **1.** Sterile objects are held above the waist of the technician.
- ☐ **2.** Sterile packages are opened with the first edge away from the technician.
- ☐ **3.** The outer inch of the sterile towel hangs over the side of the table.
- ☐ **4.** Wetness in the sterile cloth on top of the nonsterile table has been noted.

Answer: 4

Rationale: Moisture outside the sterile package contaminates the sterile field because fluid can be wicked into the sterile field. Bacteria tend to settle, so there is less contamination above waist level and away from the technician. The outer inch of the drape is considered contaminated but does not indicate that the sterile field itself has been contaminated.

Test-taking strategy: Analyze to determine what information the question asks for, which is contamination of the sterile field. The key word is "contamination," indicating that there is a break in procedure with the sterile field preparation. Eliminate options 1, 2, and 3 as proper procedure for sterile fields. Review the basics of infection control and sterile field procedures if you had difficulty answering this question.

Client needs category: Safe and effective care environment

Client needs subcategory: Coordinated care

Cognitive level: Applying

---

108. The nurse is caring for an elderly woman who reports not moving her bowels for 6 days. A cleansing enema is ordered. Which nursing interventions are most correct to perform? Select all that apply.

- ☐ **1.** Apply sterile gloves.
- ☐ **2.** Place the client in the right Sims position.
- ☐ **3.** Lubricate the enema tubing and insert 3 to 4 inches.
- ☐ **4.** Ensure the temperature of the solution is cool.
- ☐ **5.** Clamp the tubing if the client experiences cramping.
- ☐ **6.** Hold the container at least 12 inches above the client's anus.

Answer: 3, 5, 6

Rationale: The administration of an enema is a clean procedure, not a sterile one. The nurse puts on nonsterile gloves, and places the client in the left lateral position, allowing the solution to follow the natural curve of the bowel. The solution is best between 100°F and 105°F, because cooler water will cause cramping. A pause in administration, with the tubing clamped, is best if the client experiences discomfort such as cramping. The enema tubing is lubricated and advanced as the container is held above the client to enable gravity to infuse the solution. The container is held 12 to 18 inches above the client.

Test-taking strategy: Analyze to determine what information the question asks for, which is standard of care for administering an enema. Visualize the procedure for proper administration technique. Recall anatomy of the bowel and precautions to avoid trauma to the rectal tissue. Review standard protocol for enema administration if you had difficulty answering this question.

Client needs category: Physiological integrity

Client needs subcategory: Basic care and comfort

Cognitive level: Applying

109. The nurse is caring for a client on the ortho-pedic unit. Which discharge instructions should be given to a client after surgical repair of a hip fracture?

☐ **1.** "Do not flex the hip more than 30°, do not cross your legs, and get help putting on your shoes."

☐ **2.** "Do not flex the hip more than 60°, do not cross your legs, and get help putting on your shoes."

☐ **3.** "Do not flex the hip more than 90°, do not cross your legs, and get help putting on your shoes."

☐ **4.** "Do not flex the hip more than 120°, do not cross your legs, and get help putting on your shoes."

Answer: 3

Rationale: Discharge instructions should include not flexing the hip more than 90°, not crossing the legs, and getting help to put on shoes. These restrictions prevent dislocation of the new prosthesis.

Test-taking strategy: Analyze to determine what information the question asks for, which is at which angle the client should not progress past when flexing at the hip. Note that each option is the same except for the hip flexion. Recall the angle of 90° is in the mid position or a high Fowler's position with the head raised. Thus, the client should not bend forward. Review post surgical flexion restrictions if you had difficulty answering this question.

Client needs category: Safe and effective care environment

Client needs subcategory: Coordinated care

Cognitive level: Applying

---

110. The nurse is instructing young mothers of infants at a community health clinic. When instructing on mealtime activity, which activity is recommended to prevent foreign body aspiration in children during meals?

☐ **1.** Insist that children are seated.

☐ **2.** Give children toys to play with.

☐ **3.** Allow children to watch television.

☐ **4.** Allow children to eat in a separate room.

Answer: 1

Rationale: Children should remain seated while eating. The risk of aspiration increases if a child is running, jumping, or talking with food in the mouth. Television and toys are a dangerous distraction to toddlers and young children and should be avoided. Children need constant supervision and should be monitored while eating snacks and meals.

Test-taking strategy: Analyze to determine what information the question asks for, which is safety tips for mealtime. Review activities that can lead to aspiration of food if you had difficulty answering this question.

Client needs category: Safe and effective care environment

Client needs subcategory: Safety and infection control

Cognitive level: Applying

111. The nurse is assigned to care for a client following a cerebral vascular accident (CVA). The client is experiencing expressive aphasia. Which nursing interventions would assist in client communication? Select all that apply.

☐ **1.** Speak in lower tones.
☐ **2.** Face the client when speaking.
☐ **3.** Encourage client gestures to communicate ideas.
☐ **4.** Provide directions in short, simple sentences.
☐ **5.** Encourage the client to attempt verbalization.
☐ **6.** Ask the client to repeat words until ideas are clear.

Answer: 2, 3, 4

Rationale: Clients with expressive aphasia know what he or she wants to say yet has difficulty communicating it to others. Speaking facing the client enhances communication, encouraging gestures or message boards allow for basic communication of needs and providing short, simple sentences allows the client to process the instructions and determine how best to communicate the response. The client's do not have hearing difficulties thus the tone of voice does not need adjustment. Encouraging verbalization and asking the client to repeat words cause frustration.

Test-taking strategies: Analyze to determine what information the question asks for, which is strategies when working with a client with expressive aphasia. The key word is "expressive," meaning that the client is unable to express ideas. Consider strategies that would diminish frustration in communication. Review the care of clients with expressive aphasia if you had difficulty answering this question.

Client needs category: Psychosocial integrity

Client needs subcategory: None

Cognitive level: Analyzing

---

112. A client comes to the clinic for a follow-up appointment after diagnostic tests show gastroesophageal reflux disease. Which instruction should the nurse provide?

☐ **1.** "Lie down and rest after each meal."
☐ **2.** "Avoid alcohol and caffeine."
☐ **3.** "Drink 16 ounces of water with each meal."
☐ **4.** "Eat three well-balanced meals every day."

Answer: 2

Rationale: A client with gastroesophageal reflux disease should avoid alcohol, caffeine, and foods that increase acidity, all of which can cause epigastric pain. To further prevent reflux, the client should remain upright for 2 to 3 hours after eating; avoid eating for 2 to 3 hours before bedtime; avoid bending and wearing tight clothing; avoid drinking large fluid volumes with meals; and eat small, frequent meals to help reduce gastric acid secretion.

Test-taking strategy: Analyze to determine what information the question asks for, which is nursing instructions for a client with gastroesophageal reflux disease. Consider the disease process, including (1) acidity of the stomach and (2) reflux of stomach contents. Eliminate options that do not address these concerns. Eliminate options 1 and 3 as inappropriate for the disease process. Discriminate between the remaining options selecting option 2 as reducing stomach acidity. Review the nursing instructions for a client with gastroesophageal reflux disease if you had difficulty answering this question.

Client needs category: Physiological integrity

Client needs subcategory: Reduction of risk potential

Cognitive level: Applying

113. The nurse is reading the progress notes for a client who has a pressure ulcer. Based on the nurse's note in the chart below, what stage pressure ulcer does this client have?

Progress Notes	
7/9/10 0800	Client admitted to unit from long-term care facility with a pressure ulcer on coccyx approximately 2 cm × 1 cm × 0.5 cm. No drainage noted. Base has deep pink granulation tissue without visible subcutaneous tissue. Skin surrounding ulcer pink, with intact, well-defined edges. ———— Rebecca Stellato, LPN

☐ **1.** Stage I.
☐ **2.** Stage II.
☐ **3.** Suspected deep-tissue injury.
☐ **4.** Unstageable.

Answer: 2

Rationale: A stage II pressure ulcer has visible skin breaks and possible discoloration. Penetrating to the subcutaneous fat layer, the sore is painful and visibly swollen. The ulcer may be characterized as an abrasion, blister, or shallow crater. In a stage I pressure ulcer, the skin is red and intact and does not blanch with external pressure; it feels warm and firm. In suspected deep-tissue injury, the skin is purple or maroon but intact; a blood-filled blister may be present. In an unstageable pressure ulcer, the ulcer destroys tissue from the skin to possibly the bone; the base of the ulcer is covered by slough, eschar, or both.

Test-taking strategy: Analyze to determine what information the question asks for, which is stage of a pressure ulcer noted in nursing documentation. Use key words in documentation of "deep pink granulation tissue," "intact well-defined edges," and "no visible subcutaneous tissue" to determine staging. Consider that this ulcer is under the skin. Review the signs and symptoms, and pathophysiology of pressure ulcers, anatomy of skin, and stages of pressure ulcers if you had difficulty answering this question.

Client needs category: Physiological integrity

Client needs subcategory: Physiological adaptation

Cognitive level: Analyzing

114. A client in skeletal traction complains of pain even though receiving an analgesic 1 hour ago. The nurse offers an alternative pain management measure. Which measure can be implemented within the nursing scope of practice?

☐ **1.** Acupressure and shiatsu.
☐ **2.** Hypnosis and therapeutic touch.
☐ **3.** Relaxation and imagery.
☐ **4.** Swedish massage and the Feldenkrais method.

Answer: 3

Rationale: Relaxation and imagery are effective adjuncts to pharmacologic pain management that the nurse can implement without a physician's order. Although the other therapies may promote pain management, they require special training or certification.

Test-taking strategy: Analyze to determine what information the question asks for, which is complementary therapy for pain management within the nursing scope of practice. Consider which of the answers may require special training, and eliminate them as possibilities. Review complementary treatments for pain management if you had difficulty answering this question.

Client needs category: Physiological integrity

Client needs subcategory: Basic care and comfort

Cognitive level: Applying

115. A 30-year-old client experiences weight loss, abdominal distention, crampy abdominal pain, and intermittent diarrhea after the birth of her second child. Diagnostic tests reveal gluten-induced enteropathy. Which foods would the nurse instruct that she eliminate from her diet permanently?

☐ **1.** Milk and dairy products.
☐ **2.** Protein-containing foods.
☐ **3.** Cereal grains (except rice and corn).
☐ **4.** Carbohydrates.

Answer: 3

Rationale: To manage gluten-induced enteropathy, the client must eliminate gluten, which means avoiding all cereal grains except rice and corn. In initial disease management, clients eat a high-calorie, high-protein diet with mineral and vitamin supplements to help normalize the nutritional status. Lactose intolerance is sometimes an associated problem, so milk and dairy products are limited until improvement occurs. Cereal grains are the only carbohydrates this client must eliminate.

Test-taking strategy: Analyze to determine what information the question asks for, which is foods that must be eliminated to manage gluten-induced enteropathy. Focus on which food group contains gluten which is a protein composite found in foods processed from wheat and related grains such as rye and barley. Review dietary management of gluten-induced enteropathy and the gluten-free diet if you had difficulty answering this question.

Client needs category: Physiological integrity
Client needs subcategory: Basic care and comfort
Cognitive level: Applying

---

116. A 10-year-old child monitors and adjusts insulin dosage independently. Which response reflects an understanding of appropriate adjustment of insulin dosage when the child has the flu?

☐ **1.** "I won't take my insulin because I'm too sick to eat right now."
☐ **2.** "I'll take my usual dose of regular and NPH insulin."
☐ **3.** "I'll do a fingerstick test first, then figure out how much insulin to take."
☐ **4.** "I'll do a fingerstick test and record the results."

Answer: 3

Rationale: Because of the stress of illness, serum glucose will likely be elevated during an episode of the flu. Appropriate adjustment of insulin dosage based on a fingerstick reading will help prevent the child from becoming hypoglycemic or ketoacidotic.

Test-taking strategy: Analyze to determine what information the question asks for, which is correct management of diabetes and insulin dosage in times of illness. Consider the effect illness has on serum glucose levels. Recall that any stress on body systems rises blood sugars. Review management of diabetes in times of illness if you had difficulty answering this question.

Client needs category: Physiological integrity
Client needs subcategory: Physiological adaptation
Cognitive level: Analyzing

117. A client calls the nurse to his room, stating he is experiencing substernal chest pain that radiates to his jaw. The nurse records a rhythm strip and monitors the client's vital signs. Which graphic highlights the portion of the client's ECG complex that may become elevated above the baseline, indicating MI?

☐ **1.**

☐ **2.**

☐ **3.**

☐ **4.**

Answer: 1

Rationale: A change in the ST segment (option 1) may indicate myocardial damage. The ST segment typically elevates at the onset of an MI, indicating myocardial injury is occurring. Option 2 is highlighting the PR interval, option 3 is highlighting the QT interval, and option 4 is highlighting a U wave. These components do not elevate above the baseline with an MI.

Test-taking strategy: Analyze to determine what information the question asks for, which is elements of an ECG indicating an MI. Recall that the ST segment is sensitive to myocardial tissue damage and assists to determine medical treatment options. Review the components of an ECG rhythm and focus on the characteristic changes seen with an MI if you had difficulty answering this question.

Client needs category: Physiological integrity

Client needs subcategory: Physiological adaptation

Cognitive level: Analyzing

118. A nurse completes the discharge teaching for a client being treated for a sexually transmitted infection (STI) and provides him a copy of written instructions. Which comment would indicate that the client has understood the instructions?

- ☐ **1.** "I don't need condoms because I'm not allergic to penicillin. Besides, I can always come in for a shot at the first sign of infection."
- ☐ **2.** "I'll notify my sex partners and avoid having unprotected sex from now on."
- ☐ **3.** "I'll just be careful not to have intercourse with someone who has an STI."
- ☐ **4.** "I guess there's not much anyone can do to prevent it. If you're going to get it, you're going to get it."

Answer: 2

Rationale: The nurse would know that the client understands the teaching when he/she can describe preventive behaviors and good, safe health practices. The other options indicate that the client does not understand the need to take preventive measures.

Test-taking strategy: Analyze to determine what information the question asks for, which is client statement indicating an understanding of discharge instructions. The key word is "understanding," suggesting a correct client statement. Analyze each option for a correct statement regarding STIs. Review the pathophysiology of STIs and how they are transmitted if you had difficulty answering this question.

Client needs category: Safe and effective care environment

Client needs subcategory: Safety and infection control

Cognitive level: Analyzing

---

119. The nurse is working in the emergency room and is assigned to a client with necrotizing enterocolitis. When assessing the client, the nurse should expect which finding?

- ☐ **1.** Abdominal distention and gastric retention.
- ☐ **2.** Gastric retention and guaiac-negative stools.
- ☐ **3.** Metabolic alkalosis and abdominal distention.
- ☐ **4.** Guaiac-negative stools and metabolic alkalosis.

Answer: 1

Rationale: Necrotizing enterocolitis is an ischemia disorder of the gut. The cause is unknown, but it is more common in preterm neonates who have had a hypoxic episode. The neonate's intestines become dilated and necrotic, and the abdomen becomes extremely distended. Paralytic ileus develops, causing gastric retention. These retained gastric contents, along with any passed stool, will be guaiac positive. The neonate also develops metabolic acidosis, not metabolic alkalosis.

Test-taking strategy: Analyze to determine what information the question asks for, which is symptoms a client experiences when diagnosed with necrotizing enterocolitis. Use knowledge of medical terminology to link necrosis and colon. Eliminate options 2 and 4 when having no blood in the stools (negative guaiac). Review the pathophysiology of necrotizing enterocolitis and symptoms which present if you had difficulty answering this question.

Client needs category: Physiological integrity

Client needs subcategory: Physiological adaptation

Cognitive level: Applying

120. A child has been diagnosed with mumps, a viral infection that involves the parotid glands. Indicate on the illustration below where would you expect to see swelling.

Answer:

Rationale: The parotid glands are one of three pairs of salivary glands located below and in front of the ears.

Test-taking strategy: Analyze to determine what information the question asks for, which is location of the parotid glands. Recall that the gland is a salivary gland in close approximation to the mandible. Review the anatomy of the head and neck and the location of the salivary glands if you had difficulty answering this question.

Client needs category: Physiological integrity

Client needs subcategory: Physiological adaptation

Cognitive level: Analyzing